CLINICAL COACH

for

Fluid & Electrolyte Balance

Davis's

CLINICAL COACH

Series

CLINICAL COACH

for

Fluid & Electrolyte Balance

Elizabethe Westgard, RN, MSN
Albert Einstein Medical Center
Philadelphia, PA

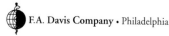

F.A. **Davis Company** • Philadelphia

F. A. Davis Company
1915 Arch Street
Philadelphia, PA 19103
www.fadavis.com

Printed in China

Last digit indicates print number: 10 9 8 7 6 5 4 3 2 1

Acquisitions Editor: Jonathan Joyce
Developmental Editor: Kim Mackey
Director of Content Development: Darlene Pedersen
Project Editors: Jamie Elfrank and Tyler Baber
Manager, Art and Design: Carolyn O'Brien

As new scientific information becomes available through basic and clinical research, recommended treatments and drug therapies undergo changes. The author(s) and publisher have done everything possible to make this book accurate, up to date, and in accord with accepted standards at the time of publication. The author(s), editors, and publisher are not responsible for errors or omissions or for consequences from application of the book, and make no warranty, expressed or implied, in regard to the contents of the book. Any practice described in this book should be applied by the reader in accordance with professional standards of care used in regard to the unique circumstances that may apply in each situation. The reader is advised always to check product information (package inserts) for changes and new information regarding dose and contraindications before administering any drug. Caution is especially urged when using new or infrequently ordered drugs.

ISBN-13:978-0-8036-2290-6
ISBN-10:0-8036-2290-2

This book is dedicated to my family and friends, who encouraged me to write, and to all of the caregivers who seek to increase their knowledge and share it with others.

Preface

Fluid, electrolyte, and acid-base–related disorders are encountered in health-care settings from community to intensive care. This text assists in translating theoretical knowledge into clinical application, reinforcing basic principles in a patient care context. This handbook also delivers concise details correlated with expected outcomes to support classroom and clinical learning.

The first chapter introduces fluids, electrolytes, and acids and bases, and it describes how these elements are transported throughout the body to maintain homeostasis. The next three chapters delve into fluid, electrolyte, and acid-base balance and imbalance. The balance and imbalance chapters include case studies and review questions to reinforce underlying theoretical principles and to develop understanding of clinical presentations that are related to imbalances. The fifth chapter addresses 13 common disorders associated with body imbalances (e.g., cancer, diabetes, etc.), and the last chapter contains a number of helpful tools for the busy clinician, including simplified equations and at-a-glance charts.

The fluid, electrolyte, and acid-base chapters are organized to enable clinicians and educators to locate essential information rapidly. The chapters begin with basic information on physiological function, dietary and parenteral intake, regulation, loss, and laboratory measures, and they continue by discussing the imbalances associated with each element. The imbalance sections of each chapter start with laboratory values, basic concepts, and etiologies. Symptoms are outlined by neurological, cardiovascular (CV), respiratory, gastrointestinal (GI), genitourinary (GU), and reproductive and/or musculoskeletal systems. The imbalance sections also discuss various assessments and actions to promote patient care, and they end with scenarios to help put the information into a clinical perspective. Pediatric and geriatric concerns are also listed at the end of each fluid and electrolyte imbalance chapter, and suggestions for health promotion and public health teaching are scattered throughout the book. Much of the information in these chapters is bullet-pointed so that answers can be found quickly, giving busy clinicians ready access to information.

Patient safety is a paramount concern, as fluid, electrolyte, and acid-base imbalances can rapidly cause life-threatening neurological, cardiac, and respiratory compromise. Clinicians are not expected to manage these changes independently; rather, critical imbalances require immediate notification and collaboration with medical or rapid response teams. The medical team should also be consulted with the onset of new or worsening symptoms or if vital signs are outside the normal range. In addition, if neurological, respiratory, or cardiac compromise occurs, clinicians are directed to call for assistance from the rapid or urgent response team or, if outside an acute care setting, to call community emergency medical services.

Directions for assessments and actions in this book are based on clinical standards. However, institutional guidelines should be consulted before providing patient care. Laboratory procedures, calculations, and assessment scales are also based on clinical standards, but these tools should be confirmed prior to initiating procedures.

Providing safe patient care requires collaboration among health-care team members and resources to inform decision making. My hope is that the information in this book will assist students and practicing clinicians in delivering safe care by promoting balance and preventing ill effects from the imbalance of fluids, electrolytes, and acids and bases.

Elizabethe Westgard, RN, MSN

Reviewers

Marilyn L. Adair, MSN, RN
Director of Nursing
South Puget Sound Community College
Olympia, WA

Janet J. Adams, MSN, RT(ARRT), RN
Instructor
Southeast Missouri State University
Cape Girardeau, MO

Rachel Adema-Hannes, RN, MSc
Professor of Nursing
Mohawk College
Hamilton, Ontario, Canada

Tamara E. Condrey, RN, MSN, CCRN
Assistant Professor of Nursing
Columbus State University
Columbus, GA

Karen Demzien Connors, RN, MSN, CNE
Nursing 1080 Level Coordinator
Central New Mexico Community College
Albuquerque, NM

Darlene Creed, RegN, BScN, MScN(C), CNCC(C)
PN Sessional Professor
Mohawk College
Hamilton, Ontario, Canada

Penelope L. Davis, BScN, MEd
Instructor
University of Manitoba
Winnipeg, Manitoba, Canada

Andrea Deakin, RN, BScN
Coordinator, Practical Nursing With Aboriginal Communities
Mohawk College
Hamilton, Ontario, Canada

Shari Gould, RN, MSN Candidate
Instructor
Victoria College
Gonzales, TX

June S. Goyne, RN, MSN, EdD
Professor
Chair, Nursing Department
Columbus State University
Columbus, GA

Regina Hanchak, RN, MS
Professor
Erie Community College
Buffalo, NY

Ruth F. Harold, AAS, AND, BSN, MSN
Faculty
Caldwell Community College & Technical Institute
Hudson, NC

Tracey L. Hodges, EdD, MSN, RN
Assistant Professor
Troy University
Montgomery, AL

Deloria Jones, RN, BSN, MSN
Faculty
Snead State Community College
Boaz, AL

Christine Kemp, RN, MSN
Instructor
North Hennepin Community College
Brooklyn Park, MN

Douglas W. Kilts, RN, MS, CEN, MBA, MPA
Assistant Professor
Borough of Manhattan Community College
Brooklyn, NY

Susan J. Lamanna, RN, MA, MS, ANP, CNE
Professor
Onondaga Community College
Syracuse, NY

Deborah Langlois, RN, BScN, Med, MBA
Clinical Instructor
Mohawk College
Hamilton, Ontario, Canada

Carrie Sue Lovel, RN, BSN
Associate Professor
Victoria College
Victoria, TX

Betsy M. McDowell, PhD, RN, CCRN, CNE
Professor
Chair, Department of Nursing
Newberry College
Newberry, SC

Stephanie McPheron, RN, MSN
Nurse Educator
Technical College of the Lowcountry
Beaufort, SC

Diane Peters, RN, MSN
Director, Associate Degree Nursing Program
Georgia Northwestern Technical College
Ringgold, GA

Joyce W. Pompey, APRN, DNP
Assistant Professor
University of South Carolina at Aiken
Aiken, SC

Darlene Sheremet, RN, BScN, MEd
Professor
Mohawk College
Hamilton, Ontario, Canada

Rose Stone, RN, BScN, MA
Professor
Mohawk College
Hamilton, Ontario, Canada

Virginia Elaine M. Sullivan, RN, MN
AD Nursing Instructor
Central Carolina Technical College
Sumter, SC

Stephanie Turner, RN, MSN, EdD
Instructor
Wallace State Community College
Hanceville, AL

Angela Vandenberg, RN, BN
Instructor
Red River College
Winnipeg, MB, Canada

Table of Contents

1 General Principles of Fluid, Electrolyte, and Acid-Base Balance and Imbalance

CHAPTER 1

General Principles of Fluid, Electrolyte, and Acid-Base Balance and Imbalance

Health-care professionals must understand the processes involved in fluid, electrolyte, and acid-base balance and imbalance in order to assist in care management of both healthy and ill individuals. Fluid, electrolyte, and acid-base balance are interdependent processes; they also depend on other factors, such as the integrity and function of body organs, the metabolism of nutrients, and the ingestion, injection, or inhalation of medications or toxins. For example, electrolytes like phosphorus, potassium, and sodium are integral to cellular membrane energy exchange. In addition, calcium, magnesium, and sodium are key to the electrical stimulation that occurs in nerves and muscles, and calcium and phosphorus are required to build and maintain a skeleton.

The movement and function of electrolytes depend on fluid and acid-base balance; conversely, acid-base and fluid balance depend on electrolytes. For example, chloride and sodium are closely linked to fluid movement, retention, and excretion, and chloride and potassium are closely related to acid-base balance because the negative charge of chloride and the positive charge of potassium cause a shift of bicarbonate and hydrogen ions. Overhydration and dehydration also have an effect on electrolyte function and availability, which subsequently impacts acid-base relationships.

Recent studies have shown that essential minerals are also key to maintaining overall balance. The function and normal distribution of some minerals are well understood, whereas others continue to be investigated for their effect on body systems and general homeostasis.

A deficit or excess of essential minerals, electrolytes, or molecules of acid-base balance may cause dramatic health problems for patients. It is essential for health-care providers to measure and follow laboratory values, intake and output measures, and signs and symptoms of imbalance. Understanding the impact of imbalance of these individual and interdependent components allows the health-care team to work together to maintain the patient's optimum health.

Examples of fluids in the human body include blood, sweat, tears, urine, gastric secretions, synovial fluid, and the fluid contained inside cells. Electrolytes are elements such as sodium, calcium, and potassium, which carry electrical charges when dissolved in water, and they are also components of cells or in fluid solutions. Acids and bases are molecules formed during metabolism that can either accept or donate excess hydrogen ions. Healthy people are generally able to take in appropriate amounts of fluids, electrolytes, and components of acid and base molecules, and they are able to maintain homeostasis of fluid, electrolyte, and acid-base balance through complex metabolic mechanisms, including excretion and release of gases.

Patients facing chronic or acute illness, trauma or surgery, or unusual environmental conditions are at risk for imbalance, which can occur rapidly or gradually. For example, these patients are at high risk for rapid and extreme shifts in their overall homeostasis. Patients with more long-term or chronic problems may experience an imbalance that occurs gradually, creating long-term complications. They may have only a fragile balance of fluids, electrolytes, and acid-base status, and they may be at risk for a sudden, dramatic shift from homeostasis to imbalance with the impact of any stressors. Most hospitalized patients will receive intravenous fluid support, and many patients will experience electrolyte imbalance as a secondary diagnosis.

This chapter introduces fluids, electrolytes, and acid-base balance and imbalance, and it describes molecular shifts in the body and the interdependency of fluids and electrolytes in maintaining homeostasis.

Fluids

Fluids in the body are water-based, so a discussion of fluids is really a discussion of the balance of water and the cells, gases, electrolytes, minerals, and other molecules that are contained in it. Water has special properties of hydrogen-binding and polarity that allow it to act as a transport medium for ions, which are particles that are able to carry electrical charges. Fluid balance and fluid movement are key to understanding the overall impact of fluids on the body.

Fluid Balance

Fluid balance depends on intake, output, and the distribution of total body water between intracellular and extracellular compartments in the body. Intracellular fluid (ICF) is the fluid in the internal compartments of cells, and extracellular fluid (ECF) is a general term used to describe any fluid outside of a cell, either in the vascular cavity or outside of both cells and the vascular cavity. Three types of ECF are:

1. Intravascular fluid: fluid in the vascular space
2. Interstitial fluid: fluid in the area surrounding cells
3. Transcellular fluid: fluid in compartments like the cerebral spinal space and the synovial cavities

ICF, interstitial fluid, and transcellular fluid are also described as extravascular fluid (EVF), as it lies outside of the vascular space. Figure 1-1 illustrates intracellular, interstitial, and intravascular movement.

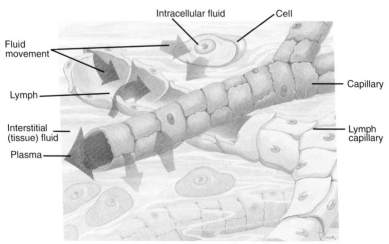

FIGURE 1-1: Intracellular, interstitial, and intravascular fluid compartments and fluid movement.

During homeostasis, about two-thirds of the body's fluid is ICF and about one-third is ECF. About one quarter of ECF is intravascular fluid, with the remainder occurring as interstitial fluid and transcellular fluid (Fig. 1-2). In healthy individuals, fluids travel between ICF and ECF compartments carrying essential nutrients, gases, and electrolytes as part of normal metabolism. Depending on chemical shifts within the body, fluid will either leave the cells or the vascular space and travel through the interstitial space toward the opposing space.

The impact of fluid intake and output on patient homeostasis will be discussed in Chapter 2. The principles, which are discussed here, of volume and the shifting of fluids between the body's intravascular and extravascular compartments are based on basic anatomy and physiology.

COACH CONSULT

Determining a patient's fluid status is key to care delivery in acute and chronic settings. It includes a physical assessment of the patient's body systems; levels of fluid intake through diet, supplements, or intravenous support; and levels of output through urine, stool, sweat, and other insensible losses.

Fluid Movement

Fluid moves in and out of cells, through interstitial spaces, and in and out the vascular space depending on chemical and biological processes. For instance, waste products leave cells and travel to the bloodstream, whereas nutrients leave the bloodstream and travel to cells. Fluid typically only leaves or enters the vascular compartment at the capillary level, which is where the cells are structured to allow for the passage of fluids, electrolytes, and some molecules; the vascular compartment at the capillary level is also where capillary pores, called *aquaporins*, allow for the passage of selected cells, such as white blood cells.

Because of fluid's special properties of hydrogen-binding and polarity, it is an ideal means of transporting not only waste and nutrients but also electrolytes, acids, and bases, which are ions. More on the transportation of these elements can be found in this chapter after the discussion of electrolytes, acids, and bases.

COACH CONSULT

An important part of fluid movement is the permeability of the capillaries of the vascular system. Trauma or other damage to large veins or arteries causes extreme fluid shifts and therefore needs to be addressed promptly.

Fluid Imbalance

In pathological states, excess fluid, cells, electrolytes, and minerals can leave the cells and flood the interstitial spaces and the interior of veins and arteries. Conversely, fluid may leave the veins and arteries and flood the interstitial

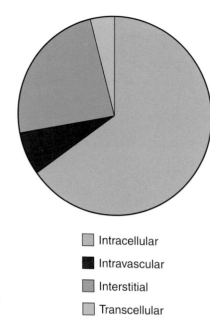

Intracellular

Intravascular

Interstitial

Transcellular

FIGURE 1-2: Normal distribution of body fluids.

space, the cavities that surround organs, or the interior of cells. Normal metabolism is negatively affected during these pathological fluid shifts if they cannot adequately process the excess fluid. For example, *edema* is the swelling that occurs when the spaces between cells and the vascular compartment become overwhelmed with fluid, usually because fluid has leaked out of its normal vascular or cellular compartments. Vascular and intracellular fluid can also accumulate in body compartments due to pathological problems, such as in *ascites*, which is the buildup of excess fluid in the abdominal cavity that occurs with liver dysfunction. Fluid can also build up around the cavities that surround the brain, heart, and lungs, putting pressure on these organs and changing the normal exchange of electrolytes and other essential molecules, such as glucose.

These collections of excess extravascular fluid can be life-threatening because they increase cavity pressure, interrupting the normal functioning of these organs. Tubes or drains may be placed to draw off excess fluid. A pathological increase in the fluid inside of cells can also occur; this is known as *fluid intoxication*. Fluid intoxication occurs with infusion or ingestion of fluids without appropriate sodium replacement or with concurrent excess loss of sodium and fluid retention. See Chapter 2 for details about fluid balance and imbalance.

Electrolytes

An *electrolyte* is an element that is able to carry an electrical charge when dissolved in water. This quality allows electrolytes to form and break bonds when exposed to chemical changes in the fluid in which they are dissolved. Common body electrolytes include calcium, chloride, magnesium, phosphorus, potassium, and sodium.

Electrolytes typically have a variety of functions within the body. They are key components of cellular structures, such as calcium in the bones and teeth. They also function as chemical messengers, components of energy pathways, and as a means of polarizing cellular membranes. Potassium, sodium, calcium, and magnesium are essential to the electrochemical processes that allow the heart muscle to contract regularly. Chloride assists with maintaining acid-base balance, and sodium is the key determinant of fluid *tonicity*, which is the potential for solutes to cause fluid to move across a membrane.

Electrolyte Balance
During normal metabolism, balance of electrolytes is maintained through adequate ingestion, hormonal regulation, chemical interactions, and regulated excretion. Transport of electrolytes depends on metabolic requirements and the amount of electrolytes in the bloodstream. At times, certain electrolytes may be pulled into the bloodstream from cells, such as calcium moving from the bones and into the vascular space during periods of low blood calcium. Conversely, electrolytes also travel into cells to support electrochemical mechanisms or, as in the case of phosphorus, as a component of the cellular membrane.

Electrolyte Imbalance
Bodily dysfunction can occur when the level of available electrolytes in the bloodstream falls below or rises above a narrow normal range. Healthcare providers routinely assess blood levels of electrolytes to screen for shifts outside of the normal range. Certain symptoms are also associated with high or low levels of certain electrolytes and can provide clues that electrolytes may not be balanced. At times, these symptoms can be specific to a certain electrolyte imbalance; for instance, delayed clotting times can be associated with low calcium levels. Often the symptoms may be of

a general nature, such as headache, lethargy, or nausea, which can be attributed to a variety of electrolyte imbalances as well as other disorders.

In many cases, electrolyte shifts occur with acute illnesses or surgery, when the patient is not able to adequately compensate for abnormal metabolism. Chronic illness can also contribute to electrolyte imbalance. In some circumstances, patients may live with chronically elevated or depleted levels of certain electrolytes. Although these patients may be able to compensate for abnormal electrolyte levels during normal periods of illness, they may be at risk for dramatic effects of electrolyte shifts if they suffer an infection or trauma with a preexisting imbalance. For more on electrolytes, see Chapter 3.

Acids and Bases

An *acid,* generally, is a substance that forms hydrogen (H^+) ions when dissolved in water. It is more accurately defined as a substance that can act as a hydrogen donor. Acids form as normal by-products of glucose, fat, and protein metabolism and the normal destruction of cells. Glucose metabolism results in the formation of carbon dioxide during normal metabolism and lactic acid during anaerobic metabolism. Fats form keto acids, and proteins with sulfur-containing amino acids form sulfuric acid.

A *base,* also known as an alkaline substance, is a substance that forms hydroxide ions (OH^-) when dissolved in water. A broader definition that includes substances such as ammonia (NH_3) describes a base as a substance that can accept a hydrogen ion. Bases such as ammonia, hydrogen phosphate, and bicarbonate are formed through metabolic processes. In addition, hydrogen phosphate can be derived from food intake or from the breakdown of molecules, such as adenosine triphosphate (ATP) or adenosine diphosphate (ADP).

In short, acids are molecules that can release hydrogen ions, and bases are molecules that can accept excess hydrogen ions. Therefore, *acid-base balance* is essentially a measure of the number of excess hydrogen ions in body fluid.

Acid-Base Balance

Acid-base balance depends on access and intake of foods, liquids, and—in some cases, like vitamin D—environmental exposure. It also depends on biological functions that influence the shift of molecules in one of three directions: between cells, into and out of intercellular spaces, and into and out of intravascular spaces. Finally, acid-base balance is affected by elimination through normal body functions that produce urine, stool, sweat, and other fluids, as well as abnormal elimination that is common with disease processes. Acid-base balance is closely linked to fluid and electrolyte balance, and it changes when certain electrolytes or the overall fluid balance is shifted.

The acid-base balance is described in a ratio called pH, and blood pH levels need to remain within normal limits (pH 7.35–7.45) for body cells to function properly. When pH shifts out of the normal range, acidosis—an excess of acids—or alkalosis—an excess of bases—can occur.

The body can compensate for normal pH shifts. For example, ammonia is formed from amino acid catabolism in the kidneys, and bicarbonate is formed in the pancreas and in the kidneys. The kidneys can reabsorb bicarbonate when pH is shifting toward acidosis, and they can excrete bicarbonate when it shifts toward alkalosis.

Acid-Base Imbalance

Buffer systems are continually acting to prevent large shifts in pH through chemical changes that turn strong acids into weak acids or strong bases into weak bases. The mechanisms for these buffering systems are explained in Chapter 4.

Shifts away from the normal range of acidosis or alkalosis can cause disturbances in cardiac, endocrine, muscle, nerve, and respiratory function. Extreme shifts result in death (Fig. 1-3). Although some patients with chronic illness—such as chronic obstructive pulmonary diseases or kidney diseases—may also have chronic acid-base imbalance, life-threatening imbalances are often associated with acute illness, trauma, and surgery. Care providers need to be aware of risk factors for and signs and symptoms

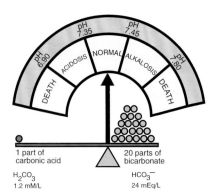

FIGURE 1-3: Dramatic shifts in acid-base balance can result in death.

of imbalance so that patients can be provided proper treatment to regain balance.

Fluid, Electrolyte, and Acid-Base Transport

To maintain homeostasis, fluids, cells, electrolytes, essential minerals, and nutrients need to pass across the capillaries of the bowel and through the capillaries of the vascular wall. Then they need to pass from the vascular space across the interstitial space and into cells. Similarly, excess fluids and electrolytes and cellular waste products need to be transported out of cells, through the interstitial space, and back into the bloodstream to be transported back to the bowels and the kidneys for excretion. Fluids can also depart the body through exocrine glands, such as sweat or tear glands, through endocrine glands in the form of hormones or other secretions, and through cells such as the mucous membranes of the gastrointestinal tract or the lining of the lungs. The transport mechanisms responsible for these processes are diffusion, facilitated diffusion, osmosis, active transport, and filtration. All these processes are illustrated in Figure 1-4.

Passive Transport: Diffusion

Diffusion is a process that is essential to electrolyte balance. It occurs when a molecule passes from an area of high concentration to an area of low concentration (see Fig. 1-4A). This is sometimes described as "downhill" movement. When the concentration is high, the movement to an area of lower concentration is rapid. When the concentration moves closer to equilibrium, the speed of diffusion slows. In addition, large molecules move slower than smaller molecules, and higher-temperature solutions diffuse faster than colder solutions.

Diffusion is considered a passive process because it does not take an expenditure of energy to move something from one compartment to the next. Diffusion of a substance requires the cellular membrane to be permeable to that substance without any energy being expended in addition to the energy that is generated by the random motion of all molecules. If substances can travel freely across the membrane, then they will move from an area of higher concentration to an area of lower concentration until the fluids on both sides of the membrane have an equal, balanced amount of the substance.

Passive diffusion can occur when the membrane allows for the diffusion of certain particles. In the body, some membranes are permeable to certain molecules while they remain impermeable to others. Also, certain membranes may be modified by chemical processes to allow for more or

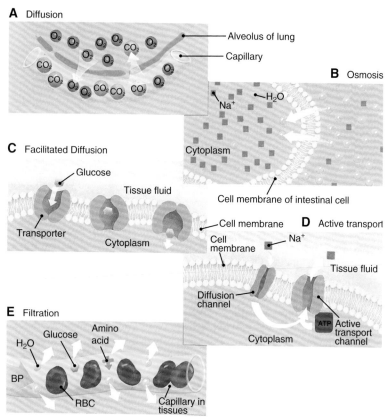

A Diffusion

O₂ ... CO₂ ... — Alveolus of lung

— Capillary

B Osmosis

Na⁺ — H₂O

Cytoplasm

Cell membrane of intestinal cell

C Facilitated Diffusion

Glucose

Tissue fluid

Transporter

Cytoplasm

Cell membrane

D Active transport

Cell membrane

Na⁺

Tissue fluid

Diffusion channel

ATP Active transport channel

Cytoplasm

E Filtration

Amino acid

H₂O Glucose

BP

RBC

Capillary in tissues

F I G U R E 1 - 4 : Cellular transport mechanisms: (A) Diffusion is the movement of solute molecules through a cell membrane from an area of higher concentration to an area of lower concentration; (B) Osmosis is the movement of fluid across a membrane from a less concentrated solution to a more concentrated solution; (C) Facilitated diffusion involves a shift in the cellular membrane that does not require energy; (D) Active transport requires energy for movement across a membrane; (E) Filtration is the movement of fluids and smaller particles from an area of high pressure to an area of low pressure.

less diffusion, depending on the body's shifting chemistry. This process whereby changes occur in the membrane or when a "carrier molecule" assists with transport is known as *facilitated diffusion* as long as no energy is expended in the process (Fig. 1-4C).

In the case of electrolytes that carry a charge, some diffusion may also be influenced by electrical charge. When one fluid compartment has a more negative or a more positive charge, negative electrolytes will move toward the positive area, and positive electrolytes will move toward the negative area. When differences in both concentration and electrical charge exist, electrolytes will move across the membrane until a balance has been created.

Osmosis

Osmosis is a key factor in fluid balance. It is the movement of fluid across a membrane from a compartment where there is a low concentration of particles to a compartment where there is a high concentration of particles (see Fig. 1-4B). During osmosis, chemical pressures pull water, which is the solvent of the human body, toward the fluid compartment that has a higher concentration of certain dissolved solutes. Water passes in and out of cells across *aquaporins*, which are specialized channels in the cellular membrane. Electrolytes can pass freely between the two parts of the ECF—the interstitial space and the vascular space—and thus normally there will be the same concentration of electrolytes on both sides of the vascular capillary membrane. However, proteins cannot pass as freely as electrolytes and will remain within the blood vessels under normal conditions, which creates an intravascular fluid osmotic force greater than the osmotic force of interstitial fluid.

Factors that limit osmosis include the permeability of the membrane, the osmotic pull of various elements, and fluid mobility.

Membrane Permeability

Human cellular membranes are considered to be selectively permeable. This means that only certain substances can cross the membrane under certain conditions. Increased fluid pressures from increased fluid volume can increase the amount of fluid leaving the vascular space. Excess fluid in the interstitial space may be inhibited from returning back across the vascular capillary membranes due to the elevated intravascular fluid volume pressures. Other factors that can contribute to increased permeability include localized or systemic inflammatory processes from infection, allergic reactions, and trauma or burns actually damaging the capillary wall.

Osmotic Pull

Whereas the ICF and ECF do not have the same electrolyte concentration, they do have a similar osmolarity. *Osmolarity* is the weight of molecules or particles that have osmotic pull: 1 osmole of a substance is equal to 1 gram of molecular weight. Osmoles on a cellular level are measured in milliosmoles (mOsm) per liter (L) of fluid. The term osmolality is also used, but this term technically represents not the weight but the *volume* of osmotic molecules. More information on osmolality is in Box 1–1. Both the ICF and the ECF contain about 275–295 milliosmoles in each liter of fluid (mOsm/L).

Albumin is a key plasma protein that contributes to normal osmotic pressures. In low albumin states, such as during malnutrition or during periods of "nothing by mouth" (NPO) status, fluid that normally moves back into the vascular space stays in the interstitial space. Other factors that can cause a loss in plasma proteins are chronic diarrhea, kidney diseases that cause renal protein losses, and liver disease that prevents the appropriate synthesis of plasma proteins.

Fluid Mobility

The ability to use intravenous fluids to increase hydration is described as tonicity and is based on the content of sodium and other molecules. In order for a substance to be an effective osmole and to be able to increase the tonicity of fluid, that substance needs to stay on one side of a membrane while fluid moves toward it. Substances that are considered effective osmoles in serum include glucose, mannitol, and sodium. While urea is used to measure osmolality, it is not considered an effective osmole.

Glucose can be an effective osmole, but it is not used to increase serum tonicity because it moves quickly into cells under normal conditions. If patients are not able to mobilize glucose properly from the bloodstream into cells, such as in case of poorly controlled diabetes, then glucose can increase vascular tonicity. High serum glucose pulls fluid out of cells and causes cellular fluid deficit.

Mannitol is used to increase serum tonicity. Sudden shifts of fluid in and out of cells can occur when the tonicity of serum is suddenly elevated or decreased. If the serum has too little water in ratio to osmolar substances, then fluid leaves cells and migrates into the bloodstream. This shrinking or dehydration of cells can be life-threatening when brain cells are affected. If serum has low tonicity (low concentration of effective osmoles), then water leaves the vascular space and may contribute to the dangerous overhydration of cells, especially brain cells. Clinically, intravenous infusion of mannitol is used to increase serum tonicity and reduce the swelling of brain cells.

COACH CONSULT

Fluid returns from cells and the intracellular compartment through the lymphatic system. Disruption of the lymphatic system can also cause fluid to stay in the interstitial spaces or in the lymph system. Lymphatic dysfunction can be caused by trauma or surgery to the lymph vessels and lymph nodes, tumors, or by infection or inflammation of the lymph system.

🗫 NURSE-TO-NURSE TIP

Patients on salt restriction may be placed on fluid restriction. In combination, salt and fluid restriction can cause a fluid deficit (dehydration). When patients who are normally on these restrictions experience episodes where their fluid demands are greater than normal—for instance, sweating due to a fever—then they may lose both sodium and fluids. Patients who breathe at a rate of 24 or more breaths per minute for more than 24 hours can lose up to 3 L of fluid through respiratory fluid loss.

Signs of dehydration include tachycardia, confusion, decreased skin and mucous membrane turgor, decreased urine output, and thirst. Patients on a sodium and fluid restriction who present with thirst should be rapidly assessed for fluid volume deficit.

Box 1–1 Osmolality

Osmolality is the measure of the total concentration of solutes in a fluid. The normal serum osmolality range is 280–295 mOsm/kg. Sodium, glucose, and urea are the main particles that determine the osmolality of serum.

OSMOLALITY AND SODIUM

Sodium is the principal extracellular electrolyte. When combined with either chloride or bicarbonate, sodium makes up 90% or more of osmotic particles and osmotic force in the ECF. The normal concentration of sodium in serum is 135–145 mEq/L (135–145 mmol/L). When there is more sodium present, more

Continued

Box 1-1 **Osmolality—cont'd**

fluid is pulled into and held in the vascular space. Too little sodium in the serum may cause a fluid shift in the extracellular space, which will present clinically as edema.

Three major pathways affect sodium and fluid balance:

1. **Renin-angiotensin-aldosterone system.** The kidney has receptor cells that sense the volume of fluid flowing through the glomerulus. If too little fluid is flowing through the kidneys, then renin is released, and a cascade is initiated to transform angiotensinogen into angiotensin I, then angiotensin II. Angiotensin II causes sodium retention in the kidneys and stimulates the adrenal cortex to release aldosterone. Aldosterone also causes sodium retention in the distal nephron of the kidneys.

2. **Vena cava receptors.** Volume sensors in the vena cava and in the heart's atria sense an increase in fluid volume flowing through the heart. This stimulates the release of atrial natriuretic factor, which in turn increases sodium excretion.

3. **Aorta and carotid sinus receptors.** Pressure receptors in the aorta and carotids sense a drop in arterial fluid volumes, causing an increase in retention of sodium by the kidneys.

For healthy individuals, the kidneys are usually able to appropriately modify the amount of sodium excreted so that ECF says in balance. However, when patients ingest or retain too much sodium, they can develop fluid overload. Patients who have weak hearts are often prescribed low-sodium diets to ensure that too much fluid does not accumulate in their veins and arteries, causing excess stress on their heart.

OSMOLALITY AND GLUCOSE, UREA

With diabetes or renal dysfunction, osmolality can increase from elevated blood glucose or blood urea nitrogen. Osmolality can also be calculated and compared with measured osmolality to determine the presence of substances such as acetone or mannitol. The formula for calculated osmolality is:

$$\text{Osmolality} = (2 \times \text{sodium concentration in mEq/L}) + \\ (\text{[glucose concentration in mg/dL]}/18) + \\ (\text{[blood urea nitrogen in mg/dL]}/2.8)$$

If measured osmolality is more than 10 mOsm/L greater than calculated osmolality, then the abnormal presence of osmotic particles is suggested. This may be a sign of methanol or ethylene glycol poisoning.

Sodium and saline solutions are also used to increase tonicity. Although sodium can cross the membranes of vascular capillaries, it is continually pumped out of cells by the sodium-potassium ATP-ase pump. An increase in sodium concentration in the blood vessels also stimulates thirst and the release of antidiuretic hormone, which causes fluid retention by the kidneys, further increasing fluids in the bloodstream.

Normal saline solution is 0.9% sodium chloride because it has a tonicity similar to that of human blood. When hypotonic solutions, such as 0.45% sodium chloride, enter the bloodstream, they dilute the sodium levels in the bloodstream and cause water to move toward the cells. Hypertonic solutions, such as 3% or 5% sodium chloride, greatly increase the concentration of sodium in the bloodstream and cause fluid to move from cells and interstitial space into the vascular space. Figure 1-5 illustrates these fluid shifts.

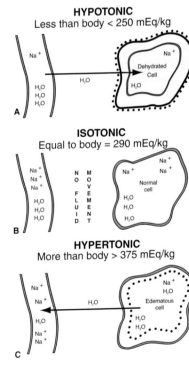

FIGURE 1-5: Hypotonic, isotonic, and hypertonic fluid shifts.

Urea is included in measures of osmolality, but it does not affect tonicity. The concentration of urea is calculated and measured but, because urea crosses capillary membranes easily, it moves to an area of lesser concentration rather than remain in the vascular space. Therefore, it does not effectively pull fluid into the vascular space and thus does not increase tonicity.

Active Transport: The Sodium-Potassium Pump

Active transport is a process that requires the expenditure of energy for movement across a membrane (see Figure 1-4,D). This process can be used to move solutes from an area of lower concentration to an area of higher concentration and is sometimes known as "uphill" movement.

Active transport requires a carrier molecule and may require a chemical reaction from an enzyme. The primary energy source is an ATP molecule, which is used to exchange sodium and potassium across the cellular membrane. Chapter 3F contains more information on the sodium-potassium pump. Energy is also available from the difference between ions on two sides of the membrane. Glucose-sodium co-transport and sodium-calcium counter-transport rely on energy from this ionic charge.

Filtration

Filtration is the movement of water or solutes across a membrane due to the force of pressure (see Fig. 1-4E). In filtration, both the solute and the solvent move together from an area of high pressure to an area of low pressure. *Hydrostatic pressure* is the pressure exerted by fluids in various body compartments. In the blood vessels, this pressure is exerted at the capillary level, pushing solutes into the interstitial space.

Fluid does not normally pass out of large veins or arteries despite high pressures, like the normal mean arterial pressure of 60 mm Hg. This is because the cellular structure of arteries and veins prevents fluids from passing across them until they decrease in size at the capillary level. When the arterial tree narrows down into its smallest branches, which are called arterioles, there is a hydrostatic pressure of approximately 18 mm Hg near the capillary bed. At this point, the interstitial space, located outside the capillary bed, has a negative hydrostatic pressure of approximately -6 mm Hg. The pressure of 18 mm Hg against a pressure of -6 mm Hg results in some fluid leaving the capillaries and migrating out into the tissues. Fluid returns into the capillary bed at the venules, which are the smallest branches of the veins.

The pressures that pull fluid back into the capillaries are osmotic pressures. An osmotic pressure of about 28 mm Hg is created by cells and molecules in the capillary bed where capillaries join the venules. The osmotic pressure of the interstitial space at this point is about 4 mm Hg. The higher osmotic pressure functions to pull fluid from the interstitial space into the capillaries. In combination, hydrostatic pressures and osmotic pressures allow for fluid exchange across the capillaries.

ALERT

Increased capillary permeability is a key pathological process with sepsis. Massive fluid resuscitation is required for the patient to maintain blood pressure and survive.

2 Fluid Balance and Imbalance

Fluids

CHAPTER 2

Fluid Balance and Imbalance

In healthy adults, fluids account for about 60% of body weight. Because fluids are a major component of most body systems, it is necessary to monitor a patient's fluid balance and to assess and respond to signs of fluid excess and fluid deficit in order to maintain health.

The basis of fluid balance and imbalance in humans is water. Approximately two-thirds of water is bound inside of cells, and approximately one-third is free to move between intravascular, interstitial, and organ cavities. The water travels across cellular and capillary membranes in conjunction with electrolytes to transport gases, nutrients, and wastes through the body's systems.

The body-weight-to-water ratio depends on body mass index and age. A 70-kg (154-lb) adult has approximately 42 L of water; of those 42 L, about 28 L is held in the intracellular space, and about 14 L is held in the extracellular space. Blood volume accounts for approximately 5 L of a 70-kg adult's body weight. Note that obese and geriatric individuals have less water by body weight because fat contains less water than muscle.

Fluid imbalances include fluid excess, fluid deficit, and fluid shift. Fluid excess and fluid deficit are usually discussed in terms of when too much fluid is held in the body (e.g., when patients do not have the ability to make urine) and when too much fluid leaves the body (e.g., during episodes of bleeding). The concept of fluid excess and fluid deficit are also discussed when fluid shifts in an abnormal manner between body compartments. In these cases, a patient may have a normal amount of fluid in the body overall, but too much of the body's fluid is in areas that normally only contain a small amount of fluid (such as in the cavities around the lungs and heart) while too little of the body's fluid is in other areas (such as with decreased blood volume in the veins and arteries). The shift of fluid into interstitial space is called "third spacing," and it occurs when a patient appears to be experiencing fluid deficit even though the overall body fluid levels are normal.

Functions

AGE-RELATED IMPLICATIONS

According to the United States Department of Agriculture (USDA), infants are about 75% water from birth to 6 months. After 6 months, males are about 60% water, and females are about 50%–56% water. Both male and female water content declines after 51 years of age to about 56% and 47% water, respectively. These differences between males and females are based on percentage of body fat.

Water functions in a variety of pathways. For example, it is a means of transportation for gases, nutrients, and wastes, and it is the basis for blood, lymph, and serous exocrine products. Water also supports gastrointestinal (GI) function, regulates body temperature, lubricates joints and eye sockets, and is a medium for flushing waste products through the kidneys and GI tract.

Transports Gases, Nutrients, and Waste

Water is used as a transport mechanism for gases, nutrients, and waste between cells and the vascular system. Mechanisms described in Chapter 1—including filtration, osmosis, diffusion, and active transport—require water as a medium for solutes and molecules to move between body tissues and fluids.

Has Unique Chemical Properties

The chemical structure of water allows for an abundance of reactions in biochemistry. Water acts as a solvent for ionic and polar substances such as acids, alcohols, and salts. Water has the ability to act as either a base or an acid in certain chemical circumstances, allowing it to function as a buffer.

Provides the Basis for Blood, Lymph, and Serous Exocrine Products

Water molecules form the basis for all body fluids, including blood, lymph, and serous fluid. Blood consists of about 45% cellular components—including red blood cells (RBCs), white blood cells, and platelets—and about 55% plasma. Plasma consists of about 90% water, carrying protein, ions, and organic substances.

Lymph is similar to plasma, traveling through the body via the lymph system and between the lymph vessels and vascular space as interstitial fluid. The lymph system is a vital part of the immune system, and lymph fluid contains white blood cells.

Serous fluid is found in body cavities, such as the pericardium; it is also secreted from certain exocrine glands, which are known as serous glands or mixed glands. Mixed glands secrete both serous fluid and mucus. Serous fluid is similar to blood serum without the blood cells or clotting factors, and it forms a basis for glandular secretions such as saliva.

Supports GI Function

The GI tract secretes about 6–8 L of fluid over 24 hours because the intestine reabsorbs about 5–6 L of GI fluid plus about 1–2 L of dietary fluid. In addition, epithelial cells that line the GI tract produce 3.5 L of fluid, and accessory gland and organ secretions, such as saliva and bile, make up the remaining amount of fluid needed to keep the GI system functioning. Epithelial secretions lubricate mucous membranes, which allows for swallowing food and passing stool. Gland and organ secretions, such as hydrochloric acid and pancreatic fluids, aid in digestive processes.

Regulates Body Temperature

Water assists in regulating body temperature in two ways: through insensible loss via respiratory vapors and skin pores and through the evaporation of sweat. Insensible losses account for about 25% of cooling, even without sweating. Sweating to such an extent that water is dripping off the skin does not contribute to heat regulation because there is no evaporation of this water. Evaporation accounts for about 900 calories of heat regulation per day versus about 60 calories of heat lost through urine and feces. In 100% humidified environments, evaporation cannot occur, and heat cannot be lost through sweat.

To maintain homeostasis, humans can sweat up to 4 L/hr but more typically will lose 1 L/hr during exposure to excessive heat. At 10% of weight loss, or 7 L for a 70-kg person, the body may become too dehydrated to maintain basic metabolic functions.

COACH CONSULT

Patients who have sustained body temperatures below 91.4°F (33°C) will lose consciousness; at 107°F (42°C), the central nervous system breaks down. Expected variations in body temperature range from cold-weather or early morning temperatures of 95°F (35°C) to very hard exercise or high level of emotions at 104°F (40°C).

Lubricates Joints and Eye Sockets

Cartilage is 80% water, and its structure allows for water to be mechanically shifted to accommodate for dynamic changes in stress that result from joint movement. In addition to intracartilage water, synovial cavities contain molecules formed from water, which add to lubrication.

The eye's anterior aqueous humor is similar to plasma and lubricates the anterior eye between the lens and the cornea. This humor is continually secreted by the ciliary body to deliver nutrients and oxygen to these structures. The vitreous humor at the posterior portion of the eye is about 98% water, but it is formed into a gel-like substance that does not exchange fluid.

Flushes Waste Products Through the Kidneys and GI Tract

About 200 L of blood circulate though the kidneys over 24 hours, creating on average 2 L of urine. Urine is composed of water and waste products, the latter of which includes metabolized cells, foods, and medicines. Decline in kidney function affects the ability of the kidneys to concentrate urine, either causing the concentration to be too high or too low, depending on the type of dysfunction. Renal disease can also create conditions in which important nutrients are lost or potentially toxic materials are retained. Kidney disorders are a special concern for the geriatric patient, who naturally loses some renal function as part of the aging process, and for any patient who is taking medication that is normally excreted from the kidneys.

Healthy feces, or stool, should be about 75% water. This measurement depends on proper hydration, health, and dietary factors. The Bristol Stool Chart (also known as the Meyers Scale) rates stool in seven categories, and some institutions use the chart to gauge proper hydration of stool. When feces are about a foot in length, smooth, and soft, they contain a proper amount of water. If a person does not have two bowel movements over a 24-hour period with this consistency, then food, cellular waste, and toxins will not be sufficiently removed from the colon.

Fluid Intake

In healthy patients, fluid intake is through dietary sources. However, many patients who are admitted to acute care facilities may require hydration via intravenous (IV) infusion or enteric tube feedings.

Dietary Intake

Dietary intake of water comes from drinking water or ingesting beverages or foods that contain water. The USDA estimates an average daily adequate dietary intake for healthy adults between the ages of 19 and 30 years to be 3.7 L for men and 2.7 L for women. In the U.S. population, approximately 80% of water intake is through water and beverages, with about 20% from food. However, the USDA cautions that hydration needs can vary from individual to individual and from day to day. The primary factors creating the variation are diet, level of physical activity, and weather. Acutely ill patients may be unable to obtain sufficient quantities of water due to lack of independence, increased metabolic needs, or excessively dry indoor environments.

Fluid Regulation

According to the USDA, the body is normally able to self-regulate fluid input and output (I&O). Thirst is the primary mechanism that induces drinking. Receptors in the vascular system are stimulated when intravascular fluid levels are low. A loss of about 1% of body weight, which is about 0.7 kg or 700 mL of fluid, stimulates thirst.

Primary regulation of water excretion is through the kidneys. The USDA cautions that fluid intake in excess of 700 mL/hr can exceed the kidney's ability to excrete water, even in healthy individuals, and cause water toxicity.

Abnormal ingestion or excretion of water may result in fluid deficit or fluid loss. However, with acute or chronic illness, a patient with an overall normal body fluid volume may experience a shift of the ratio of fluid between body spaces. This is sometimes called third spacing, which describes an abnormal amount of fluid outside of the vascular or intracellular spaces.

Fluid Loss

Fluid loss depends on exposure to heat and the requirement to cool the body through sweat and respiratory losses.

For healthy people at rest and under temperate conditions, the USDA cites average fluid losses at 1000–2000 mL/day. Less fluid, about 500 mL/day, is lost through urine when fluids are needed to cool the body from exercise, exposure to hot weather, or fever.

Normal breathing patterns result in 250–350 mL/day of fluid losses for people with no respiratory problems in temperate climates. With exercise, tachypnea, or changes in the climate, this loss can be up to 700 mL/day. Respiratory therapists can aid in determining the need for humidification of oxygen sources for patients who are tachypneic but are breathing unhumidified room air.

In addition to sweat and respiratory losses, about 100 mL of fluid is lost each day through feces when no bowel dysfunction is present. Unexpected fluid losses can occur through the respiratory, integumentary, GI, and urinary systems, as well as through burns, sepsis, and trauma.

COACH CONSULT

Fluid losses can be estimated using the formula of 1 kg in body weight = 1 L in fluid. Losses in body weight from limited caloric intake of foods are rarely above 350 g/day, so weight loss exceeding 350 g should be considered fluid loss.

Vascular fluid loss is also a concern. If fluid collects in organ cavities, then the function of these organ systems may be compromised. Fluid collection in the thoracic cavity is serious because a pleural or pericardial effusion can lead to rapid respiratory or cardiac decline and death. Fluid accumulation in the abdomen or pelvis can lead to compression of blood vessels and vital organs and create excess pressures in the thoracic cavity. If a patient appears to be losing vascular fluid without an evident source, then a thorough assessment of these organ systems should be conducted with a suspicion of hemorrhage or effusion.

With an acute illness, it may be difficult for the medical team to establish whether the patient is experiencing fluid excess, fluid deficit, or fluid shifts. In these cases, a careful review of I&O and of serum and urine laboratory values is required. However, even with comparison of fluid volumes and evaluation of laboratory studies, a pulmonary artery catheter may be placed at times when the medical team believes that accurate fluid assessment can be measured only by obtaining data from within the heart and major blood vessels, such as during shock or sepsis. This catheter is designed to provide computerized pressure readings of the fluid flowing through the chambers of the heart. These measures can be used to estimate a patient's fluid status and modify a fluid balance treatment plan.

COACH CONSULT

Patients who are experiencing fluid loss may maintain a normal-to-high blood pressure. The physiological mechanisms that increase blood pressure during fluid loss can be sustained for only a brief time. The nurse should anticipate a drop in blood pressure if there is a known source of fluid loss or shifting of fluid to extravascular spaces.

Laboratory Measures

Serum samples are drawn to assess for dehydration or overhydration. *Serum osmolality* is the primary indicator of hydration. It is a measure of the number of particles in a solution, and it can be compared with urine osmolality to help form a diagnosis. Bicarbonate, chloride, glucose, sodium, and urea contribute to serum osmolality. Normal serum osmolality for patients from 2 months to adult is 275–295 mOsm/kg.

When hemoconcentration occurs due to *fluid deficit*, certain serum laboratory values become elevated, including electrolytes, blood urea nitrogen (BUN), creatinine, and total protein. A slow drop in hemoglobin (Hgb) and hematocrit (Hct) levels may indicate active bleeding; a rapid elevation indicates hemorrhage due to hemoconcentration.

Laboratory values that are consistent with *overhydration* include decreased serum electrolytes and total protein. Common results for these tests are listed below:

- BUN levels for people 14–90 years are 8–21 mg/dL. BUN measures are considered in ratio to creatinine and within the context of the overall clinical picture. They can be elevated with renal insufficiency, which causes fluid excess, or they can be decreased due to fluid excess.
- Normal creatinine levels for males >10 years are 0.6–1.2 mg/dL and for females >10 years are 0.5–11 mg/dL.
  - Critical levels are greater than 7.4 mg/dL; chronic renal insufficiency is 1.5–3 mg/dL; chronic renal failure is 3 mg/dL.
  - Creatinine estimates renal function and is also compared with urine creatinine to provide enhanced estimates of the glomerular filtration abilities in the kidneys.
- Normal total protein levels for adults >19 years are 6–8 g/dL. Protein becomes diluted in states of fluid excess. Decreased protein levels also cause fluid to move out of the vascular space and into interstitial spaces.
- Urine osmolality is used to evaluate renal function with a random test, a "first morning void," or a 24-hour collection. The normal urine range from 2 months to adult is 250–900 mOsm/kg.
  - When urine osmolality is near the range of normal serum osmolality, this reflects an inability of the kidneys to concentrate

urine. The expected ratio for normal kidney function is *urine osmolality:serum osmolality* in the range of 0.2–4.7 (i.e., urine osmolality is 0.2–4.7 times the osmolality of serum).

- With fluid excess, serum osmolality and urine osmolality are both decreased. With fluid deficit, serum osmolality is normal or increased, and urine osmolality is increased.
- Urine specific gravity normally ranges 1.002–1.028 g/mL. An increase reflects fluid deficit, and a decrease reflects fluid excess. Urine specific gravity correlates with serum osmolality when specific gravity is 1.010 g/mL and serum osmolality is 285 mOsm/kg. Specific gravity may be measured in the laboratory or on the nursing unit using a hydrometer (Fig. 2-1). See Chapter 6 for a chart of normal electrolyte levels.

Serum Specimen Collection

Serum for BUN, creatinine, electrolytes, osmolality, and total protein is collected by phlebotomy in a red- or tiger-top tube. Serum for complete blood count (CBC), including Hgb and Hct levels, is drawn from a lavender-top tube. Standard phlebotomy procedure requires that the nurse avoid drawing blood from the same arm with IV access. This is particularly important so as to avoid contamination of the specimen by infused or instilled fluids. To avoid processing errors, ensure that the specimen is delivered within the time frame of your laboratory's guidelines.

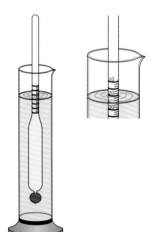

FIGURE 2-1: Specific gravity may be measured in the lab or on the nursing unit using a hydrometer. The hydrometer floats in urine and specific gravity is read at the surface level.

Urine Specimen Collection

Urine is collected by clean catch or from the tubing of an indwelling catheter. Urine may be ordered for "first morning void" in order to see the most concentrated urine or for a 24-hour collection to measure the overall ability of the kidneys to concentrate urine over that period. Patients and family members should be instructed on how and where to collect a 24-hour urine specimen, which is often kept on ice.

Fluid Excess

Fluid excess can occur due to increased fluid intake or fluid retention.

Laboratory Values

Serum osmolarity < 275 mOsm/kg indicates fluid excess, especially with concurrent urine osmolality < 500 mOsm/kg. Other indicators may be:

- BUN < 7 mg/100 mL or creatinine < 0.5 mg/dL. However, BUN and creatinine values may also be elevated in renal failure, which could be the cause of fluid overload.
- Total protein < 6 mg/dL and urine specific gravity < 1.002 g/mL can be caused by fluid excess.
- Decreases in electrolytes can also indicate overhydration, although this is not always a true indication of fluid status.
- Prolonged prothrombin time (PT) can indicate liver disease, which can cause fluid retention.
- Elevated serum amylase indicates pancreatitis, which may be associated with abdominal fluid collections.
- Elevated bilirubin level can indicate liver-related causes of fluid overload.

COACH CONSULT

Hct level can be used to estimate vascular fluid loss if the loss is not due to hemorrhage. An increase in one point from the baseline Hct percentage reflects approximately 100 mL of intravascular fluid loss and 400 mL of interstitial fluid loss.

COACH CONSULT

Fluid loss—through hemorrhage, diuresis, or diaphoresis—or fluid retention can be estimated by comparing the patient's baseline weight with current weight: 1 kg is roughly equal to 1 L of fluid. A 70-kg (154-lb) patient who has rapidly lost or gained 1 kg (2.2 lb) in weight over less than 24 hours can be assumed to have lost or gained 1 L of body fluid. Blood volume is estimated at roughly 5 L.

Basic Concepts

Fluid excesses may be intravascular, intracellular, or interstitial. Electrolytes should always be measured when evaluating fluid levels because overhydration of vascular spaces may cause critical decreases in circulating electrolytes.

Etiology

Fluid excess can be caused by:

- Cardiac disease, especially cardiac failure
- Endocrine dysfunction, including Cushing's syndrome (excess cortisol levels have an effect similar to that of aldosterone on the kidneys, causing sodium and fluid retention) and syndrome of inappropriate antidiuretic hormone (increasing antidiuretic hormone is released, related to underlying disease or as part of the stress response [e.g., secondary to major surgery, trauma] or head injury)
- Hepatic or liver disease, which can cause vascular, interstitial, and peritoneal fluid excess
- Renal insufficiency or renal failure

Iatrogenic causes, which are common and should be carefully observed, include:

- Overinfusion of fluids or blood products, especially for patients with impaired kidney function
- Medications, including steroid use
- Medication failure; note that decreased absorption of diuretics can be a cause of and can cause fluid overload when the GI tract is overloaded and/or when absorption of medications is poor

Symptoms

Symptoms of fluid excess often stem from dilution of electrolytes. Refer to the electrolyte chapters of this book for symptoms associated with low serum electrolyte levels.

- **Neurological:** Confusion or decreased level of consciousness related to electrolyte changes
- **Cardiovascular (CV):** Edema of extremities or dependent areas of trunk occurring with 2 L or more of excess fluid; tachycardia; distended neck veins (jugular venous distention [JVD])
- **Respiratory:** Respiratory insufficiency or distress; pleural effusion; orthopnea; cough; pink, frothy sputum; pulmonary edema

causing wheezing and brochospasm; rales/crackles; third heart sound: gallop

- **GI:** Rapid weight gain of more than 0.5 kg/24 hours, hepatomegaly, ascites, failure to thrive, malnutrition due to hepatic overload, nausea or vomiting related to electrolyte changes
- **Genitourinary (GU):** Decreased or increased urination can be signs of fluid overload because the body's inability to excrete excess fluid can cause fluid overload, and frequent or large volumes of urination can indicate excess fluid being diuresed
- **Musculoskeletal:** Weakness, tremors, or cramping related to electrolyte shifts

Assessment and Actions

Fluid, electrolyte, and acid-base imbalances can rapidly cause life-threatening neurological, cardiac, and respiratory compromise, requiring immediate notification of the medical or rapid response team. Consult the medical team if any new onset occurs, or if worsening symptoms or vital signs occur that are outside the normal range. If neurological, respiratory, or cardiac compromise occurs, call for assistance from the rapid or urgent response team or, if outside of an acute care setting, call community emergency medical services (EMS).

Patient History

Review for clues to cause of fluid excess. The following conditions may be associated with or cause fluid volume excesses:

- Acute or chronic metabolic process such as:
  - Acute renal disease or dysfunction
  - Acute heart failure related to myocardial infarction or trauma
  - Acute biliary dysfunction related to kidney stones
  - Acute pancreatitis related to infection or injury
- Chronic health problems, including:
  - Endocrine diseases
  - Congestive heart failure (CHF)
  - Chronic hepatic or liver disease
  - Chronic pancreatic disease
  - Chronic renal disease

Iatrogenic intervention may also be causative, including unintended fluid overload. Note that IV fluids should be delivered via infuser pump or rate controller, especially with patient populations at high risk for fluid overload, such as pediatric patients, chronically ill patients, and seniors.

Laboratory Assessment and Actions

If serum osmolarity is < 275 mOsm/kg, anticipate the need for correction:

- Anticipate orders for an electrocardiogram (ECG) to evaluate for possible cardiac insufficiency related to myocardial infarction, insufficient perfusing rhythm, heart block, or heart failure. If the ECG demonstrates abnormal findings, consult the medical team for treatment plan, including potential admission to continuous cardiac monitoring or emergency care.
- Anticipate orders for patient to undergo echocardiogram to evaluate for heart failure, and teach the patient that this is a noninvasive examination.
  - B-type natriuretic peptide (BNP), a hormone that is synthesized primarily in the atria and left ventricle, is released in response to fluid overload and is measured to rule out CHF. Normal BNP is < 100 pg/mL. If it is over 100, heart failure is suggested, with severity increasing as levels increase to above 900, which indicates severe heart failure.
- Anticipate orders for chest x-ray.
  - Check for potential pregnancy prior to examination.
  - If x-ray demonstrates pulmonary edema, or if echocardiogram or BNP elevated > 100 pg/mL indicates heart failure, then anticipate administration of oral or IV diuretics.
    - Because diuretics can cause fluid shifts and subsequent dehydration, patients should be observed closely for increased electrolyte levels and signs of dehydration. For example, rapid diuresis can cause rapid potassium loss; therefore, patients should be observed carefully for signs of hypokalemia.
      - Oral loop diuretics—in particular, furosemide (Lasix)—are commonly prescribed medications for fluid overload. Caution must be used to ensure that potassium shifts do not occur with these medications.
      - In cases where edema is severe or other symptoms do not resolve with oral diuretics, IV furosemide may be ordered. Preparations of IV furosemide may be light-sensitive, and IV furosemide is not compatible with many

MED INFO ℞

IV furosemide infusions are usually started with a loading dose of 40–80 mg, slow IV push. Rapid infusion can cause ototoxicity and should be slow, over no more than 4 mg/min.

medications. Do not use an IV furosemide preparation if the medication has turned yellow. Check for compatibility with other medications before connecting through a Y site.

- Oral and IV furosemide should induce diuresis within 30–60 minutes and have peak action in 1–2 hours. Overall effects will be completed in 6–8 hours.
- Patients with decompensated heart failure may be prescribed IV nesiritide (Natracor), which is a purified DNA recombinant peptide.
- Anticipate orders for restriction of sodium to 2 g/day and water to less than 2 L/day.

If excess fluid is causing low concentrations of electrolytes, then:

- Prepare for cautious IV administration of electrolytes (see Chapter 3 subchapters for information on IV administration of each electrolyte).
- Watch carefully for signs of dehydration and other electrolyte shifts from fluid deficits.

Note that liver function tests can demonstrate low albumin and protein levels and help identify liver disease as a causative agent. If liver enzymes are elevated (which means that aspartate aminotransferase is >80 units/L for men or 70 units/L for women, or that alanine aminotransferase is >1750 units/L), then:

- Evaluation should be made with the medical team of the source of liver dysfunction.
- In the presence of abdominal distention, girth and weight should be measured to establish a baseline.
- Anticipate preparing the patient for sterile needle or catheter paracentesis

MED INFO

Some patients are not responsive to oral or IV furosemide due to underlying disease, such as kidney or liver disease. These patients may require other diuretic medications such as oral or IV bumetanide (which is 40 times more potent than furosemide), oral metolazone (which is 10 times more potent than hydrochlorothiazide), or oral chlorothiazide (which potentiates furosemide).

COACH CONSULT

Some patients with CHF routinely return to the hospital for nesiritide administration.

COACH CONSULT

Alternative methods for fluid removal may be used in a critical care setting. One example includes *slow, cautious dialysis* through a prescribed continuous dialysis machine or other device that is able to pull fluid off the patient without requiring insertion of a hemodialysis catheter; instead, these devices use specialized large-bore catheters.

(Fig. 2-2) to drain excess fluid, especially if the patient is experiencing any respiratory insufficiency.

- If ascities is not severe, then:
  - Anticipate orders for sodium and fluid restriction. Plan for patient teaching.
  - Anticipate administration of diuretics.

Note that serum creatinine that is 1.5–3 mg/dL or above indicates chronic renal disease. Creatinine >7.4 mg/dL is considered a critical

NURSE-TO-NURSE TIP

Paracentesis is performed with aseptic technique at the bedside or under radiology or ultrasound. Pregnancy must be ruled out prior to performing paracentesis. Due to a high potential for anticoagulation related to liver disease, serum coagulation studies are usually measured. Removing large volumes of fluid from the abdomen can cause severe fluid shifts of vascular fluids into the abdomen. Fluid is usually removed at up to 4 L/hr. In addition, if over 4 L is removed, anticipate orders to replace intravascular volumes with IV fluids. Furthermore, patients undergoing any type of cavity drain should be closely observed for any signs of re-effusion or loss of vascular fluid, such as hypotension or tachycardia. Infection and bowel and bladder puncture are additional complications that require nursing surveillance for fever, excess bleeding from puncture site, severe pain, heat or errythmia at site, or blood in the urine.

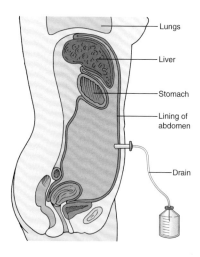

F I G U R E 2 - 2 : Paracentesis may be ordered to drain acites. A drain is placed by a surgeon into the peritoneal cavity and fluid is slowly drained into a sterile container to prevent dramatic fluid shifts.

value. Creatinine is also related to BUN. A BUN/creatinine ratio of greater than 20:1 indicates decreased blood flow to the kidneys. A ratio between 10:1 and 20:1 is considered normal, and a ratio of less than 10:1 indicates renal damage. Discuss with the medical team the most likely cause for renal insufficiency, including acute versus chronic renal disease:

- If creatinine is <2 mg/dL, anticipate use of thiazide diuretics.
- If creatinine is >2 mg/dL, anticipate use of loop diuretics or initiation of dialysis.
- If dialysis is ordered, then:
  - Continue to monitor I&O, and restrict fluids as ordered.
  - Closely monitor vital signs and level of consciousness for signs of uremia, which range from lethargy to coma due to the buildup of urea and other waste products in the blood.
- Teach patient about the need for placement of a short-term dialysis catheter, the process of dialysis, and safety concerns around catheter and dialysis.
  - If patient has known chronic renal disease and a preexisting dialysis regime, then:
    - Anticipate preparing patient for typical dialysis course.
    - Assess patient's baseline knowledge of dialysis and typical response, and reinforce baseline knowledge.
  - If patient has an indwelling peritoneal dialysis catheter, assess catheter for integrity, and prepare supplies per agency policy.
  - If patient has an indwelling arterial-venous fistula or graft or a preexisting dialysis catheter (Fig. 2-3), then:
    - Assess for a bruit with auscultation and a thrill with light palpation in the fistula or graft or integrity of indwelling catheter. Do **not** attempt to access indwelling catheter because this catheter is to be managed only by a nurse certified in hemodialysis.
    - Report any abnormal assessment of access to the medical team.
    - Review agency policy for ordering prophylactic type, and screen for blood products in advance of dialysis.

COACH CONSULT

It is essential to adhere to aseptic technique when administering peritoneal dialysis because peritonitis is a common problem, which can make future dialysis through the peritoneal membrane impossible. Fever, nausea, and vomiting are complications that require consultation with the medical team.

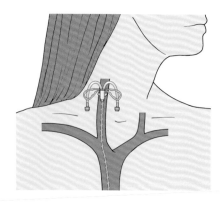

FIGURE 2-3: Indwelling hemodialysis catheter.

Serum sodium should be measured. If sodium is >145 mEq/dL, then:

- Anticipate 2 g/day sodium restriction in diet and IV fluids.
- Cautiously continue to monitor for signs of hyponatremia because electrolyte shifts often occur with diuresis.
- Measure weights, and report increases of more than 0.5 kg over 24 hours.

Systems Assessment and Actions

If laboratory values are pending, but fluid excess is suspected, proceed with a systems assessment. **Immediately consult the medical team at the onset or worsening of any of the symptoms that are listed in the following section.**

Neuro-Musculo-Skeletal

If lethargy, weakness, malaise, or decreased level of consciousness occurs, then:

- Evaluate patient on Glasgow Coma Scale (see Chapter 6), and continually reevaluate patient's ability to follow instructions.
- Consult the medical team to discuss the need for one-on-one continuous observation and for patient restraints and restraining side rails.
- Continue close monitoring, and provide safety supports, such as:
  - Assistance to reach desired objects
  - Assistance to ambulate to bathroom
  - Placement of bed in lowest position

If anxiety is present, evaluate for hypoxemia related to fluid overload, and provide supplemental oxygen as ordered.

Respiratory

If respiratory insufficiency, shortness of breath, frothy white or pink sputum, rales/crackles, or wheezing is noted, then:

- Measure oxygen saturation.
- Raise head of bed to high Fowler's position to facilitate breathing.
- Place emergency respiratory equipment at bedside, including ambu-bag, oral airway, and suction equipment. Closely monitor I &O, and communicate need for accurate I&O measures to all ancillary staff.
- Consult the medical team to discuss:
  - Possible transfer to emergency care.
  - The need for supplemental oxygen; *Note:* Caution should be used before administering supplemental oxygen because supplemental oxygen is not always indicated if removal of excess fluids is successful.
  - Orders for chest x-ray to evaluate potential pneumonia, CHF, or pulmonary edema or effusion:
    - Prepare for transport with emergency equipment and personnel if patient must leave unit for testing.
    - All female patients should be evaluated by the medical team for potential pregnancy.
    - Prepare for administration of diuretics.
    - Closely monitor respiratory symptoms for improvement from baseline by measuring initial height of rales/crackles and height of rales/crackles after administration of diuretics.

CV

If symptoms such as tachycardia, S_3 gallop, JVD, or bounding pulses are present, then:

- Consult the medical team:
  - Anticipate orders for continuous cardiac monitoring, and discuss with the medical team preferred leads and alarm setting for monitoring of fluid-related electrocardiogram (ECG) changes.
  - Anticipate orders for frequent blood pressure measures.
- Prepare for administration of diuretics.

If edema is present in lower legs, elbows, genitalia, or hips, then:

- Elevate extremities, protect skin and tissue from excess pressure, and provide support to dependent aspects of the trunk to help fluid return to circulation and prevent pressure ulcers.

- Cautiously observe for fluid shifting from extremities to central circulation into the lungs.

If chest, neck, arm, or thoracic pain; cyanosis; diaphoresis; or decreased capillary refill is present, then:

- Consult the medical team for evaluation of possible myocardial infarction.
- Anticipate obtaining 12-lead ECG, drawing laboratory tests for cardiac enzymes, and obtaining orders for nitroglycerin, with special attention to blood pressure to observe for hypotension.

GI

If abdominal distention is present, measure abdominal girth and report increases to the medical team:

- Closely monitor I&O, and communicate need for accurate I&O measures to all ancillary staff.
- Anticipate orders for oral or IV diuretics or preparing to assist with paracentesis to relieve congestion.

If nausea or abdominal pain is assessed, then:

- Place suctioning equipment at bedside.
- Stay with patient. If vomiting occurs, attempt to protect airway from aspiration by maintaining the patient's head at a 30° angle. If patient loses consciousness, place patient in the left lateral recumbent position (recovery position).
- Provide oral care with water-based moisture solutions and soft swabs.
- Consult the medical team to:
  - Evaluate for thoracic or abdominal sources of discomfort.
  - Administer antiemetics as ordered. Note that GI symptoms may not resolve until electrolytes are stable, despite use of antiemetics.
  - Follow orders for nasogastric tube insertion.

GU

With any signs of fluid deficit, closely monitor I&O, and communicate need for accurate I&O measures to all ancillary staff. Anticipate orders for repeated urine samples to assess effect of diuresis on electrolyte imbalance:

- Collect specimen with caution to avoid contamination with water or soap. If drawing from a catheter, make certain to draw urine from the collection tube rather than the collection bag, because urine in the bag will start to biologically degrade.
- Note that <30 mL/hr may point to renal insufficiency, which may be causative agent of fluid excess.

Vital Signs

If vital signs are persistently above or below a patient's baseline or if they are outside of the normal adult ranges (see Chapter 6), then:

- Consult the medical team.
- Anticipate potential need to call for rapid response with significant decline of patient's status.
- Anticipate orders for transfer of patient to a critical care environment for continuous neurological, respiratory, and cardiac monitoring.

Prevention

Teach at-risk populations to monitor for:

- Signs and symptoms of fluid overload.
- Appropriate dietary intake of fluids and sodium.
- Weight: obtain weights at least three times a week, on the same scale at the same time of day, and report increases of more than 0.5 kg (1.1 lb) over 24 hours or 2–3 kg (4.4–6.6 lb) over a week.
- Medications: take medications as prescribed, and inform the medical team if unable to obtain medications.
- Appointments: attend dialysis appointments, or self-administer dialysis as prescribed, and inform the medical team if dialysis schedule is interrupted.

When advocating for public health, note that:

- Patients with chronic cardiac and renal disease and diabetes are at high risk for fluid overload.
- Populations that have decreased cognition or decreased access to medications, transportation, proper diet, or caregiver or health provider support are at high risk for hospital admission or death related to fluid overload.
- Special populations at risk for fluid overload include endurance athletes (for more information on athletes, see Chapter 3F), heroin addicts, alcohol abusers, and those with pre-eclampsia related to pregnancy.

Fluid Deficit

A fluid deficit can exist in the whole body due to bleeding, diuresis, diaphoresis, surgery, trauma, burns, or lack of ingestion. Individual organs may be affected when trauma, surgery, or disease is isolated within one organ or body system. A fluid deficit may be present intracellularly, intravascularly, or both.

DIAGNOSIS: FLUID EXCESS

Mr. De Jesus is a 65-year-old patient with a known diagnosis of cardiac insufficiency and a measured ejection fraction of 45% at last echocardiogram. Three days ago, he walked his daughter down the aisle, sparing no expense. Today, he presents to his physician's office for a regular visit with complaints of shortness of breath. Upon auscultation, the nurse practitioner explains that she would like to transport Mr. De Jesus to the hospital by ambulance. Both Mr. De Jesus and his wife are upset, but both state that they expected he was back in heart failure.

Upon arrival in the emergency room, vital signs are T 97.5, respirations 28, pulse 114, blood pressure 156/88, and SaO_2 90%. Oxygen is ordered at 2 L, and serum chemistry, CBC, and BNP are drawn. Cardiology is asked to consult the medical team, and an ECG and echocardiogram confirm Mr. De Jesus's known left bundle branch block with a mild sinus tachycardia and a new, lower ejection fraction of 35%. Laboratory tests return with following: serum osmolality at 265 mOsm/kg, urine osmolality at 450 mOsm/kg, BNP 500, creatinine 2 mg/dL, BUN 7 mg/dL, K^+ 3.5, Na^+ 149, Cl^- 109, CO_2 21, glucose 115, Hgb 13 g/dL, and Hct 40%.

Orders placed for IV push furosemide 40 mg were followed. The nurse instructed Mr. De Jesus to void in the urinal and keep the head of his bed elevated to 90%; 20 mEq of potassium was ordered in a 50-mL bag of normal saline and run through a peripheral IV line over 2 hours. Hourly urine volumes and reporting of physical assessment findings were ordered hourly, and a repeat complete blood chemistry was ordered for 1 hour after the potassium completed its infusion. Mrs. De Jesus was asked to stay at the bedside to help decrease Mr. De Jesus's anxiety, and she was asked to report any subtle changes in Mr. De Jesus's level of consciousness to the nurse.

A half hour after furosemide administration, Mr. De Jesus produced 400 mL of urine and continued to diurese at about 100 mL/hr for 6 hours. His vital signs came back into his normal range, and his oxygen saturation rose to 94%. Assessment confirmed a decrease in jugular vein distention and a resolution of most of his pulmonary rales/crackles to barely auscultated at bilateral bases. The nurse included a referral to a support group for patients with chronic CHF in Mr. De Jesus's discharge plan.

1. What does the laboratory value of a BNP of 500 indicate for Mr. De Jesus?
2. Given Mr. De Jesus's laboratory values, what types of foods does the nurse anticipate focusing on when teaching Mr. De Jesus about diet management?
3. When assessing Mr. De Jesus's respiratory status, what does the nurse expect to hear after diuresis begins?

Basic Concepts

It is essential to determine the source of fluid loss and the relationship of this loss to the electrolytes that govern movement of fluid between the body's extracellular and intracellular spaces. The key electrolytes in fluid loss are sodium and chloride (for more information, see Chapter 3). Fluid resuscitation or the correction of fluid deficits is governed by what type of fluid is lost, where the loss occurs, and where a counterbalance of fluid retention may be in place.

Etiology

Fluid deficit can be caused by:

- Fluid shift from the vascular space into cells or interstitially (interstitial movement is commonly called third spacing)
- Hemorrhage, which can occur due to surgery, trauma, or coagulation problems
- "Silent" hemorrhage, which can occur in body cavities and is dangerous because it may be difficult to detect until large volumes of blood have moved out of the vascular space
- Iatrogenic losses, which occur when:
  - Patients are placed on "nothing by mouth" (NPO) status without proper IV support
  - Patients are mechanically unable to obtain fluids due to disability, language barriers, or fluid or mobility restriction
  - There is a lack of replacement of underestimated losses, e.g., due to diaphoresis or tachypnea
  - Medical equipment, such as specialty beds, overheat
  - There is overuse or overprescription of diuretics
- Infection, which can cause a state where fluids are used to cool the body and manufacture essential white blood cells, causing dehydration
- Neurological or psychiatric diseases, where patients are unable to determine their need for oral intake

Symptoms

With extravascular fluid volumes of approximately 14 L for a 70-kg (154-lb) patient, symptoms may not appear until after a 5% fluid loss of about 700 mL, and even dehydration may be demonstrated only as poor skin turgor. At a loss of 10% or 1400 mL, shock may be impending.

- **Neurological:** Decreased cognition, confusion, disorientation, fatigue, headache, dizziness, irrational behavior, irritability, sleepiness, sunken eyes, convulsions

- **CV:** Flushing of face, dry and warm skin or excessive diaphoresis, tachycardia, weak pulses, hypotension
- **Respiratory:** Tachypnea, deep breathing
- **GI:** Extreme thirst, dry mouth and tongue, thick saliva, nausea and vomiting, weight loss of 3%–5% over 30 days
- **GU:** Oliguria, dark amber color of urine
- **Musculoskeletal:** Decreased motor control, muscle weakness, or cramping

COACH CONSULT

Nausea and vomiting can be symptoms of dehydration and can also interfere with oral rehydration. Correction of dehydration is usually initiated with small amounts of fluids.

COACH CONSULT

Rapid fluid loss or shift is often associated with electrolyte imbalance. Symptoms may stem from dehydration or from relative vascular electrolyte excess or deficiency. The underlying cause of symptoms should be determined based on patient history and laboratory values.

Assessment and Actions

Fluid, electrolyte, and acid-base imbalances can rapidly cause life-threatening neurological, cardiac, and respiratory compromise, requiring immediate notification of the medical or rapid response team. Consult the medical team if any new onset occurs or if worsening symptoms or vital signs occur that are outside the normal range. If neurological, respiratory, or cardiac compromise occurs, call for assistance from the rapid or urgent response team or, if outside an acute care setting, call community EMS.

Patient History

Review for clues to cause. The following conditions may be associated with or cause fluid deficit.

- Acute or chronic metabolic processes may cause low fluid volumes, including:
  - GI losses from vomiting, fistulas or diarrhea
  - Fever-inducing states, such as influenza, pneumonia, or other infection
  - Bleeding from trauma or anticoagulated states
  - Wounds from surgery or pressure ulcers, especially if actively draining from interventional drain or wound VAC
- Chronic health problems may be associated with dehydration, including:
  - Constipation
  - Dementia, developmental delay, or depression related to inability to access water

- Diabetes mellitus or diabetes insipidus
- Dysphagia or alternative means of nutrition such as tube feeding
- Urinary tract infections
- History of dehydration or GI bleeding
- Excess ingestion of medications may result in low fluid levels, including:
  - Antibiotics causing diarrhea
  - Diuretics
  - Angiotension-converting enzyme (ACE) inhibitors

Laboratory Assessment and Actions

Anticipate frequent serum laboratory draws, based on frequency and effect of interventions. If electrolyte levels are low, anticipate orders for correction of electrolytes through oral or IV repletion (see Chapter 3 for more information on correcting electrolyte values).

Elevated serum glucose can point to the cause of vascular fluid deficit as osmotic diuresis. If glucose is elevated above 160 mg/dL, also called the "renal threshold," fluid will leave the kidneys with excess glucose and cause a sympathetic nervous system and adrenal gland cycle of glucose production in an effort to maintain blood pressure. If serum glucose levels are elevated, then:

- Anticipate frequent measures of blood glucose by finger stick, alternating with serum blood assessment for glucose levels.
- Discuss with the medical team potential orders for insulin administration.
- Observe for symptoms of hypoglycemia as glucose migrates out of bloodstream and back into cells. Symptoms include weakness, somnolence, hunger, confusion, irritability, trembling, diaphoresis, or tachycardia.

COACH CONSULT

Serum sodium is measured in cases of suspected dehydration to assist in identification of the source. If both sodium and water are lost together, the loss is termed *isotonic dehydration*. If sodium is lost in greater ratio than water, it is considered a primary sodium deficit and called *hypotonic dehydration*. If more water is lost in ratio to sodium, it is termed *hypertonic dehydration*.

If serum osmolality is normal or increased from the range of 275–295 mOsm/kg, Hct level is >50%, BUN is >21 mg/dL, creatinine is >1.2 mg/dL, or urine specific gravity is >1.028, then:

- Anticipate measures of urine osmolality, which will be increased with fluid deficit to >900 mOsm/kg.

- Calculate BUN/creatinine ratio. A ratio of over 25:1 should be assessed as a sign of dehydration. Elevated BUN with a normal creatinine or slightly elevated creatinine level indicates fluid volume deficit.
- Anticipate correction with oral solutions or IV crystalloids. According to the American Medical Directors Association, goals for fluid replacement should be correcting half of the deficit in the first 24 hours and replacing the balance of deficit over the following 48–72 hours.

- Oral solutions: Oral administration (PO) is the preferred route in non-emergent situations, if the patient can tolerate PO. Oral electrolyte solutions are the most common form of replacement in noncritical situations. These contain 2% glucose and 50–90 mEq/L of sodium.
  - Most commercial sports drinks contain too much glucose to qualify for this ratio of solutes. Without the proper ratio, glucose can interfere with transport of water to the cells.
  - Tablets or packets of electrolytes and glucose may be ordered to be mixed in a specific ratio of water. Improper dilution can cause serious health problems related to electrolyte shifts.
  - Patients with nausea or vomiting may not tolerate drinking fluids until electrolytes have been corrected:
    - Consult the medical team to evaluate cause of nausea and vomiting, anticipate orders to attempt to rehydrate with 5 mL every 5 minutes.
    - If electrolyte losses have been severe from GI or renal sources, anticipate orders to reverse fluid and electrolyte losses through IV fluids before introducing oral fluids.
    - If patients are unable to swallow or take oral fluids, discuss with the medical

team the possibility of nasogastric intubation or placement of gastrostomy tube for hydration.

- Most institutions have policies about which personnel may place what type of nasogastric, gastric, or jejunal access device (see Chapter 6).
- Surgical placement of a gastric or jejunal device requires normal surgical procedures, except that in some cases it may be conducted at the bedside under conscious sedation.

- IV crystalloids: If patients are unable to tolerate rehydration or electrolyte replacement via oral solution, anticipate orders for IV crystalloids.

  - Crystalloids include lactated Ringer's solution, dextrose solutions, and saline solutions. Administer fluids cautiously because adverse effects can include rapid electrolyte shifts, rapid fluid overload, and hyperchloremia-induced acidosis or—in the case of dextrose administration—dilution of serum sodium, leading to extravascular fluid shift.
  - If an IV device is currently in place, assess the device for patency, the condition of the vein, the stabilizing dressing, and the correct size for ordered infusion. Anticipate orders for insertion of a large-bore, 16- or 18-gauge IV angiocatheter or assistance with sterile insertion of a central vein IV line:
    - A large-bore angiocatheter may be placed in the cephalic, basilic, or antecubital veins. Proper insertion

MED INFO

For mild dehydration, anticipate orders for 50 mL/kg oral solutions over 4 hours; for moderate dehydration, 100 mL/kg solutions are given over 4 hours. After 4 hours, the medical team reassesses hydration and, if dehydration persists, the dosing is repeated. After rehydration, less concentrated solutions may be used to maintain hydration.

ALERT

Nasogastric tube insertion is contraindicated for patients with facial trauma. Tube insertion should be halted if any signs of respiratory irritation or decline occur, because those signs mean that the tube was most likely passed into lungs.

COACH CONSULT

A new IV catheter should not be placed in the same vein as an existing IV access device. Documentation of insertion should be clear on the medical record,

Continued

COACH CONSULT —CONT'D

including any special considerations and the number and location of unsuccessful attempts at insertion of a catheter.

requires confirmation of physician order, hand hygiene, patient teaching, vein assessment, and proper training in intravenous access.

- Nurses certified in IV catheter insertion or peripherally inserted central catheter (PICC) placement may insert these catheters in institutions where policy permits.
- Physicians are responsible for other types of central line placement (Box 2–1). Figures 2-4 and 2-5 show peripheral veins of the arm and hand. Figure 2-6 shows sites for placement of PICC.

Box 2–1 Central Lines: Application and Maintenance

Central lines allow for faster infusion of fluids because they will mix more quickly into the fast-flowing blood of large veins. However, rapid infusion can still put the patient at risk for fluid or electrolyte overload, with hypertonic or blood solutions pulling fluids away from cells and into the vascular space. Remember that:

- Central lines include PICCs, triple-lumen short catheters, medicine ports, long-term catheters (Hickman, Broviac), and hemodialysis catheters. Hemodialysis catheters are accessed only by a nurse who is certified in hemodialysis. Indwelling, long-term medicine ports are accessed by a nurse certified in this procedure. After access, the Huber needle extension can be used as a central line by a nurse trained in the proper use.
- Central lines require special attention because of the high rate of septic infection associated with these lines. During states of acute fluid deficit, a central line may be placed under emergency conditions. When this occurs, the line should be changed as soon as the patient has become stable or within 24 hours.
- Central lines placed in the internal jugular, subclavian, or femoral area are typically secured with sutures and covered with a special dressing designed to prevent infection. A mask, sterile gloves, and sterile drape should be used to change dressings when they are no longer intact. The lines should be changed with any sign of infection.
- All central lines should be accessed with caution. Some institutions require that all personnel in the room during access don sterile gloves, a gown, and a mask before accessing the line.

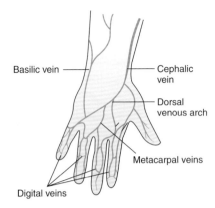

FIGURE 2-4: Peripheral veins of the hand.

Basilic vein

Cephalic vein

Dorsal venous arch

Metacarpal veins

Digital veins

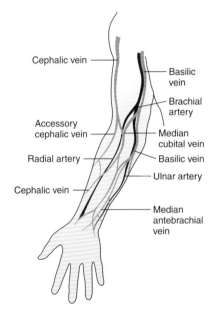

FIGURE 2-5: Peripheral veins of the arm.

Cephalic vein

Basilic vein

Brachial artery

Accessory cephalic vein

Median cubital vein

Radial artery

Basilic vein

Ulnar artery

Cephalic vein

Median antebrachial vein

- Remember to educate the patient on the need for hydration fluids and the process for IV insertion.
- If peripheral access cannot be obtained or if central access is required for administration of medications that may be

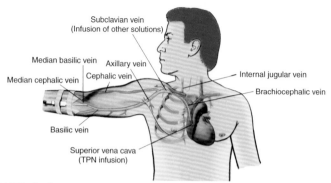

Subclavian vein
(Infusion of other solutions)

Median basilic vein

Axillary vein

Median cephalic vein

Cephalic vein

Internal jugular vein

Brachiocephalic vein

Basilic vein

Superior vena cava
(TPN infusion)

FIGURE 2-6: Insertion points for PICC line placement.

delivered only through a central vein, a central venous access device may be ordered. Note that:

- Central venous catheters and central venous tunneled catheters are placed by physicians. These catheters can be single-lumen or double-lumen, but typically they are triple-lumen, allowing for up to three incompatible fluids to be infused at the same time into a large central vein. In triple-lumen central venous catheters (Fig 2-7):
  - The distal (or "CVP") port is typically the first choice for high-volume or viscous fluid administration.
  - The proximal port is reserved for blood administration and blood sampling.
  - The medial port is reserved for total parenteral nutrition (TPN) administration.
  - An (optional) smaller-gauge extra-infusion port can be used for medication or fluid administration.

- Peripherally inserted central venous catheters may be placed by nurses certified in this procedure, either in the patient's room or during the radiology examination. For PICC lines, the nurse should compare and document the distance from the insertion site and the hub of the catheter to the distance documented in the insertion record to ensure that the hub has not migrated before beginning an infusion.

COACH CONSULT —cont'd

insertion of a small-bore catheter may be used for initial low-rate IV administration until the veins distend enough for insertion of a large-bore catheter. If patient is unstable, a central line or external jugular catheter may be placed by the medical team.

- After catheter placement, the nurse should confirm a physician's order allowing the device to be accessed (based on radiological confirmation of placement) before attempting to infuse fluids or flush the line. Stability of the line and dressing and the integrity of the site should be documented.

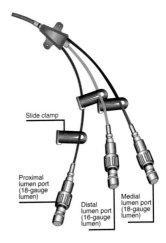

Slide clamp

Proximal lumen port (18-gauge lumen)

Distal lumen port (16-gauge lumen)

Medial lumen port (18-gauge lumen)

FIGURE 2-7: Triple-lumen central venous catheter. Depending on the manufacturer, the ports are labeled or color-coded according to gauge and use. Distal may be blue and 16-gauge. Medial may be white for TPN and 18-gauge. Proximal may be red or brown for blood and 18-gauge.

- If the catheter is in place and the insertion site is free of problems, the line access hub must be cleansed based on agency procedures with 70% isopropyl alcohol, 2% chlorhexidine, or a combination of both. Once the cleansing has air-dried, the hub may be flushed with 5 mL of 0.9% saline solution and fluid administration initiated.
- All central line flushes should be delivered via a syringe of 10 mL or larger. If medications are provided in a smaller-gauge syringe, the nurse should transfer the medication to a larger syringe before accessing the line to prevent line rupture from the increased pressure generated from smaller syringes.
- PICC lines are supplied by a variety of manufacturers and may require special techniques for flushing. Refer to manufacturer guidelines to ensure proper maintenance of pressures in these lines to prevent blood backflow and clotting.
- Once IV access is established, then:
  - Check the medical team's order for solution, route, volume, rate, duration, and reason for infusion.
  - Follow institutional guidelines regarding labeling and replacing tubing used for IV fluid administration. Note that tubing that is used to infuse fluids or medications that are highly incompatible with other solutions should be labeled at each Y site and at the end of the tubing where it connects to the access device hub; this labeling will remind other nurses of the primary solution at the drip chamber.
  - Continually reassess patient for signs of irritation or injury at insertion site because hypertonic solutions, blood, and electrolyte solutions can be irritating to veins and cause injury more readily than isotonic or hypotonic solutions.
    - Assess proximal to and at the insertion site for signs of inflammation (including redness or swelling), coolness, or heat.
    - Ask the patient about pain or tenderness, and instruct the patient to report any symptoms that develop during infusion, including a sensation of burning or tingling.

If serum sodium is low and hypotonic dehydration is assessed, then:

- Consult the medical team to ensure that cause of low sodium is fluid loss (**not** fluid excess) due to risk of unintentional increase of water overload in hyponatremic states.
- Anticipate orders for administration of normal saline solution (NSS), also known as 0.9% saline.

If serum sodium is high, hypertonic dehydration is assessed, and blood pressure is normal, anticipate orders for administration of hypotonic saline, also known as 0.45% saline solution.

If serum sodium is high, hypertonic dehydration is assessed, but blood pressure is low, anticipate administration of NSS.

If the patient's hydration status is stabilized, review etiology of factors for correction of metabolic states or iatrogenic causes of dehydration, and consult the medical team to correct factors that may contribute to dehydration.

If fluids are delivered to correct dehydration, assess patient for signs of response through frequent laboratory measures and physical assessments:

- Veins of the hand should become more visible, skin turgor should improve to become more elastic, mucous membranes should appear moist, and the patient should report less thirst.
- Urine output of 0.5–1.0 mL/kg/hr is desired for patients with healthy kidney function.
- Blood pressure and mean arterial pressure (MAP) can be used, but they may be inaccurate due to fluctuations in blood pressure

NURSE-TO-NURSE TIP

The safest method of IV administration is via an infusion pump or controller. However, if fluid hydration is ordered to be delivered rapidly and no pump is available, a "macro" drip IV set should be used, and the nurse should remain with the patient over the duration of the infusion to prevent air embolus unless the control set has a device to stop the flow of air once the chamber is empty. Read the manufacturer's instructions carefully to determine if this safety mechanism is available. The calculation for macro drip tubing rates is:

X gtt/min = mL/hr × drop factor/60 minutes.

in relationship to compensatory vasoconstriction. A MAP of 60–80 mm Hg is considered an indication of adequate perfusion of coronary arteries, brain, and kidneys.

If Hgb and Hct levels are high and rising, then:

- Consult the medical team to determine if the increase is related to vascular fluid deficit.
- Anticipate orders for administration of IV crystalloids for direct hydration or colloids or other blood products to pull fluid back into the vascular space from the interstitial space.

If Hgb and Hct levels are low and falling, consult the medical team to evaluate if changes are related to an acute source of bleed or a chronic health condition. The American Red Cross recommends that Hgb levels above 10 g/dL are unlikely to require transfusion, whereas levels below 6 g/dL often require transfusion. If Hgb falls below 6 g/dL, anticipate orders to transfuse RBCs. One unit of RBCs should increase Hgb by 1 g/dL and Hct by 3% in adults if no active bleed is present. See Boxes 2–2, 2–3, and 2–4 for the safe administration of blood products.

Box 2–2 Safe Administration of Blood Products: General Information

According to the American Red Cross (ARC), blood products should not be used to correct hypovolemia or fluid deficit unless the deficit is related to blood loss. Hgb and Hct levels are measured along with oxygen-carrying capacity. Caution should be used when evaluating Hgb during fluid deficit and excess because the relationship with fluid may not be reflected in Hgb counts. The ARC recommends that mixed venous oxygen levels drawn from a pulmonary artery catheter or oxygen extraction ratios calculated from arterial and venous blood draws be used to measure the tissue availability and use of oxygen as a gauge for the need of RBC transfusion.

Each institution has a procedure for safe administration of blood products. *Follow the procedure carefully.* Note that, because of risks from blood transfusions (e.g., hemolysis, hypothermia, or infection), a written consent is usually required from a physician before administration unless it is an emergency. The ARC process includes:

- Checking for a physician order, including indication for transfusion (usually infusion of platelets or plasma)
- Checking for informed consent documentation

- Performing identification checks (when receiving blood from the blood bank and at the point of delivery) against patient's verbal confirmation of name, birth date, blood type if known (if unknown, type O blood is used in emergency transfusions until a type and crossmatch are available), and ID band confirmation of medical record number
- Completing blood bank documentation, including blood product unit identification numbers, times of transfusion initiation and completion, times and results of vital sign measures, and reactions, if any
- Monitoring of patient's vital signs and cardiovascular and respiratory status
- Assessing outcome of clinical and laboratory goals

Box 2–3 **Safe Administration of Blood Products: Preparing the Patient for a Transfusion**

To prepare the patient for a transfusion:

- Check for history of blood transfusion or pregnancy because transfusion reactions can occur more commonly in these populations. Report this history to the medical team.
- Check patency or insert a new IV of at least 20-gauge. For large-volume transfusion, an 18- or 16-gauge IV is preferred. Gauges smaller than 20 will crush RBCs.
- Send a sample of the patient's blood to the blood bank for crossmatching with ABO and Rh typing and direct crossmatch with transfusion.
- Obtain a set of baseline vital signs prior to administration. Report any signs outside the patient's normal range or any fever to the medical team before requesting blood.
- Assess the patient for any rash or itching, and report any positive findings to the medical team prior to requesting blood.
- Prepare specialized blood tubing that has a filtering mechanism with isotonic NSS.
- Prepare a second, new IV line of isotonic saline solution to have on hand in case of transfusion reaction, but do not connect to the patient's IV access. This line should not be contaminated by the patient's blood or the transfusion blood.
- Note that two licensed professionals should check the transfusion at the patient's bedside. In some states or institutions, blood may be checked only by registered nurses and doctors.
- Confirm that patient identifiers, including correct spelling for full name, birth date, blood type, and medical record number, match patient's verbal confirmation, arm band, transfusion label, and transfusion documentation.

Continued

Fluid Balance and Imbalance **51**

- Confirm that unit number and blood type on transfusion bag match transfusion documentation record.
- Verify that blood should be infused using specialized blood administration tubing over no more than 4 hours per unit.

Box 2–4 **Safe Administration of Blood Products: The Transfusion**

During the infusion, obtain the patient's vital signs every 5 minutes for the first 15 minutes of the infusion. Stay next to the patient, and observe for any signs of transfusion reaction (e.g., wheezing or rash). The first 15 minutes of each bag or bottle is the most likely time that a reaction may occur. If signs or symptoms of transfusion reaction occur, then:

- Immediately stop the transfusion
- Anticipate orders to draw stat CBC for microscopic examination of RBCs and platelets and orders for plasma exchange.
- Educate patient on causes of bleeding and procedure of plasma exchange. Exchange is typically done over 3 hours through two, temporary large-bore IVs in the patient's room or in the hemodialysis suite. Pain is not usually associated, but allergic responses can occur, including wheezing or rash. Low calcium can occur due to anticoagulants added to the plasma (see Chapter 3A).
- Anticipate delivery of supportive medications, including steroids, folic acid, hepatitis B vaccine, and aspirin after platelets have returned to normal thresholds.

ALERT

Blood must be delivered through special IV tubing that contains a filter. New tubing should be used for every unit of blood because mixing blood could interfere with determining the cause of any transfusion reaction.

If acute disseminated intravascular coagulation (DIC) is demonstrated through medical team analysis of a DIC blood panel with concurrent active bleeding, then:

- Anticipate orders for fresh-frozen plasma (FFP), platelets, or cryoprecipitate:
  - DIC is a life-threatening cascade of clotting and bleeding simultaneously, leading to organ failure and massive hemorrhage associated closely with cancer or sepsis.

- If no active bleed is present, blood products should not be given.
- Cryoprecipitated antihemophilic factor, also known as cryoprecipitate, contains concentrated levels of several acellular coagulation factors; therefore, ABO compatibility should be evaluated.
- Transfuse within 6 hours of thawing for single units and 4 hours for pooled multiple units.
- Anticipate dosing orders based on laboratory studies prior to and after administration, coagulation of the factor being treated, and the patient's weight. Each unit of coagulation factor is 5–10 mL, with a usual dose of 6–10 units.
- Anticipate use of cryoprecipitate with (1) a massive transfusion, when fibrinogen levels are < 100 mg/dL or (2) when volumes from FFP may put patient in fluid overload.

If blood or blood products have been transfused, monitor closely for reactions:

- Observe for 2–14 days for hemolytic destruction of RBCs, which usually occurs during infusion.
- Monitor laboratory values for decreased Hgb or Hct and a positive direct antiglobulin test.
- Observe patient for increase in temperature, tachycardia, hypotension, chills, dyspnea, chest and/or back pain, abnormal bleeding including hematuria, or descent into shock.
- Prepare for orders to stabilize blood pressure with NSS and vasopressors; treat coagulation problems such as DIC arising from the transfusion reaction.
- Keep urine blood flow > 30 mL/hr to prevent kidney failure.

ALERT

Blood should never be infused with any product except NSS. The NSS bag used to prime the blood tubing should be opened at the time of administration and connected to new sterile tubing.

ALERT

No other solution or medication except sterile, normal saline should ever be infused into the same peripheral vein as the blood. In an emergency, blood may be infused through a dedicated port of a double- or triple-lumen central line at the same time as emergency medications are being delivered, but antibiotics should never be administered concurrently with blood, and the infusion of other drugs should be avoided in order to properly assess for potential complications from the blood itself.

COACH CONSULT

The most common cause of transfusion reaction is misidentification during the chain of blood product preparation and administration.

- Observe for immune-mediated cell destruction, known as alloimmunization.
  - Patients with prior infusions of blood products or previous pregnancy can develop human leukocytic antigen antibodies.
  - Alert blood bank if patient has had previous transfusions so that serological tests can be completed on patient's blood to reduce incidence of this reaction.
  - Observe for febrile, nonhemolytic reaction.
- Note that temperature elevates $1\,°C$ or $2\,°F$ in about 1% of transfusions and more frequently in patients who have previously received blood transfusions or have been pregnant.
- Anticipate orders for antipyretics.
- Anticipate orders for leukocyte-reduced blood products for patients at risk for immunocompromise.
- Observe for allergic reactions ranging from itching to anaphylaxis. If allergic reactions occur, anticipate orders for treatment with antihistamines, corticosteroids, and/or epinephrine.
- Observe for 7–10 days for post-transfusion purpura (PTP), which occurs after the transfusion when the patient's own natural platelets are typically destroyed. If PTP occurs, anticipate orders to treat with high-dose immune globulin intravenous (IGIV). IGIV has many critical side effects, including renal failure, stroke, or other clotting disorders.
- Observe for 6 hours after transfusion for transfusion-related acute lung injury. Anticipate emergency respiratory support as fluid and proteins leak into alveolar and interstitial spaces.
- Observe for signs of sepsis or circulatory collapse immediately after transfusion due to bacterial or endotoxin contamination. If sepsis is suspected, then:
  - Suspend transfusion
  - Anticipate medical orders for sepsis treatment including:
    - Anticipate placement of two large-bore IV catheters.
    - Infuse NSS for fluid resuscitation at 20 mL/kg (about 1.5 L for a 70-kg adult).
    - Draw CBC, lactate levels, prothrombin time with International Normalized Ratio, partial thromboplastin time, D-dimer,

arterial blood gas (ABG), amylase and lipase, basic metabolic panel (chemistry-7).
- Draw blood cultures from two locations.
- Infusions of broad-spectrum antibiotics.
- Take stat chest x-ray.
- Transfer to emergency care if signs of sepsis proceed to severe sepsis or septic shock:
  - Send blood back to blood bank with any suspected reaction.
  - Draw a patient's blood sample from limb other than the one that is the transfusion site.
- Observe for circulatory overload due to excessive volumes or rapid infusion; elderly and chronically anemic patients are at higher risk as are patients who are already fluid-overloaded.
- Observe for citrate-induced hypocalcemia due to use of citrate anticoagulant, especially for patients with liver disease or circulatory compromise who are unable to metabolize increased levels of citrates.
  - If signs of hypocalcemia are present, anticipate orders to draw laboratory tests for ionized calcium or look for ECG changes associated with

COACH CONSULT

Patients with special needs may require blood that has been treated by centrifuge, radiation, or other methods to reduce the amounts of preservatives, anticoagulants, cytomegalovirus, and competitive white blood cells. Check the label to ensure that blood is prepared based on medical team orders before infusion.

hypocalcemia (see Chapter 3A for more information on hypocalcemia). Also observe for citrate-induced acidosis or alkalosis (see Chapter 4 for more information on acidosis and alkalosis).

Systems Assessment and Actions

If laboratory values are pending but fluid deficit is suspected, proceed with a systems assessment. **Immediately consult the medical team at the onset or worsening of any of the symptoms that are listed in the following section.**

Neuro-Musculo-Skeletal

If level of consciousness is decreased or if the patient complains of headache, dizziness, sleepiness, or appears confused or irrational, then:

- Anticipate frequent measures of neurological status using the Glasgow Coma Scale.
- Maintain safety measures, including bed in lowest position and call bell in reach.
- Continually reevaluate patient's ability to follow instructions.
- Consult the medical team to discuss the need for one-on-one supervision and patient restraints and side rails.
- Continue close monitoring, and provide safety supports, such as assistance to reach desired objects and for all ambulation and transfers.

Respiratory

Check for rate and depth of respirations. If respirations are greater than 20, if patient complains of any shortness of breath, or if the use of accessory muscles is noted, then:

- Measure oxygen saturation, and anticipate orders for supplemental oxygen.
- Raise head of bed to high Fowler's position to facilitate breathing.
- Place emergency respiratory equipment at bedside, including ambu-bag, oral airway, and suction equipment.
- Consult the medical team to discuss the need for supplemental oxygen and orders for chest x-ray:
  - Caution should be used because supplemental oxygen is not always indicated if removal of excess fluids is successful.
  - If patient must leave unit for testing, prepare for transport with emergency equipment and personnel.
  - Note that all female patients should be evaluated by the medical team for potential pregnancy.

CV

If dry or warm skin, excessive diaphoresis, tachycardia, weak pulses, or hypotension present, then:

- Closely monitor I&O, and communicate the need for accurate I&O measures to all ancillary staff.
- Anticipate orders for:
  - Continuous cardiac monitoring. Consult the medical team for preferred leads and alarm settings for monitoring of fluid excess and fluid deficit—related ECG changes.
  - IV infusion with crystalloid solutions to increase blood pressure.
  - Drawing of stat laboratory tests to evaluate for source of deficit and potential electrolyte imbalances, including sepsis, hemorrhage, or other acute or chronic metabolic processes.

GI

If vomiting, volumes of suction, or gastric drainage from interventional intubation or fistulas are present, then:

- Closely monitor I&O, and communicate need for accurate I&O measures to all ancillary staff.
- Anticipate volume replacement with crystalloids:
  - Note that fluid orders are typically based on a milliliter-for-milliliter replacement.
  - Provide oral care with water-based moisture solutions and soft swabs.
  - Observe carefully for any bleeding.
- Administer antiemetics as ordered. Note that GI symptoms may not resolve until electrolytes are stable, despite use of antiemetics:
  - Place suctioning equipment at bedside.
  - Stay with patient:
    - If vomiting occurs, attempt to protect airway from aspiration by maintaining the patient's head at a 30° angle.
    - If patient loses consciousness, place patient in the left lateral recumbent position (recovery position).

GU

Closely monitor I&O, and communicate need for accurate I&O measures to all ancillary staff. If urine is < 30 mL/hr or > 125 mL/hr, then:

- Consult the medical team because the patient may be descending into renal failure or may be experiencing inappropriate diuresis.
- Anticipate orders for hydration with crystalloid solutions.

- Anticipate orders for repeated urine samples to assess effect of fluid loss on electrolyte imbalance:
  - If urine specimens are ordered, use caution to avoid contamination with water or soap.
  - If drawing from a catheter, make certain to draw urine from the collection tube rather than the collection bag, because urine in the bag will start to biologically degrade.
- Discuss with the medical team orders to give or hold diuretics to balance fluid loss in overhydration with potential extended loss of chloride.

Vital Signs

If vital signs are persistently above or below the patient's baseline or outside the normal adult ranges (see Chapter 6), then:
- Consult the medical team.
- Measure vital signs frequently.
- Anticipate potential need to call for rapid response due to significant decline of patient's status.
- Anticipate orders for transfer of patient to a critical care environment for continuous neurological, respiratory, and cardiac monitoring.

Prevention

Teach at-risk populations:
- Signs and symptoms of fluid deficit and symptoms of infection and diabetes
- Signs and symptoms of fluid retention, e.g., edema, shortness of breath, weight gain
- Appropriate fluid ingestion
- Safe use of diuretics and antibiotics
- Medications: take medications as prescribed, and inform the medical team if unable to obtain medications
- Appropriate ingestion of fluids in normal temperatures and during periods of excess heat and exercise

Regarding public health:
- Advocate for patients with physical disability, developmental delay, mental health issues, or dementia to be provided appropriate fluids by caregivers.
- Educate population on risks associated with uncontrolled diabetes, and test vulnerable populations.
- Provide information to organizers of sporting events on proper hydration.

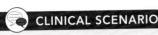

CLINICAL SCENARIO

DIAGNOSIS: FLUID DEFICIT

Mrs. Artise is a 72-year-old grandmother who lives alone, but her family visits weekly. Due to a history of CHF, she takes an ACE inhibitor and a diuretic every day. She weighs herself three times a week and knows to notify her physician if she gains any weight or becomes short of breath.

In July, Mrs. Artise's family goes away for a week to a reunion, but Mrs. Artise is not up to the travel. On Wednesday, Mrs. Artise's daughter calls a neighbor to ask her to look in on Mrs. Artise. When the neighbor knocks on the door, no one answers. The neighbor calls Mrs. Artise, but Mrs. Artise seems confused to the neighbor, who quickly calls Mrs. Artise's daughter, who then calls 911. Paramedics break down the door because Mrs. Artise is too weak to open it. They find her lying on the couch under a blanket, despite the fact that the closed and dark living room feels like 120°F. There is no air conditioning, and the windows are nailed shut. A fan circulates heated air throughout the room. Mrs. Artise is able to answer basic orientation questions, but she does not know the exact day or when she had her last drink of water. Her temperature is 95°F (35°C), her heart rate is 120, her blood pressure is 90/60, her respirations are at 24, and her oxygen saturation is 91%. Her diagnosis and medications are listed on a medical alert bracelet on her wrist. The paramedics assess extreme dehydration with potential urosepsis.

On the way to the hospital, 500 mL of NSS was given, with concern over Mrs. Artise's underlying heart disease. After the first 500 mL, her heart rate decreased to 90 bpm. Oxygen was placed, her respirations decreased to 18, and her oxygen saturation increased to 96%. Mrs. Artise states she feels better but, when she arrives at the emergency department, the staff initiates sepsis protocols due to her continually low blood pressure, low temperature, and inability to make urine.

Stat laboratory tests are ordered and drawn, including a complete metabolic panel and electrolytes, lactic acid, coagulation levels, liver enzymes, pancreatic enzymes, and a CBC. Blood cultures are drawn, another 18-gauge IV line is placed, 500 mL more of NSS is hung, a 12-lead ECG is done, and Mrs. Artise is placed on continuous cardiac monitoring. Due to suspicion of sepsis, broad-spectrum antibiotics are given, and a Foley catheter is placed. An ABG, BNP levels, chest x-ray, and echocardiogram are ordered stat to evaluate the status of her CHF.

Shortly after the delivery of antibiotics, Mrs. Artise's temperature has come up to 96.8°F (36°C), and she states she is feeling much better. The nurse adds planning for proper hydration to compensate for both heat exposure and patient CHF to Mrs. Artise's discharge plan.

1. What is the significance of weight gain or shortness of breath to Mrs. Artise's disease process?
2. What factors likely combined to cause Mrs. Artise's dehydration?
3. If Mrs. Artise is overheated, what is the likely reason her temperature is so low?

Fluid Balance and Imbalance **59**

Fluid Shift (Intravascular Fluid Deficit/Interstitial Fluid Excess, "Third Spacing")

Both acutely ill and chronically ill patients may be at risk for fluid volume shifts. When this occurs, fluid may leak into interstitial spaces or organ cavities. This shift commonly occurs with increased capillary permeability, but it can also be caused when fluid leaves cells due to trauma or burns. Caloric restriction or NPO status can also contribute to fluid shifts.

Due to either loss of proteins from the vascular space or low caloric intake, the body will burn fat and muscle. With each gram of fat or muscle burned, the body releases 1 mL of fluid. The water from fat has no salts, and the water from muscle has potassium salts and other salts that travel easily into interstitial and cellular spaces. Therefore, while the patient becomes dehydrated in the vascular space, the fluid from the vascular space will tend to move into the cells, and symptoms will arise from cells swollen beyond their normal capacity.

Laboratory Values

In most cases, vascular fluid remains isotonic to interstitial fluid, and serum electrolytes are within normal limits. However, serum electrolytes may be elevated due to the hemoconcentration that can occur when fluid leaves the vascular space. These values are dependent on the permeability of the membranes between fluid cavities, the presence of molecules that cause osmotic shifts in fluid, and the availability of electrolytes in the body.

Basic Concepts

Abnormal fluid shifts occur because of the disruption of membranes that normally separate fluid compartments. Surgery or trauma can cause mechanical interruption of membranes, including those surrounding the heart, lungs, and abdominal organs. Infection, inflammatory processes, or burns can cause a disruption of vascular capillary or cell wall structures and increase permeability. Proteins and other molecules that typically cannot escape their compartments travel more freely out of the vascular space and cells. Fluids follow the molecular or electrolyte shift due to a change in concentration.

Etiology

Fluid shifts, or "third spacing," can be caused by:
- Burns, which cause damage to and dilation of capillaries so that plasma leaks interstitially
- Chronic cardiac, hepatic, or renal disease, which causes inappropriate fluid retention or low protein states

- Compartment syndrome of soft tissues, which can be secondary to burns or trauma
- Iatrogenic infusion of high volumes of hypotonic fluids, which cause osmotic shifts interstitially
- Infection, which leads to sepsis, inflammation, and capillary permeability, causing fluids to migrate interstitially
- Malnourished states, anorexia, and diseases of malabsorption, which decrease available proteins in the vascular space and allow fluid to leak extravascularly
- Pancreatitis and pancreatic cancer, which lead to malabsorption or which allow the escape of pancreatic enzymes from the GI tract, causing proteins to shift interstitially and fluids to follow the proteins
- Surgery, especially abdominal surgery, which may cause leakage of fluids into cavities to the point where normal pressures are elevated; the presence of excess fluid in cavities is called *third spacing*
- Trauma, where similar mechanisms to surgery cause fluid shifts

Symptoms
Third spacing has some symptoms that are independent from decreased vascular fluid volumes. However, many of the symptoms, assessments, and treatments are similar (see the Symptoms section of Fluid Deficit).

- **Neurological:** Decrease in mental status due to decreased perfusion, edema of the eyes due to fluid shifts, pain with pancreatitis, burns, trauma, and compartment syndrome
- **Respiratory:** Tachypnea due to decreased perfusion, shallow breathing related to increased intra-abdominal or intrathoracic pressures
- **CV:** Hypotension, tachycardia, increased capillary filling time, decreased pulses, cool extremities due to decreased perfusion; edema in dependent portions of the body, such as lower legs or elbows, genitalia, and hips if the patient is on bedrest (see Chapter 6 for edema assessment scale)
- **GI:** Increased abdominal girth, weight gain, nausea, or vomiting related to increased pressures or pancreatitis; left upper quadrant or radiating pain related to pancreatitis
- **GU:** Concentrated urine due to fluid deficit

Assessment and Actions
Fluid, electrolyte, and acid-base imbalances can rapidly cause life-threatening neurological, cardiac, and respiratory compromise, requiring immediate

notification of the medical or rapid response team. Consult the medical team if any new onset occurs or if worsening symptoms or vital signs occur that are outside the normal range. If neurological, respiratory, or cardiac compromise occurs, call for assistance from the rapid or urgent response team or, if outside an acute care setting, call community EMS.

Patient History

Acute or chronic metabolic processes, including burns, infections, surgery, or trauma, may result in:

- Permeability of capillaries
- Rapid filling of organ cavities or soft tissues with fluids

Chronic health problems may be associated with fluid overload, fluid retention, or low albumin state fluid shifts, including:

- Cardiac disease, with unrestricted dietary fluid intake
- Cancers, including liver cancer, sarcoma, amyloidosis, multiple myeloma
- Infections, such as urinary tract infections, pericarditis, peritonitis, pancreatitis, parasitic infestation
- Renal disease
- Inflammatory bowel or rheumatic diseases
- Chronic pancreatic or GI disease, leading to malabsorption states
- Hepatic disease or biliary obstructive disease, leading to ascites
- Cushing's disease or syndrome
- Thyroid dysfunction

Laboratory Assessment and Actions

See the Laboratory Assessment and Actions section of this chapter for a discussion of laboratory values pointing to fluid loss. Note that an elevated anion gap, high lactic acid value, elevated white blood cell count, and low albumin value indicate acidosis related to sepsis. Regarding specimen collection:

- A white blood cell count is collected in a lavender-top tube.
- Lactic acid may be collected in a gray, sodium fluoride tube or a green, lithium heparin tube that is transported in an ice slurry.
- Low albumin levels are found with malabsorption, inflammatory, or septic states. However, intravascular fluid deficits can raise albumin levels, and therefore albumin is often compared with pre-albumin, which elevates in chronic renal failure or in patients receiving steroids to combat inflammation. Pre-albumin levels decrease with untreated inflammation, hepatic disease, malnutrition, and tissue death. Both albumin and pre-albumin are collected in a red- or tiger-top tube.

If electrolyte levels are low, anticipate orders for IV correction of electrolytes. Chapter 6 has a chart of normal electrolyte values.

If blood urea nitrogen, creatinine, osmolality, and total protein are high, anticipate orders for infusion of intravenous crystalloids. The Fluid Deficit section of this chapter contains more information on IV crystalloids.

If Hgb and Hct levels are high and rising, anticipate orders for administration of IV crystalloids, colloids, or other blood products. The Fluid Deficit section of this chapter contains more information on Hgb.

If the anion gap is high, lactic acid levels are high, and the white blood cell count is high, then anticipate communication with the medical team for suspected sepsis. Also anticipate transfer of patient to emergency care for pulmonary artery catheter placement, potential respiratory intubation and ventilation, and IV infusion of antibiotics and crystalloids. Normal albumin and pre-albumin levels are listed in Table 2–1.

If albumin or pre-albumin is low, anticipate delivery of albumin or fluids to halt or reverse third spacing. Controversial methods of halting or reversing third spacing include delivery of albumin versus delivery of NSS, application of Ringer's lactate, and delivery of plasma. Refer to your institutional policies, and consult the medical team regarding fluid infusion during third

SEPSIS

Sepsis is the leading cause of death in hospitals, with a 29% mortality rate. Be alert for systemic inflammatory response syndrome, which is an early warning sign of sepsis. Symptoms include the elevation of two of four measures: temperature, heart rate, respirations, or white blood cell count.

Table 2–1 Normal Albumin and Pre-Albumin Levels

PATIENT AGE	NORMAL LEVELS
Albumin	
1–40 yr	3.7–5.1 g/dL [SI units 37–51 g/L]
40–60 yr	3.4–4.8 g/dL [SI units 34–48 g/L]
60–90 yr	3.2–4.6 g/dL [SI units 32–46 g/L]
Pre-Albumin	
6 yr to adult	12–42 mg/dL [SI units 120–420 mg/L]

spacing. Refer to infusion guidelines in Blood and Fluid Deficit section of this chapter. Note that:

- In general, albumin is *ordered* for: acute peritonitis, pancreatitis, mediastinitis, cellulitis, acute liver failure, shock with oncotic deficit, and burns after 24 hours of large-volume crystalloid infusion.
- In general, albumin is *not ordered* for: chronic nephrosis, chronic cirrhosis, malabsorption, pancreatic insufficiency, or malnutrition.
- In general, albumin is *contraindicated* for CHF, renal insufficiency, or stable chronic anemia. An absolute contraindication to albumin administration is a history of allergic reaction to albumin.

If human albumin is ordered to mobilize fluids from interstitial spaces back into vascular spaces, note that albumin infusions require concurrent infusion of a crystalloid solution to prevent dehydration of cells and rapid electrolyte shifts. Due to its viscous nature, albumin must be infused via a large-bore IV line. During albumin infusions, monitor patient for:

- Dehydration induced by insufficient concurrent intravenous fluid support
- Hypertension or hypotension from induced fluid shifts
- Increased or decreased electrolyte states due to fluid shifts
- Hypersensitivity response

Stop infusion with signs of reaction, including:

- Hypersensitivity response: tachycardia, fever, hypotension
- Vascular overload: rales/crackles, dyspnea, hypertension

Systems Assessment and Actions

If laboratory assessment is not definitive or results are pending, proceed with a systems assessment. **Immediately consult the medical team at the onset or worsening of any of the symptoms that are listed in the following section.**

MED INFO **Rx**

Albumin dosing depends on medical team orders. Treatment for hypoproteinemia in adults usually requires 0.5–1 g/kg, with a maximum dose of 250 g over 48 hours by IV infusion; 25% dilutions are administered as 12.5g in 50 mL of NSS over 30 minutes or 25 g in 100 mL of NSS over 1 hour. If low albumin levels are concurrent with fluid losses, 5% solutions are administered as 12.5 g in 250 mL of NSS over 30–60 minutes or 25 g in 500 mL over 1–3 hours. The unused portion must be discarded after 4 hours. Albumin does not require crossmatching for blood typing.

Neurological

If a decrease in mental status is assessed, then:

- Evaluate patient on Glasgow Coma Scale (see Chapter 6).
- Continually reevaluate patient's ability to follow instructions.
- Consult the medical team to discuss the need for one-on-one continuous observation and the need for patient restraints and restraining side rails.
- Provide safety supports, such as assistance to reach desired objects and to ambulate to bathroom and placing bed in lowest position.

Respiratory

If *tracheal deviation* is noted, reduced breath sounds are auscultated, chest expansion is asymmetrical, or dullness is percussed over thoracic cavities, then:

- Communicate suspicion of pleural effusion with medical team.
- Prepare patient for transfer to emergency care for potential pleurocentesis.
- Monitor patient for rate, rhythm, and depth of respirations, and report changes to the medical team.
- Measure oxygen saturation.
- Raise head of bed to high Fowler's position to facilitate breathing.
- Place emergency respiratory equipment at bedside, including ambu-bag, oral airway, and suction equipment.
- Consult the medical team to discuss the need for supplemental oxygen and orders for a chest x-ray:
  - Caution should be used because supplemental oxygen is not always indicated if removal of excess fluids is successful.
  - Prepare patient for transport with emergency equipment and personnel if patient must leave unit for testing.
  - Note that all female patients should be evaluated by the medical team for potential pregnancy.

If rales/crackles or diminished breath sounds are present, anticipate orders for oral or IV diuretic administration. Closely monitor I&O, and communicate need for accurate I&O measures to all ancillary staff.

CV

If distant heart sounds are auscultated, JVD is noted, and hypotension is measured (Beck's triad), then:

- Communicate with the medical team suspicion of pericardial effusion and cardiac tamponade.
- Measure blood pressure for signs of pulses paradoxes, which is a drop of at least 10 mm Hg of systolic pressures on inspiration.

- Anticipate orders for continuous cardiac monitoring, and discuss with the medical team preferred leads and alarm setting for monitoring of ST segment changes.
- Prepare patient for transfer to emergency care for potential pericardial centesis.
- Monitor patient's pulses and blood pressure for signs of shock or pulseless electrical activity.

If concurrent fluid overload is determined by symptoms such as pulmonary rales/crackles, S_3 gallop, JVD, peripheral edema, ascites, hypertension, or bounding pulses, then communicate with the medical team to determine fluid load (see description of diuretic use in the earlier section on Fluid Excess).

If concurrent dehydration is determined by hypotension, tachycardia, increased capillary filling time, decreased pulses, decreased skin turgor, and cool extremities, anticipate orders for slow, cautious rehydration. More information on rehydration can be found in the earlier Fluid Deficit section.

If edema is apparent in dependent areas, such as lower legs or elbows, genitalia, and hips, elevate extremities, and protect skin and tissue from pressure.

GI

If bowel sounds are diminished, dullness is percussed over abdomen, or increase in girth is noted, then:
- Assess for Cullen's sign (a bruising near the umbilicus), which can indicate abdominal hemorrhage.
- Assess for Grey Turner's sign (bruising on the flanks), which can indicate acute pancreatitis or retroperitoneal hemorrhage.
- Anticipate orders to draw serum laboratory tests to evaluate for peritoneal hemorrhage.
- Monitor patient closely for decreased respiratory capacity, increased pulses, or hypotension, and report changes to the medical team.

GU

If flank sensitivity or Grey Turner's sign is noted, anticipate orders to draw serum laboratory tests to evaluate for retroperitoneal hemorrhage.

If urine is dark amber or demonstrates frank blood or sedimentation, anticipate orders to collect/direct patient to collect a urine specimen for osmolality, blood, and protein analysis.
- Elevated urine protein may indicate nephrotic syndrome.
- Blood in the urine may indicate nephritic syndrome.

With any signs of fluid deficit, closely monitor I&O, and communicate need for accurate I&O measures to all ancillary staff. More than 125 mL/hr without concurrent volume replacement may indicate inappropriate diuresis.

Cautions for Special Populations

Pediatrics

According to the USDA, infants are about 75% water for up to 6 months. After 6 months, males are about 60% water and females about 50%–56% water.

Signs of infant dehydration can include sunken fontanels and absence of tears on vigorous crying. Note that infants younger than 3 months cannot concentrate urine, so they will naturally have a lower specific gravity and osmolality. All IV fluids for pediatrics should be delivered via controller or infuser pump.

It can be difficult to obtain IV access in pediatric emergencies. In these cases, intraosseous infusions may be an option. A trained medical team can access the tibia with a short, specialty 16– to 20–gauge needle for children up to 6 years of age. Complications of intraosseous access include abscess, cellulitis, compartment syndrome, fat embolus, fractures at the insertion sight, osteomyelitis, and necrosis of tissue.

Pediatric Dietary Intake (FDA/Adequate Intake)

Healthy breastfed infants should meet dietary requirements through normal human milk intake:

- 0–6 months: 0.7 L/day
- 7–12 months: 0.8 L/day
- 1–3 years: 1.3 L/day
- 4–8 years: 1.7 L/day

Geriatrics

Water content for males and females declines after 51 years of age to about 56% and 47%, respectively. Geriatric individuals have less water by body weight because fat contains less water than muscle.

Due to a decline in their ability to concentrate urine, seniors may lose more fluid in their urine than younger adults who take in the same volumes of fluids. This increase in fluid loss puts geriatric individuals at more risk for dehydration. Note that all IV fluids for geriatric patients should be delivered via controller or infuser pump.

In addition to an increased potential for dehydration, changes in the urinary tract, kidneys, and immune system make seniors with urinary or renal problems susceptible to septic infections. GU symptoms should alert nurses to assess for infectious processes. Kidney disorders are also a special concern for the geriatric patient, who naturally loses some renal function as part of the aging process.

In the geriatric population or with trauma or infection, the eye's vitreous humor can lose its gel structure and become more liquid, causing visual problems. This is an example of fluid shift.

Geriatric Dietary Intake (FDA/Adequate Intake):
- 50–70 years: 3.7 L/day
- 70 years: 3.7 L/day

Review Questions

1. During exposure to excessive heat, such as during a heat wave, how much fluid can a patient lose per hour?
2. Why is it important for nurses to evaluate stool production?
3. Which particles are usually included in the measurement of serum osmolality?
4. How is the hematocrit used to evaluate vascular fluid loss?
5. When a patient experiences polydipsia, what volume should alert the nurse to the possibility of water toxicity?
6. Why is it dangerous to administer IV fluids through an IV line controlled only by a roller clamp?

3 Electrolyte Balance and Imbalance

CHAPTER 3

Electrolyte Balance and Imbalance

lectrolytes are ions that become charged when they are dissolved in water. A well-known example is uncharged sodium chloride (NaCl), which when dissolved in water dissociates into a positively charged sodium ion (Na^+) and a negatively charged chloride ion (Cl^-). The common electrolytes are sodium, chloride, potassium, phosphorus, calcium, and magnesium. Normal and critical serum levels for these electrolytes are in Table 3–1.

Common minerals, also known as essential micronutrients, interact with fluids and electrolytes. Some common minerals are boron, chromium, copper, fluoride, iodine, iron, manganese, molybdenum, selenium, and zinc.

This chapter begins by giving an overview of electrolyte physiology. It is further organized into seven subchapters detailing the normal function, balance, and imbalance of specific electrolytes. The subchapters are Calcium (3A), Chloride (3B), Magnesium (3C), Phosphorus (3D), Potassium (3E), Sodium (3F), and Essential Minerals (3G), which provide the effects of common minerals on body chemistry.

Electrolyte Physiology

Electrolyte charges are measured by milliequivalents. A milliequivalent (mEq) is equal to the number of charges in a given weight of an electrolyte or a compound. Most electrolytes have a specific number of valences (charges) assigned to it. If that number is 1, as in sodium, then a milliequivalent is equal to 1 millimole. If the number is other than 1, such as calcium, whose assigned valence is 2, then millimoles are not equal to

Table 3-1 Serum Electrolyte Levels

	CRITICAL LOW	NORMAL RANGE	CRITICAL HIGH
Calcium	<7 mg/dL	8.2–10.2 mg/dL	>12 mg/dL
Chloride	<80 mEq/L	97–107 mEq/L	>115 mEq/L
Magnesium	<1 mEq/L	1.32–2.14 mEq/L	>4 mEq/L
Phosphorus	<1 mg/dL	2.5–4.5 mg/dL	>5 mg/dL
Potassium	<2.5 mEq/L	3.5–5.0 mEq/L	>6.5 mEq/L
Sodium	<120 mEq/L	135–145 mEq/L	>160 mEq/L

milliequivalents. Because calcium is a divalent ion (Ca^{2+}), 1 mEq of calcium is equal to 0.5 millimoles. It is not essential to memorize chemical valences and units of measure. Instead, health-care providers should use caution when prescribing, preparing, and delivering medications to ensure that the levels measured and prescribed are in the same units.

Electrolytes can also be measured as millimoles, which is equal to the molecular weight of the substance. Millimole measurements are more common in health care outside the United States. When delivering electrolytes as intravenous or oral medications, it is essential to be aware whether electrolytes are being ordered in milliequivalents or in millimoles so that the patient receives the correct dosing. Calcium, magnesium, and phosphate are three examples of electrolytes where millimoles and milliequivalents are not equal, and therefore they require special attention to ensure that medical orders and pharmacy preparations are in the same chemical dosing.

ALERT

Millimoles and milliequivalents are not necessarily equal values, and they require special attention to ensure that medical orders and pharmacy preparations are in the same chemical dosing.

Diffusion is the process that transports electrolytes and other charged particles across cellular and vascular membranes. In diffusion, positively charged elements move toward a negatively charged area. Positively charged elements can be exchanged for other positively charged elements, and negatively charged elements can be exchanged for other negatively charged elements. These positive-positive and negative-negative exchanges are particularly important for balancing acids and bases with electrolytes. For example, positively charged hydrogen ions (H^+) may be exchanged for other positively charged ions, such as potassium (K^+), thus reducing hydrogen concentration and acidity. Similarly, bicarbonate (HCO_3^-), a base, can be exchanged for negatively charged chloride ions (Cl^-), shifting fluid pH back toward alkaline levels.

Sodium Properties With Chloride and Potassium

Sodium and chloride ions bond as cations and anions to form an ionic compound. Cations are positively charged ions, and anions are negatively charged ions.

In contrast to sodium and chloride, sodium and potassium are cations. Sodium is the major extracellular cation, and potassium is the major intracellular cation. The *sodium potassium pump* is an active transport mechanism that maintains the ratio between sodium and potassium in the body, which creates an electrical resting membrane potential. The pump is a cellular enzyme known as adenosine triphosphate-ase (ATP-ase), and it exchanges three sodium ions to the outside of the cell for every two potassium ions pumped into the cell. When fluid builds up inside the cell, the pump activates and transports water with sodium ions outside of the cell. The shift of sodium outside of the cell allows for glucose, amino acids, and other elements to move across the cellular membrane into the cell.

Calcium, Magnesium, and Phosphorus

Calcium, magnesium, and phosphorus have similar characteristics: they are divalent cations, which means that they have a valence (charge) of 2; they are mainly held in the bones, though smaller amounts of each cation are present inside of cells and very small amounts circulate in the extracellular fluid; and they are regulated and balanced by the actions of vitamin D and the parathyroid hormone. While each electrolyte has its own function and properties (to be discussed later in this chapter), they are highly interdependent.

Endocrine Regulation

Some hormones have an impact on more than one electrolyte. For instance, aldosterone will cause sodium retention while increasing potassium excretion, parathyroid hormone causes calcium retention while increasing phosphorus excretion, and calcitonin causes excretion of both calcium and phosphorus. When reviewing the etiology of electrolyte shifts, it is important to evaluate loss or excess in relationship to the underlying pathology as well as the status of other electrolytes.

3A Calcium

Calcium

Calcium (Ca$^+$) is the body's most abundant positively charged ion (cation), with 98%–99% stored in teeth and bones. In serum, calcium is either bound or free. Bound calcium is linked to proteins, such as albumin, or to anions like bicarbonate, citrate, phosphate, or lactate. Unbound calcium, also known as ionized calcium, is active in metabolic functions. In addition, protein levels in the blood affect overall serum calcium levels. Therefore, when patients have altered albumin levels, ionized calcium levels are measured to evaluate available serum calcium.

Extracellular calcium far outbalances intracellular calcium with a ratio of 10,000:1. Because of this imbalance, when calcium channels in the cellular membrane open, calcium quickly travels into cells and stimulates calcium-dependent functions. Calcium channels are known to be voltage-dependent or voltage-gated, which means that chemical shifts causing electrical excitation trigger these channels to open or close. An open channel allows calcium to travel into cells, and a closed channel ensures that the calcium remains stored in the channel.

Serum calcium is also evaluated in relationship to serum phosphorus. When calcium levels in the blood rise, phosphorous levels decrease; likewise, when phosphorous levels rise, gastric calcium absorption is inhibited. The relationship between calcium and phosphorus is due to (1) the hormone feedback cycle of the parathyroid hormone and calcitriol and (2) the binding of calcium by phosphorus (see the later section, "Regulation").

Changes in anions, such as bicarbonate, citrate, phosphate, and lactate, can cause changes in serum calcium levels. Serum pH also affects available calcium. For example, in alkaline states, calcium binds to proteins in the serum, whereas in acidotic states, calcium leaves proteins and raises ionized or free calcium levels.

Functions

Calcium provides structural support for bones and teeth, promotes movement across the cellular membrane via calcium channels, and helps to activate coagulation. In addition, calcium triggers nerve and muscle activity and promotes immune function.

Provides Structural Support for Bones and Teeth

Of the body's calcium, 98%–99% provides structural support for bones and teeth. Calcium is constantly involved in a cycle of releasing (resorption) from and depositing into bones. Bones are about two-thirds minerals and are made up mostly of calcium and phosphorus in a crystalline form called hydroxyapatite. Hydroxyapatite is taken from the extravascular fluid and transformed into bone by cells called osteoblasts. The rest of bone consists of proteins, such as collagen and water. Minerals are removed from bone structure by cells called osteoclasts.

Until about age 30 years, minerals are added to and removed from bone structure in a continuous cycle. After age 30, remodeling changes so that less bone is added than removed. At this time, osteoporosis can occur if excess amounts of bone are removed. Areas of bone that are stimulated by weight-bearing and other stresses grow stronger under normal conditions. Weight-bearing exercise can also decrease decline in bone mass related to osteoporosis. In Paget's disease, which is a genetically linked disease, abnormal processes cause the bone that is formed to be brittle, which in turn causes high risk for fractures and deformities.

Promotes Movement Across Cellular Membranes via Calcium Channels

High-voltage channels are found in cellular membranes. At rest, they are normally closed. On depolarization, they open and allow calcium to pass into the cell. Typical cell types include muscles, neurons, cells that regulate DNA and RNA production, and cells that prepare and release hormones and neurotransmitters. Calcium binds to a protein called calmodulin, which allows for product release and assists with ciliary movement and cell reproduction.

Helps to Activate Coagulation

Coagulation is a complex system of molecular activation and stimulation. Calcium is one of the components of the tenase complex, which activates factor X. It is also active with phospholipid in the common pathway, where it helps convert prothrombin to thrombin and activate factor XIII, which

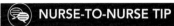
stabilizes and thickens fibrin clots. Blood levels of calcium are rarely low enough to stop the coagulation process.

Triggers Nerve and Muscle Activity

Calcium triggers the release of chemical-signaling neurotransmitters between neurons in a process called exocytosis. Low levels of calcium decrease nerve function. Calcium also binds troponin C, allowing for actin-myosin binding in muscle cells, which in turn allows for contraction. Muscle cells pump calcium back out of cells to allow for relaxation.

Promotes Immune System Function

Proteins on a cell membrane sense microbes and stimulate the movement of calcium into white blood cells. Within the cell, the endoplasmic reticulum is also stimulated to release calcium. A defect in these calcium channel proteins can cause serious immune dysfunction, such as Bubble Boy disease, in which patients lack all immune function.

Intake

In healthy patients, intake is through dietary sources. However, some patients who are admitted to acute care facilities may require supplemental oral or intravenous infusion of calcium.

Dietary Intake

Due to differences in bone formation, adequate intakes are significantly different between age groups (see pediatric concerns at the end of this chapter).

For adults over 19 years old, recommended adequate calcium intake is 1000 mg/day. Adults over 51 years should ingest 1200 mg/day because of a decreased ability to absorb dietary calcium. Dietary sources of calcium include dairy products, seaweed, nuts, seeds, oranges, figs, tofu, sardines, salmon, and vegetables such as okra, broccoli, and kale. A typical 8-oz serving of dairy products, such as milk or yogurt, has about 10 times the amount of calcium as a typical half-cup serving of green vegetables. It is difficult to obtain the recommended levels of calcium with a non-dairy, non-fish diet unless the patient carefully chooses foods that are fortified with calcium. Calcium absorption may also be decreased with certain vegetables that contain phytic acid and oxalic acid, including spinach, collard greens, sweet potatoes, beans, rhubarb, and cereals.

Intravenous Intake

Calcium chloride or calcium gluconate can be administered intravenously if required. However, this must be done with extreme caution in critical situations. It is essential to read the orders carefully for the type and dosage of calcium that is ordered because calcium chloride and calcium gluconate are not of equal strength (see the later section on hypocalcemia).

Regulation

Serum calcium is regulated strongly by the thyroid and parathyroid glands and the kidneys. Special proteins sense calcium levels in the blood. If calcium levels are high, *calcitonin* is released from the thyroid gland to stimulate calcium return into the bones. If blood calcium is low, *parathyroid hormone* is released to stimulate calcium release from the bones. Decreased parathyroid levels can occur with sepsis, burns, low magnesium levels, or other cellular disruption. Increased parathyroid levels can occur with thiazide diuretics, and they can also occur if certain types of cancers stimulate the gland. *Calcitriol*, also known as activated vitamin D, is another hormone that works in conjunction with the parathyroid hormone to regulate intestinal calcium absorption and bone calcium release and resorption.

Calcitonin

Calcitonin is produced by the thyroid gland's parafollicular cells (C cells) in response to high calcium levels. Calcitonin lowers serum calcium and serum phosphate by stopping the release of calcium from the bones and decreasing osteoclast activity, thus inhibiting the delayed release of calcium and phosphorus. It also inhibits absorption of calcium from the gastrointestinal (GI) tract and reabsorption of calcium from the renal system. Calcitonin can be provided by injection as a medication to decrease serum calcium levels.

Parathyroid Hormone

The parathyroid hormone (PTH) stimulates calcium release from bone into serum, and it increases the renal activation of vitamin D so that more calcium is absorbed from food sources by the intestines. PTH stimulates immediate release of calcium from bone cells and a delayed release of calcium and phosphorus into the serum by stimulating increased osteoclast activity. Because the release of phosphorus together with calcium may cause undesirable serum phosphate levels, PTH also affects renal reabsorption of both electrolytes. PTH increases reabsorption of calcium while decreasing renal reabsorption of phosphorus, thus keeping serum levels within a desired range.

Calcitriol

Calcitriol, also known as activated vitamin D, is the third major hormone that regulates calcium. Calcitriol is initially activated from vitamin D, which is ingested from animal or plant sources or formed in the skin. Vitamin D travels to the kidneys where it awaits signaling from circulating PTH. When PTH activates calcitriol, the calcitriol helps PTH mobilize calcium from the bone, and it sends a signal back to the parathyroid gland to stop production of PTH when there is enough circulating calcium. When PTH first appears in the circulation, it causes the kidneys to excrete phosphorus. When calcitriol is activated, it stops the kidneys from losing phosphorus. Vitamin D increases the absorption of dietary calcium and acts to stimulate ostoblast bone building and osteoclast removal of calcium from bone. PTH stimulates vitamin D production in the kidneys. Low parathyroid levels increase vitamin D production, whereas calcitonin decreases renal vitamin D production.

Loss

Calcium is added to the body through bone deposits until about age 30 years, when bone loss begins to occur. Postmenopausal women experience overall calcium loss, putting them at risk for osteoporosis. Weight-bearing exercise has been shown to decrease bone loss.

Renal excretion of calcium is about 200 mg/day, and foods high in sodium and protein increase calcium excretion. About 200 mg of calcium is lost through bile per day. Alcohol reduces both the absorption of calcium and the activation of vitamin D in the intestines; caffeine also has a negative effect on calcium absorption, and it increases calcium excretion. Calcium is also lost through sweat at about 25 mg/day.

Laboratory Measures

Serum levels are drawn to assess for calcium, both bound and unbound, in the blood. The normal serum range for calcium in adults is 8.4–10.2 mg/dL.

Serum calcium should be evaluated in relationship to serum albumin. For each gram of serum albumin, < 4 g/dL, calcium levels should be adjusted downward by 0.8 mg/dL per gram. For each gram of albumin greater than 4 g/dL, calcium should be adjusted up by 0.8 mg/dL.

Ionized calcium measures in adult serum should be 4.12–4.92 mg/dL.

COACH CONSULT

When albumin is 4 g/dL or below, use the following formula to estimate serum calcium: Serum calcium + 0.8 (4 –serum albumin) = corrected serum calcium

Serum Specimen Collection

Serum calcium and ionized calcium are collected by phlebotomy in a red- or tiger-top tube, but it may also be drawn in a green-top, heparinized tube. Standard phlebotomy procedure requires avoiding drawing blood from the same arm with intravenous access. Use of a tourniquet can elevate calcium levels. Calcium levels change depending on time of day, so serial specimens should be drawn at the same time of day for comparison. To avoid processing errors, ensure that the specimen is delivered according to your laboratory's guidelines.

Special Tests: Urine Calcium

Urine may be collected at random, using a clean-catch or catheter-obtained specimen, or over 24 hours (see Chapter 6 for collection method). Levels of urine calcium vary with dietary intake. High sodium diets can cause excessive excretion of calcium. The normal adult range for urine calcium is 100–300 mg/24 hours.

Urine calcium can be compared with creatinine. The normal calcium-to-creatinine ratio in mg/dL ratio is less than 0.14:1. The test is also used to assess for kidney stones and to evaluate renal losses. Increased urine calcium renal losses occur with acromegaly, cancer, diabetes, Fanconi's syndrome, excess glucocorticoids, hyperparathyroidism, hyperthyroidism, sarcoidosis, excess vitamin D, bone loss related to immobilization, osteitis deformans, osteoporosis, Paget's disease, and renal disease, including Wilson's disease and renal tubular acidosis. Decreased excretion occurs with hypoparathyroidism, hypothyroidism, nephrosis, nephritis, ostomalacia, pre-eclampsia, renal ostodystrophy, rickets, and vitamin D deficiency.

Hypocalcemia

Hypocalcemia occurs when there is a calcium deficit in the body.

Laboratory Values
- Serum calcium < 8.2 mg/dL
- Ionized serum calcium < 4.64 mg/dL

Basic Concepts
Hypocalcemia must always be considered in relationship to overall body calcium and to calcium stored in serum proteins. When assessing calcium levels, serum albumin < 4 g/dL should decrease calcium estimates by 0.8 mg/dL for each decrease in albumin by 1 g/dL. For instance, calcium of 10 mg/dL with an albumin of 4 g/dL is calculated as 9.2 mg/dL with an albumin level of 3 g/dL. Calcium's close relationship with magnesium and phosphorus requires evaluation of these two electrolytes as well. Alkalosis causes calcium to bind to albumin, causing less calcium to be available as serum ionized calcium and therefore demonstrating serum hypocalcemia.

> **ALERT**
>
> Hypocalcemia occurs when serum calcium is <8.2 mg/dL or when ionized serum calcium is <4.64 mg/dL. *Critical* hypocalcemia occurs when serum calcium levels are <7 mg/dL or when ionized serum calcium is <3.2 mg/dL. These critical low serum levels can lead to electrocardiogram changes and convulsions.

Etiology
Hypocalcemia can be caused by:
- Alkalotic states
- Dietary insufficiency or GI disturbances that decrease absorption of calcium, proteins, or vitamin D
- Vitamin D deficiency or metabolic impairment that results from lack of exposure to ultraviolet light (including sunlight), poor dietary absorption, or hepatic cirrhosis
- Leprosy
- Osteomalacia
- Pancreatitis related to low albumin levels

- PTH deficiency resulting from accidental PTH removal or destruction during thyroid surgery or treatments, hypomagnesemia, or congenital or idiopathic causes
- Renal failure or renal tubular disease related to decreased vitamin D and hyperphosphatemia
- Iatrogenic losses that can induce hypocalcemia, including:
  - Infusion of blood products preserved with citrate
  - Surgical removal of the parathyroid gland or portions of the stomach or small intestines
  - Medications, including:
    - Antineoplastic medications: mithramycin and cisplatinum
    - Albuterol
    - Aminoglycosides
    - Antacids with aluminum or magnesium
    - Anticonvulsants
    - Diuretics
    - Glucagon
    - Glucocorticosteroids
    - Glucose
    - Insulin
    - Laxatives
    - Magnesium
    - Methicillin
    - Phosphates
    - Tetracycline
    - Trazodone

Symptoms

- **Neurological:** Confusion, mood changes, anxiety, memory loss, increased excitability of sensory and motor tracts, paresthesia in extremities and face, seizures
- **Cardiovascular (CV):** Arrhythmias, ECG changes including prolonged QT interval and prolonged ST segment (Fig. 3A-1), delayed clotting associated with prolonged partial thromboplastin time and prolonged prothrombin time
- **Respiratory:** Laryngeal and bronchial spasms, which may lead to airway closure
- **GI:** Abdominal muscle spasms
- **Musculoskeletal:** Cramping, tremors, increased reflexes, Trousseau's sign, Chvostek's sign (Fig. 3A-2), tetany

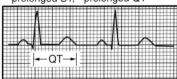

FIGURE 3A-1: Hypocalcemia ECG tracing. Note lengthened ST segment and lengthened QT interval.

Assessment and Actions

Fluid, electrolyte, and acid-base imbalances can rapidly cause life-threatening neurological, cardiac, and respiratory compromise, requiring immediate notification of the medical or rapid response team. Consult the medical team if any new onset occurs or if worsening symptoms or vital signs occur that are outside the normal range. If neurological, respiratory, or cardiac compromise occurs, call for assistance from the rapid or urgent response team or, if outside an acute care setting, call community emergency medical services (EMS).

Patient History

The following conditions may be associated with or cause hypocalcemia:

- Acute or chronic metabolic processes, which may result in alkalotic states, excess renal excretion, impaired GI absorption, low albumin levels, hypomagnesemia, or vitamin D deficiency

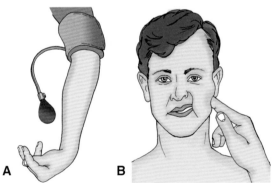

FIGURE 3A-2: Trousseau's (A) and Chvostek's (B) signs.

- Chronic health problems may be associated with hypocalcemia, including:
  - Alkalosis associated with anemia, hypotension, and respiratory diseases, including reduced lung expansion related to chronic, neuromuscular disease, pregnancy, or liver failure
  - GI diseases relating to poor calcium, albumin, or vitamin D absorption, including anorexia, Crohn's disease, pancreatitis, gastric or intestinal obstruction
  - Primary or secondary parathyroid deficiency
  - Renal diseases that cause hyperphosphatemia, such as renal insufficiency or renal failure
- Excess ingestion or infusion of citrates in blood transfusions or medications

Laboratory Assessment and Actions

Serum calcium <8.2 mg/dL or ionized serum calcium <4.64 mg/dL reflects hypocalcemia that may need correction. Serum calcium at 9 mg/dL or below with an albumin level of 4 g/dL or below may also need correction. If symptoms are present or critical values of serum calcium <7 mg/dL or ionized serum calcium <3.2 mg/dL, then:

MED INFO ℞

Oral calcium is prescribed in divided doses because absorption decreases in the presence of high doses. Calcium is available in several forms: calcium acetate (used in the presence of hyperphosphatemia related to end-stage renal disease and should be given before meals), carbonate (used as an antacid and may cause constipation; given with meals to increase absorption), chloride, citrate (easily digested and can be taken on an empty stomach and with proton pump inhibitors), gluconate, lactate; and tricalcium phosphate. Onset, peak, and duration of oral preparations is unknown.

- Anticipate frequent blood calcium, magnesium, potassium, and phosphorous levels, based on frequency and effect of interventions.
- Anticipate oral administration of calcium in doses of 1–2 g/day as a supplement. Supplements should not be taken with milk in order to prevent milk-alkali syndrome. Anticipate prescription of vitamin D with calcium to increase absorption.
- Anticipate IV administration containing calcium if oral administration is not effective or if vitamin D deficiency is present. Doses are 2.25–16 mEq for symptomatic hypocalcemia, including cardiac standstill, tetany, hyperkalemia and hypermagnesemia. These solutions should be infused via a large-bore intravenous (IV) line into a large or central vein.
  - Anticipate orders for frequent, rapid serum laboratory tests to assess effects.

- Rate for calcium chloride should not be >0.7 mEq/min. Calcium gluconate should not infuse faster than 200 mg/min. Typical dosing is a bolus of 100 mg, then 1–5 mg/kg/hr. Do not confuse (1) chloride and gluconate and (2) mEq and mg when preparing and infusing calcium. Calcium carbonate has approximately three times the bioavailability of calcium gluconate.

- Onset and peak are immediate.
- Duration is 0.5–2 hours.
- Risk for extravasation is high, resulting in cellulitis, necrosis, and skin sloughing. If infiltration occurs, anticipate orders for treatment with normal saline, procaine HCl, or hyaluronidase.
- Infusion should be stopped if tingling, warmth, or metal taste is reported. After consultation with the medical team, calcium restart may be ordered, although at a slower rate and close observation.

- Patients should remain lying down for at least 30 minutes after administration.

Systems Assessment and Actions

If laboratory test results are pending, but hypocalcemia is suspected, proceed with a systems assessment. Immediately consult the medical team at the onset or worsening of any of the symptoms that are listed in the following section.

Neurological

If confusion, mood changes, anxiety, memory losses, nerve excitability, paresthesias, or seizures occur, then:

- Anticipate frequent measures of neurological status using the Glasgow Coma Scale.
- Maintain safety measures including bed low, padded side rails in place, and call bell in reach.

- Continually reevaluate patient's ability to follow instructions.
- Consult the medical team to discuss need for one-on-one supervision.
- Anticipate orders for antiseizure medications.

CV

If ECG changes occur, then:

- Anticipate orders to initiate continuous cardiac monitoring.
- Consult with the medical team to establish preferred leads and alarm settings to detect calcium-associated changes.

If clotting times are prolonged, then:

- Anticipate orders for transfusion of blood or clotting products (see Chapter 2 for information on blood transfusions).
- Educate patient on bleeding precautions.
- Observe transfusion site for bleeding or bruising.

Respiratory

If laryngeal or bronchial spasms develop, then:

- Immediately consult the medical or rapid response team for advanced airway management.
- Keep respiratory support equipment readily available (ambu-bag, oral airway, suction, and oxygen).
- Measure oxygen saturation, and anticipate orders for supplemental oxygen.
- Raise head of bed to facilitate airway clearance.

GI

If abdominal spasms or pain occur, hold all oral intake, and consult medical or rapid response team immediately due to potential for laryngeal spasm.

Musculoskeletal

If cramping, tremors, increased reflexes, Trousseau's or Chvostek's sign, or tetany occurs, then:

- Institute standard safety precautions.
- Maintain patient on bedrest.
- Assist patient with all activities of daily living, ambulation, and transfers.

Prevention

Teach at-risk populations:

- Signs and symptoms of hypocalcemia
- Appropriate calcium ingestion and provide a list of dietary sources
- Signs of poor clotting, including bruising and bleeding

To advocate for public health:

- Health providers should ensure that at-risk patients are aware of sources of vitamin D in diet and with sunlight exposure.
- Osteoporosis (weak bones) and osteopenia (low bone mass) are common problems resulting in approximately 1.5 million fractures a year. Increased loss is associated with postmenopausal women who are inactive, smoke, take alcohol, and have a familial history. Those at risk should be encouraged to maintain adequate intake of calcium and vitamin D and participate in weight-bearing exercises.
- Use of hormone replacement therapy for postmenopausal women has become controversial due to a potential increase in health problems, including cancer. Instead, medical providers may prescribe bisphosphonates to slow bone loss.
- Adequate intake of dietary calcium is associated with lower blood pressure, based on research from the National Institutes of Health *Dietary Approaches to Stop Hypertension*.
- The "female athlete triad" has been identified as disordered eating, amenorrhea, and osteoporosis, resulting in stress fractures. Women in the military are at increased risk.
- Patients with lactose intolerance are at high risk for lack of calcium ingestion with a typical American diet. Adult population risks are significantly higher for Asians and African Americans than for whites.

 CLINICAL SCENARIO

DIAGNOSIS: HYPOCALEMIA FROM VITAMIN D DEFICIENCY

Mrs. Albert is diagnosed with calcium deficiency related to low vitamin D. Mrs. Albert works in an office and, due to a family history of skin cancer, always covers her skin when she is outside. Additionally, she has a long-standing seizure disorder and takes phenytoin, which binds vitamin D.

Her medical team has prescribed vitamin D supplements and has recommended increased vitamin D from food sources. The nurse reviews sources of dietary vitamin D with Mrs. Albert, including egg yolks, fortified dairy products, cereals, and fatty fish including salmon, tuna, and mackerel. She was also reassured that she could obtain sufficient amounts of vitamin D with about a half hour of sunshine three or more times a week, with a little more sun exposure in the winter due to a decrease in the intensity of the sun.

Continued

CLINICAL SCENARIO—cont'd

1. What are Mrs. Albert's long-term risks from low calcium levels?
2. Which other electrolyte might be compromised by low levels of vitamin D?
3. With Mrs. Albert's medical history, if seizure activity is noted, then what laboratory tests would you anticipate in addition to measuring serum phenytoin levels?

Hypercalcemia

Hypercalcemia occurs when there is an excess of calcium in the body.

Laboratory Values
- Serum calcium >10.2 mg/dL
- Serum ionized calcium >5.28 mg/dL

> **ALERT** !
>
> Hypercalcemia occurs when serum calcium is >10.2 mg/dL and when serum ionized calcium is >5.28 mg/dL. *Critical* hypercalcemia occurs when serum calcium is >12 mg/dL and ionized serum calcium is >6.2 mg/dL. Critical high values of calcium can lead to ECG changes and coma.

Basic Concepts
When addressing hypercalcemia, the health practitioner should keep in mind the potential for occult disease processes, such as hyperparathyroidism and cancer. Calcium needs to be evaluated with albumin levels. Low albumin levels that occur when serum calcium is in the normal range are actually an indication of excess calcium in the serum.

Etiology
Hypercalcemia can be caused by:
- Acidosis, including chronic acidosis, which may result in osteoporosis
- Acromegaly
- Cancers, including primary lymphomas, leukemia, myeloma, squamous cell carcinoma, kidney cancer, or metastasis to the bone
- Dehydration states
- Endocrine dysfunctions such as Addison's disease, in which dehydration occurs
- Hyperparathyroidism
- Immobility
- Lung diseases that cause overactivation of vitamin D, including tuberculosis and histoplasmosis

- Paget's disease
- Pheochromocytoma
- Thyrotoxicosis

Iatrogenic causes include:
- Overinfusion of calcium
- Renal transplant
- Medications including:
  - Anabolic steroids and corticosteroids
  - Calcitriol
  - Lithium
  - Overinfusion or ingestion of calcium
  - Parathyroid hormone
  - Tamoxifen
  - Thiazide diuretics (inducing hypercalemia and hypercalciuria)
  - Vitamin A
  - Vitamin D toxicity

Psuedohypercalcemia occurs when fluid volumes are low. Calcium is more concentrated due to the low fluid volumes in the body. It can occur with dehydration states and with polycythemia vera.

Symptoms
- **Neurological:** Lethargy, apathy, headache, confusion, decreased level of consciousness leading to coma
- **CV:** Shortened ST segment, shortened QT interval on ECG (Fig. 3A-3)
- **Respiratory:** Tongue twitching
- **GI:** Constipation, anorexia, nausea, reflux, elevated pancreatic enzymes
- **Genitourinary (GU):** Polyuria
- **Musculoskeletal**: Weakness, hyperreflexia

Assessment and Actions
Fluid, electrolyte, and acid-base imbalances can rapidly cause life-threatening neurological, cardiac, and respiratory compromise, requiring immediate notification of the medical or rapid response team. Consult the medical team if any new onset occurs or if worsening symptoms or vital signs occur that are outside the normal range. If neurological, respiratory, or cardiac compromise occurs, call for assistance from the rapid or urgent response team or, if outside an acute care setting, call community EMS.

Hypercalcemia:
- shortened ST, -shortened QT

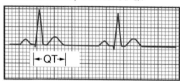

FIGURE 3A-3: Hypercalcemia ECG tracing. Note shortened ST segment and shortened QT interval.

Patient History

Review for clues to cause. The conditions listed below may contribute to hypercalcemia:

- Acute or chronic metabolic processes, such as acidosis from respiratory or other sources, dehydration states, or bone demineralization
- Chronic health problems, including:
  - Acromegaly from concurrent PTH tumor or overgrowth
  - Cancers related to PTH stimulation by certain tumors
  - Endocrine diseases, such as Addison's disease, hyperparathyroidism, thyrotoxicosis
  - Respiratory or systemic diseases, such as tuberculosis and histoplasmosis
  - Paget's disease
  - Pheochromocytoma
  - Iatrogenic intervention may be causative, including:
    - Infusion or ingestion of calcium or medications that increase calcium absorption or decrease secretion
    - Loop diuretics
    - Renal transplant

Laboratory Assessment and Actions

Serum calcium >10.2 mg/dL or serum ionized calcium >5.28 mg/dL reflects hypercalcemia that may need correction. Anticipate treatment for hypercalcemia with symptoms or critical values of serum calcium >12 mg/dL or ionized serum calcium >6.2 mg/dL.

- Anticipate orders for frequent blood and urine measures of calcium levels based on the effect of interventions.
- Anticipate orders for frequent blood measures of other electrolytes, ions, and albumin throughout the course of therapy.
- Anticipate orders for IV administration of normal saline solution with or without the addition of loop diuretics to increase

renal excretion of calcium. Diuretics should not be given until volume depletion has been corrected. IV furosemide requires (1) slow IV administration to protect the patient from ototoxicity and (2) protection from light sources to prevent degradation of the medication.

- Anticipate orders for administration of intramuscular or subcutaneous calcitonin, which prevents calcium from leaving bones and promotes renal excretion of calcium.
- If the cause of hypercalcemia is related to parathyroid stimulation from cancer, anticipate orders to administer corticosteroids, which decrease bone loss and GI absorption. Prednisolone is typically given in divided doses up to 30 mg/day. Caution must be used when administering corticosteroids to prevent rebound steroid insufficiency.

Systems Assessment and Actions

If laboratory test results are pending but hypercalcemia is suspected, proceed with a systems assessment. Immediately consult the medical team at the onset or worsening of any of the symptoms that are listed in the following section.

Neuro-Musculo-Skeletal

If lethargy, apathy, headache, confusion, decreased level of consciousness, tongue twitching, weakness, or hyperreflexia is present, then:

- Perform frequent neurological assessments for decreased level of consciousness, hyperreflexia, or weakness.
- Anticipate frequent measures of neurological status using the Glasgow Coma Scale.
- Maintain safety measures including bed low, padded side rails in place, and call bell in reach.
- Continually reevaluate patient's ability to follow instructions.
- Consult the medical team to discuss need for one-on-one supervision.

MED INFO

Calcitonin doses start at 4 units per kg every 12 hours and may increase every 1–2 days if necessary. A calcitonin sensitivity test is sometimes ordered when sensitivity is suspected. Vials should be stored in refrigeration. Salmon calcitonin has 100 times the potency of human calcitonin. Calcitonin is also used long-term to treat Paget's disease and postmenopausal osteoporosis. Calcitonin in available in a nasal spray, but this use is normally for long-term treatment.

COACH CONSULT

Oral phosphate therapy is limited; if a dose is >2 g/day, it often causes diarrhea. IV biophosphonate (pamidronate or etidronate) administration is dangerous because phosphate binds with calcium and forms mineral deposits in lungs, kidneys, and blood vessels, which can be fatal.

CV

If ECG changes are noted, including shortened ST segment or shortened QT interval, anticipate orders to initiate continuous ECG monitoring, and consult medical team to establish preferred leads and alarm settings to detect calcium-associated changes.

Respiratory

If tongue twitching is noted, raise the head of the bed to facilitate airway clearance, and keep respiratory support equipment readily available (ambu-bag, suction, oral airway, suction equipment, and oxygen).

GI

If constipation, anorexia, or nausea occur, then:

- Hold all oral intake, and consult the medical team due to potential for dysphagia.
- Anticipate orders for antiemetic medications (may not be effective until electrolyte imbalance has been corrected).
- Consult the medical team for hydration or medications to address constipation.

GU

If polyuria is measured, then:

- Measure fluid volumes (>125 mL/hr without concurrent volume replacement may point to inappropriate diuresis).
- Communicate need for accurate intake and output measures to all ancillary staff.
- Anticipate repeated urine samples to assess effect of fluid loss on electrolyte imbalance. Collect specimen with caution to avoid contamination with water or soap. If drawing from a catheter, draw urine from the collection tube rather than the collection bag, because the bag is where urine starts to biologically degrade.

Prevention

Teach at-risk populations:

- Signs and symptoms of hypercalcemia
- Appropriate dietary intake and supplement levels

To advocate for public health:

- Ensure that clients who are taking digitalis and calcium are aware of enhanced effects of digoxin and risk of life-threatening bradycardia.

- Ensure that patients with renal failure, cancers, and chronic lithium, steroid, and thiazide diuretic use are aware of risk of hypercalcemia.
- Educate patients with chronic low states of hypercalcemia that immobility may dangerously increase hypercalcemia.

 CLINICAL SCENARIO

DIAGNOSIS: HYPERCALCEMIA ASSOCIATED WITH OSTEOPOROSIS AND HYPERPARATHYROIDISM

Mrs. Woods is a 62-year-old widow who lives alone. Her primary activities include knitting and watching television because she lives in a somewhat dangerous urban neighborhood and has no private transportation. She has been recently diagnosed with osteoporosis related to primary hyperparathyroidism. The nurse reviews Mrs. Wood's diet and finds a deficiency in calcium intake, which is verified by the patient when Mrs. Woods complains that it is difficult for her to transport heavy milk, cheese, and fresh vegetables from the grocery store. She mostly purchases dried foods and breads and drinks coffee. The nurse explains that, without an adequate source of calcium, her overactive parathyroid gland is forcing calcium to leave her bones.

Her medical team has decided to take a "wait-and-see" approach to her parathyroid secretion due to her healthy kidneys and mild osteoporosis. However, they prescribe 1200 mg of calcium with 1000 units of vitamin D per day with the goals of improving her bone density. Her diet was also reviewed. Calcium bone loss from caffeine had been shown, but Mrs. Woods is advised that adding milk may offset the effect. She strategized with the nurse for assistance in grocery shopping, including contacting a shopping service for seniors. The nurse discussed ideas for access to weight-bearing activities. Mrs. Woods identified a local church group that walked together on nice days.

Mrs. Woods asks about a nasal spray her friend uses, calcitonin. The medical team tells her this is typically used as a second-line medication after other drugs have failed. The team prescribes an oral bisphosphonate, alendronate (Fosamax). Mrs. Woods is cautioned to report any GI irritation, signs of hypocalcemia, or muscle or bone pain. She is also told to take it 30 minutes before breakfast and with a full 8-ounce glass of water. Further cautions for Mrs. Woods include sitting upright after taking the medication and stopping the drug and informing the medical team if swallowing problems, vomiting, diarrhea, chest pain, heart burn, blurred vision, eye pain or swelling, or prolonged periods of immobility occur. The nurse will follow up with Mrs. Woods in a month to check on the progress of her entire treatment plan. Mrs. Woods will also continue to have radiological bone scans to confirm halting or reversal of her osteoporosis.

Continued

1. What factors contributed to Mrs. Wood's bone demineralization?
2. How will ingestion of calcium affect Mrs. Wood's elevated calcium?
3. How will walking affect Mrs. Wood's calcium levels?

Cautions for Special Populations

Pediatric

The normal ranges of serum levels for pediatric patients after early infancy are higher because of the formation of bones during normal childhood growth.

- 11 days to 2 years: 9.0–11.0 mg/dL
- 3–12 years: 8.8–10.8 mg/dL
- 13–18 years: 8.4–10.2 mg/dL

Pediatric Dietary Intake

Pediatric dietary intake (FDA/adequate intake) of calcium is:

- 0–6 months: 210 mg/day
- 7–12 months: 270 mg/day
- 1–3 years: 500 mg/day
- 4–8 years: 800 mg/day
- 9–18 years: 1300 mg/day

Healthy breastfed infants should meet dietary requirements through normal human milk intake.

Geriatric

Adults older than 90 years have decreased levels of serum calcium in the range of 8.2–9.6 mg/dL. The geriatric dietary intake (FDA/adequate intake) of calcium for adults 51 + years is 1200 mg/day.

Review Questions

1. When a patient has low albumin levels, how is calcium accurately measured?
2. What is the effect of high serum calcium on serum phosphorus?
3. What effect does acidosis have on serum calcium levels?
4. Where is most of the body's calcium stored?
5. What is the effect of calcium channel blocking medications on vascular smooth muscle?
6. How should orders for calcium chloride and calcium gluconate be written?

3B Chloride

Chloride

C hloride (Cl⁻) is the major negatively charged ion (anion) in extracellular fluid (ECF). The normal range is 97–107 mEq/L. Minimal
amounts of approximately 3–4 mEq/L are found intracellularly.
The chlorine atom's unbound state is a highly toxic gas. In nature, it is
most commonly bonded to another element to form a salt. In the body,
chloride is most commonly bound with sodium, so it is typically assessed
or treated in the form of sodium chloride (NaCl). However, chloride does
have an independent role in maintaining acid-base balance in the blood
and tissues. Even if sodium levels are normal, chloride imbalance should
not be ignored.

Functions

Chloride establishes acid-base balance, maintains fluid balance, and aids
in digestion and nutrient absorption. It also promotes nerve and muscular activity, and it supports red blood cell neutrality.

Establishes Acid-Base Balance

Chloride and bicarbonate (HCO_3^-) compete to bind with sodium (Na^+) to
form either sodium chloride or sodium bicarbonate ($NaHCO_3$). When the
body is in a state of acidosis, the kidneys excrete sodium chloride and reabsorb bicarbonate. With a state of alkalosis, the kidneys reabsorb sodium
chloride. If hydrogen ions are lost and serum chloride levels are low
(hypochloremia), sodium combines with the bicarbonate that has been reabsorbed by the kidneys. This increase of sodium bicarbonate into the
blood creates metabolic alkalosis (pH levels over 7.45).

Maintains Fluid Balance

Osmotic pressure, which is the pressure created by solutions on either side of a cellular membrane, is affected by the concentration of ions in that solution. In the human body, molecules such as proteins and ionic compounds affect osmotic pressures. Chloride functions with sodium to maintain osmotic pressure in the blood. Sodium chloride moves easily across cellular membranes, and water follows the sodium chloride shifts in and out of cells.

Aids Digestion and Nutrient Absorption

Chloride is required for activation of digestive enzymes; it is also required to combine with hydrogen (H^+) to form hydrochloric acid in the stomach. Hydrochloric acid activates digestive enzymes and increases the absorption of iron and other nutrients. Without hydrochloric acid, iron and nutrient absorption decreases.

Promotes Nerve and Muscular Activity

Along with sodium, potassium, and other ions, chloride creates an action potential and works with the chemical electric cascade that occurs with nerve stimulation and muscle action.

Supports Red Blood Cell Neutrality

Chloride shift is a process of ion exchange involving chloride (Cl^-), hydrogen, carbon dioxide (CO_2), water (H_2O), and hemoglobin (Hgb). Normally, the body's cells produce carbon dioxide as a waste product. A small amount of carbon dioxide is dissolved in plasma or bound as carbamino-hemoglobin. Most of the carbon dioxide works together with water to form carbonic acid (H_2CO_3), which then disassociates into bicarbonate and hydrogen (H^+). Carbon dioxide within red blood cells also binds to hemoglobin as carbamino-hemoglobin. As more carbon dioxide enters the bloodstream, the level of bicarbonate within red blood cells increases.

Chloride shift begins when high concentrations of bicarbonate cause bicarbonate to diffuse out of the red blood cell and into the plasma, which is a shift of a negatively charged molecule out of the cell. To balance this charge, negatively charged chloride ions (Cl^-) enter the red blood cell. When blood passes through the lung capillaries, carbon dioxide is lost to the atmosphere, which decreases the level of circulating carbonic acid. Therefore, chloride functions to balance the shifting of bicarbonate in and out of red blood cells so that the waste product, carbon dioxide, can leave tissue cells and be transported by red blood cells to the lungs for release by the aveoli.

Intake

In healthy patients, chloride intake is through dietary sources. However, many patients who are admitted to acute care facilities may require sodium chloride by intravenous (IV) infusion.

Dietary Intake

Dietary chloride is mostly bound to sodium as table salt (NaCl) or to potassium as potassium chloride (KCl). One teaspoon or 5 mL of table salt contains about 1.5 g of chloride. Adequate chloride intake for people age 9–50 years is 2.3 g/day.

Dietary sources include many foods that list sodium chloride in their ingredients and salt substitutes that list potassium chloride as an ingredient. Sodium chloride is easily absorbed in a healthy small intestine. Cheeses, milk, fish, and dates are also sources of chloride.

IV Infusion

Sodium chloride and potassium chloride are commonly delivered in IV fluids. Because safety precautions require that potassium chloride be premixed or added by a pharmacist, standard mixtures are prepared for the nursing unit. Electrolytes should always be delivered via IV controller pump, and potassium chloride may never be administered as a direct IV push because improperly diluted solutions or too rapid infusions can be lethal.

Regulation

Chloride is reabsorbed by renal tubules, and excess chloride is excreted in urine. Because chloride is closely bound to sodium, mechanisms that regulate sodium, such as the renin-angiotension-aldosterone system, also affect chloride.

Loss

About 90% of excreted chloride is through urine, with minimal loss from gastric hydrochloric acid (HCl) and sweat. In healthy individuals, urine

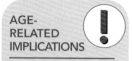
chloride loss is almost equivalent to chloride intake. Abnormal chloride loss occurs most commonly with patients who have prolonged episodes of vomiting or gastric drainage through nasogastric intubation.

Laboratory Measures

Serum levels are drawn to assess for anion levels with suspected electrolyte or acid-base imbalance. Hyperchloremia may cause metabolic acidosis or, if chloride is normal, will point to another source of imbalance.

The normal chloride serum range from age 2 months to adult is 97–107 mEq/L (100-110 mmol/L).

Serum Specimen Collection

Serum is collected by phlebotomy in a red- or tiger-top tube. Standard phlebotomy procedure requires avoiding drawing blood from the same arm that has IV access. This is particularly important in order to avoid contamination of the specimen by infused or instilled sodium chloride. To avoid processing errors, ensure that the specimen is delivered according to your laboratory's guidelines.

Chloride Sweat Test

Chloride is excreted in sweat. The normal range of chloride in sweat is 0–40 mEq/L. A measurement of >60 mEq/L is consistent with a diagnosis of cystic fibrosis (CF). An absolute diagnosis of CF requires a review of the patient's history and symptoms. Conditions that affect overall electrolyte balance can interfere with obtaining accurate test results. Poor collection technique can also significantly affect results; therefore, the test should be performed after competencies are demonstrated by the clinician.

Hypochloremia

Hypochloremia occurs when the body has a deficit of chloride.

Laboratory Values
- Serum chloride <97 mEq/L

Basic Concepts

Hypochloremia is typically a sign that patients are ill and that other electrolytes should also be measured. Low chloride levels may be true low levels due to loss or lack of ingestion, or they may only be a reflection of hemoconcentration. *Pseudohypochloremia* can occur when extracellular fluids are diluted. Hypochloremia correlates, in symptoms and management, with "chloride responsive" metabolic alkalosis, which is alkalosis that can be corrected with chloride replacement.

Etiology

Hypochloremia can be caused by:

- Addison's disease: adrenal insufficiency
- Acidotic states, including diabetic ketoacidosis, which typically result in hyperchloremia or hypochloremia
- Cystic fibrosis: with this congenital disease, less secretion occurs from the pancreas, intestines, and lungs, resulting in thickened, obstructive mucus
- Dietary intake deficiencies, which can be caused by anorexia or failure to thrive
- Gastrointestinal (GI) losses from diarrhea, fistula, nasogastric suction, vomiting, and gastric surgery, all leading to chloride loss
- Renal loss, typically either from salt-wasting nephritis or diuretic losses
- Sweating or diaphoresis, which causes losses through the skin
- Respiratory problems that increase carbon dioxide, which causes increased bicarbonate; increased bicarbonate causes chloride extracellular dilution by water and chloride movement intracellularly; some related respiratory problems include:
  - Chronic respiratory acidosis
  - Chronic obstructive pulmonary disease
  - Pneumonia

EVIDENCE-BASED PRACTICE

According to the United States Department of Agriculture, symptoms of hypochloremia were well documented by the Centers for Disease Control in the 1980s when infants were mistakenly given formula low in chloride and developed metabolic alkalosis.

Iatrogenic losses can induce hypochloremia, including:

- Use of diuretics
- Paracentisis
- Infusion of IV dextrose 5% in water (D_5W) with no electrolytes

Pseudohypochloremia exists when the body has enough chloride but the chloride is diluted by fluids. Pseudohypochloremia states can result from:

- Burns—ECF dilution
- Congestive heart failure
- Overhydration/water intoxication
- Syndrome of inappropriate antidiuretic hormone (SIADH)

Symptoms

- **Neurological:** Twitching/tremors, convulsions, paresthesias, hyperactive deep tendon reflexes, lethargy
- **CV:** Low blood pressure, cardiac dysrhythmias
- **Respiratory:** Slow and shallow, may lead to respiratory arrest
- **GI:** Anorexia, failure to thrive
- **GU:** Highly concentrated urine
- **Musculoskeletal:** Low body mass index, tetany, muscle cramps

COACH CONSULT

With vomiting or altered chloride reabsorption, metabolic alkalosis can stimulate excess urinary potassium losses. This can cause systemic hypokalemia and the accompanying symptoms.

Assessment and Actions

Fluid, electrolyte, and acid-base imbalances can rapidly cause life-threatening neurological, cardiac, and respiratory compromise, requiring immediate notification of the medical or rapid response team. Consult the medical team if any new onset occurs or if worsening symptoms or vital signs occur that are outside the normal range. If neurological, respiratory, or cardiac compromise occurs, call for assistance from the rapid or urgent response team or, if outside an acute care setting, call community emergency medical services (EMS).

Patient History

Review for clues to etiology. The following conditions may be associated with or cause hypochloremia:

- Acute or chronic metabolic processes, which may result in gastric loss, renal loss of sodium, excessive loss of sweat, or SIADH

- Chronic health problems, including:
  - Endocrine disease (Addison's disease, cystic fibrosis, uncontrolled diabetes)
  - Congestive heart failure, especially risk for fluid overload with low sodium chloride diet
  - Chronic obstructive pulmonary disease
- Excess ingestion or infusion of fluids or competitive medications (e.g., bicarbonate), which may result in low chloride levels
- Trauma or burns, which can cause direct loss of chloride
- Infectious disease, which can result in chloride shifts related to respiratory compromise

Laboratory Assessment and Actions

Values < 97 mEq/L reflect hypochloremia that may need correction. Anticipate treatment for hypochloremia with symptoms or critical values < 80 mEq/L:

- Anticipate frequent blood and urine measures of chloride levels, based on frequency and effect of interventions.
- Anticipate arterial blood gas (ABG) draw to determine pH measures. If results show metabolic alkalosis, pH > 7.45, and HCO_3 > 28, anticipate orders for acidifying treatments. ABG sampling is typically restricted to qualified nurses, respiratory therapists, and physicians (see Chapter 4 for further information).
- Anticipate oral administration of chloride:
  - Electrolyte solutions are the most common form of replacement in noncritical situations.
  - Tablets may be ordered to be mixed in a specific ratio of water.
  - Patients with nausea or vomiting may not tolerate drinking fluids until electrolytes have been corrected. In these cases, IV fluids must be introduced to reverse fluid and electrolytes losses before introducing oral fluids.

AGE-RELATED IMPLICATIONS

The American Academy of Pediatrics recommends rehydration in gradual steps (see the section on Fluid Balance and Imbalance in Chapter 2 for details).

COACH CONSULT

All IV electrolyte solutions should be administered via an infusion control pump. Additional safeguards include multiple small-volume IV bags and volume control administration sets for intermittent administration.

- Anticipate administration of IV fluids containing chloride if oral administration is not effective or possible:
  - There is controversy over best practices for IV solution for chloride imbalance, so close consultation with the medical team and hospital pharmacy policies is required.
  - Hypertonic saline solution of 3% or 5% may be recommended. These solutions should be infused via large-bore IV (16- to 18-gauge) or central line access.
  - Reevaluate patient's condition after 100 mL of solution. Frequent, rapid serum laboratory samples should be drawn. Caution should be exercised to observe for and prevent hypernatremia from sodium chloride infusions.
  - The rate should not be greater than 100 mL/hr or 1 mEq/kg/hr.
  - Onset is within minutes.
  - Peak is at the end of the infusion.
  - The duration is unknown.
  - Isotonic solution or lactated Ringer's solution may be ordered in some cases.
  - In rare instances, ammonium chloride can be ordered for IV administration to reverse metabolic alkalosis, but only if the liver is shown to be able to convert ammonia. See Box 3B–1 for more information.

ALERT

Caution must be exercised for unintended shift of other electrolytes and/or shift to acidotic state.

Systems Assessment and Actions

If laboratory test results are pending but hypochloremia is suspected, proceed with a systems assessment. Immediately consult the medical

---

Box 3B–1 **Critical Care Medications: Ammonium Chloride**

Ammonium chloride (NH_4^+) can be administered IV to reverse metabolic alkalosis if the liver is able to convert ammonia. This frees hydrogen and chloride to increase acidosis.

Use **extreme caution** with this medication. Thoroughly read the package insert and administration directions. Dosing is weight-based. Ammonium chloride has metabolic contraindications for kidney or liver failure, sodium loss, and primary respiratory acidosis. Bicarbonate levels are measured after initial test dose.

Ammonia toxicity and metabolic acidosis are severe side effects of ammonium chloride administration. Signs can include confusion, seizure, coma, nausea, vomiting, twitching, and hyperventilation. Alkalizing agents should be on hand.

team at the onset or worsening of any of the symptoms that are listed in this section.

Neurological

If neurological irritability, restlessness, tetany, decreased level of consciousness, or convulsions are present, then:

- Institute seizure precautions.
- Anticipate frequent measures of neurological status using the Glasgow Coma Scale.
- Maintain safety measures including bed low, padded side rails in place, and call bell in reach. Note that four rails up may be a restraint in some settings. Follow your institutional restraint policies.
- Continually reevaluate the patient's ability to follow instructions.
- Consult the medical team to discuss need for one-on-one supervision.
- Anticipate orders for anti-seizure medications.
- Keep respiratory support equipment readily available (ambu-bag, suction, oral airway, suction equipment, and oxygen).

CV

If concurrent fluid overload is determined by symptoms such as pulmonary rales/crackles, S_3 gallop, jugular venous distention, peripheral edema, ascites, hypertension, or bounding pulses, then:

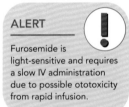

ALERT

Furosemide is light-sensitive and requires a slow IV administration due to possible ototoxicity from rapid infusion.

- Consult the medical team to determine fluid load. Urine chloride > 20 mEq/L points to serum dilution of chloride by high fluid volumes.
- Prepare for oral or IV diuretic use. Use caution with diuresis due to increased loss of chloride.

If concurrent dehydration is present, prepare for slow, cautious rehydration:

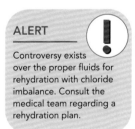

ALERT

Controversy exists over the proper fluids for rehydration with chloride imbalance. Consult the medical team regarding a rehydration plan.

- Anticipate repeated orders for phlebotomy laboratory samples to assess the effect of fluid loss on electrolyte imbalance. Concurrent dehydration symptoms are decreased skin turgor and dry mucous membranes; urine chloride < 10 mEq/L, which indicates concurrent fluid and chloride loss; and tachycardia, hypotension, and thready pulses.

- Anticipate orders for ABG for blood pH measures:
  - pH >7.45, HCO_3 >26, and CO_2 >32 mEq/L demonstrate metabolic alkalosis.
  - ABG sampling is typically restricted to qualified nurses, respiratory therapists, or physicians (see Chapter 6 for procedure).

Respiratory

Check for rate and depth of respirations. If rhonchi, wheezing, rales/crackles, or diminished breath sounds are present, then:

- Measure oxygen saturation, and anticipate orders for supplemental oxygen.
- Raise head of bed to facilitate airway clearance.
- Prepare patient for chest x-ray to assess for pneumonia, congestive heart failure, pulmonary edema, or effusion. Check for potential pregnancy prior to examinations.
- Keep respiratory support equipment readily available (ambu-bag, suction, oral airway, suction equipment, and oxygen).
- Anticipate orders for bronchodilators with wheezing and antibiotics with diagnosis of pneumonia.

COACH CONSULT

Several diuretics are incompatible with many medications. Cautiously review compatibility of ordered medications. Anticipate orders for multiple IV catheter access if multiple IV medications are ordered to run concurrently.

GI

If vomiting, volumes of suction, or gastric drainage from interventional intubation or fistulas is present, then:

- Measure and document all intake and output.
- Discuss with medical team clamping of GI drainage.
- Anticipate volume replacement.
  - Note that fluid orders are typically based on a milliliter-for-milliliter replacement.
  - Communicate need for accurate intake and output measures to all ancillary staff.
- Administer antiemetics as ordered. GI symptoms may not resolve until electrolytes are stable, despite use of antiemetics.

GU

Measure fluid volumes; >125 mL/hr without concurrent volume replacement may indicate inappropriate diuresis. If fluid losses are high, hypochloremia may be the result of concurrent losses. If volumes are <30 mL/hr, consult the medical team for alternative causes.

When hypochloremia is a result of fluid loss, anticipate repeated urine samples to assess effect of fluid loss on electrolyte imbalance. Collect specimens with caution to avoid contamination with water or soap. If drawing from a catheter, make certain to draw urine from the collection tube rather than the collection bag, because urine in the bag will have started to biologically degrade.

If overhydration is diagnosed, discuss orders with the medical team to give or hold diuretics. When diuretics are used to correct overhydration, they may also lead to extended loss of chloride.

Musculoskeletal

If parasthesias or muscle cramping occurs, assist with all activities of daily living, ambulation, and transfers in order to prevent injury.

Prevention

Teach at risk populations:

- Signs and symptoms of hypochloremia
- Signs and symptoms of fluid retention, e.g., edema, shortness of breath, weight gain
- Appropriate fluid ingestion (see Chapter 2)
- Appropriate chloride ingestion (approximately 1.5 teaspoons of sodium chloride per day for adults) and provide a list of dietary sources

To advocate for public health, communicate that rehydration requires electrolyte support with proper oral solutions.

 CLINICAL SCENARIO

DIAGNOSIS: HYPOCHLOREMIA FROM VOMITING AND ACCOMPANYING METABOLIC ALKALOSIS

Mrs. Henninger is brought to the emergency department (ED) after a 911 call due to intractable vomiting over 24 hours. She denies any chronic health conditions or recent acute illness, except a head cold for several days. She reports current, extreme vertigo in which motion, loud noise, or talking induces vomiting. The ED nurse assesses Mrs. Henninger and observes a temperature of 99°F, regular respirations at 14 breaths per minute, regular heart rate in the 90s, BP of 95/65, SaO_2 of 98%, and dry mucous membranes. The nurse draws stat chemistry and hematology laboratory samples and places an 18-gauge IV catheter at the same time, noting that Mrs. Henninger's veins are difficult to palpate. Mrs. Henninger is placed on a continuous cardiac monitor, which demonstrates a normal sinus rhythm.

Continued

While waiting for Mrs. Henninger's laboratory results, the nurse conducts a head-to-toe assessment, with no further relevant findings except for abdominal muscle pain, which Mrs. Henninger reports is from persistent vomiting. After the medical team examines Mrs. Henninger, scopolamine subcutaneous (SQ) and transdermal is ordered. The nurse informs Mrs. Henninger that the SQ dose will have an onset of 30 minutes and will last approximately 4–6 hours, whereas the transdermal patch will not start working for 4 hours and will last for 3 days. The nurse also asks Mrs. Henninger to inform the team of any new onset eye pain, which is a symptom of acute angle-closure glaucoma that can be an adverse effect of the scopolamine patch.

The nurse continues to observe Mrs. Henninger for neurological or respiratory symptoms associated with hypochloremia and metabolic alkalosis and administers a Glasgow Coma Scale test every 15 minutes. To decrease sensitivity, the lights are dimmed, and a "Quiet" sign is placed outside the room. The nurse instructs Mrs. Henninger on a clean collection of urine and provides a basin for nausea. Mrs. Henninger comments that she is too dry to urinate or make any more emesis.

Mrs. Henninger's laboratory tests show hypochloremia and hypokalemia. Potassium chloride 20 mEq in 250 mL of normal saline solution (NSS) is ordered over 1 hour, and the infusion is placed on a pump, which has controls to regulate electrolyte administration. Mrs. Henninger is instructed to let the nurse know if any irritation occurs at the site of insertion.

After 1 hour of infusion, Mrs. Henninger reports feeling less vertigo. Laboratory samples are again measured and, with symptoms resolving and electrolytes returning toward normal ranges, NSS is ordered at 50 mL/hr, and Mrs. Henninger is scheduled to be transferred to a telemetry unit for observation.

1. Which of Mrs. Henninger's vital signs points to dehydration?
2. Why does the nurse place an 18-gauge IV catheter?
3. The nurse anticipates difficulty in obtaining an 18-gauge IV line because Mrs. Henninger's veins are difficult to palpate. What steps can be taken?

Hyperchloremia

Hyperchloremia occurs when the body has an excess of chloride.

Laboratory Values
• Serum chloride >107 mEq/L

Basic Concepts
High chloride levels may be true high levels due to excess ingestion or they may only be a reflection of hemoconcentration. In low fluid states, the body

holds a normal amount of chloride, but in ratio to fluid levels it appears as *pseudohyperchloremia*. Hyperchloremia correlates closely with metabolic acidosis in symptomatology and management .

Hyperchloremic acidosis is typically distinguished from other sources of acidosis as normal ion gap acidosis. However, hyperchloremic states can exist as a result of other pathologies, typically called high ion gap acidosis. Causes of both types of acidosis can be similar. GI fluid and bicarbonate losses through ostomies or diarrhea and renal losses are commonly associated with normal ion gap acidosis. Normal physiology is interrupted, and kidneys absorb chloride instead of bicarbonate.

> **ALERT**
>
> Hyperchloremia occurs when serum chloride is >107 mEq/L. *Critical* hyperchloremia occurs when chloride serum level is >115 mEq/L. High values of chloride can lead to respiratory arrest and coma.

Etiology

Hyperchloremia can be caused by:

- Metabolic acidosis (high ion gap acidosis), including:
  - Ketoacidosis, which can be induced by diabetes, alcohol abuse, or starvation
  - Lactic acidosis, which can be induced by respiratory compromise, shock, or seizures
  - Renal tubular acidosis, in which hydrogen secretion and bicarbonate absorption are impaired
  - Toxicity, which can result from alcohols (ethanol, methanol, ethylene glycol) or salicylates (aspirin and other nonsteroidal anti-inflammatory drugs)
- Acute renal failure, which results in decreased urine output and decreased renal acid excretion
- Cushing's syndrome (hypercorticism), in which chloride is retained in ratio to sodium retention
- Head injuries, which can result in hypothalamic stimulation from trauma or tumors and cause retained chloride
- Poisoning/intoxication from alcohol or salicylate sources should be considered, such as:
  - Ethanol taken as drinking alcohol, although doing so has a low incidence of hyperchloremia
  - Ethylene glycol poisoning with antifreeze
  - Methanol poisoning with industrial solvent or fuel

> **ALERT**
>
> Acid states with a pH <7.10 may not show acidosis symptoms if patients have chronic processes causing slow onset of acidosis.

- Salicylate sensitivity or overexposure to skin and hair products, topical pain relief medications, food preservatives, toothpaste, and antiseptics. *Note:* Cross-sensitivities are noted with patients with asthma.

Iatrogenic causes are common and should be carefully observed, including:

- Overinfusion of chloride as calcium chloride, sodium chloride, or potassium chloride in health-care settings
- Medications, including:
  - Ammonium chloride (used as an acidifier)
  - Sodium polystyrene (Kayexalate)
  - Magnesium sulfate
  - Acetazolamide as a diuretic and antiseizure medication
  - Lysine for herpes simplex, osteoporosis, and rheumatoid arthritis

Psuedohyperchloremia occurs when fluid volumes are low, which causes chloride to become more concentrated as in dehydration states and diabetes insipidus.

Symptoms

- **Neurological:** Weakness, headache, lethargy, possible coma
- **CV**: Peripheral vasodilation, hypotension, ventricular arrhythmias, shock
- **Respiratory:** Deep, rapid breathing, Kussmaul's respirations
- **GU:** Decreased urine output
- **Musculoskeletal:** Chronic states may induce bone loss, e.g., osteomalacia, osteopenia, rickets
- **Serum:** Hypernatremia >145 mEq/L, pH <7.35, HCO_3 <22 mEq/L

Assessment and Actions

Fluid, electrolyte, and acid-base imbalances can rapidly cause life-threatening neurological, cardiac, and respiratory compromise, requiring immediate notification of the medical or rapid response team. Consult the medical team if any new onset occurs or if worsening symptoms or vital signs occur that are outside the normal range. If neurological, respiratory, or cardiac compromise occurs, call for assistance from the rapid or urgent response team or, if outside an acute care setting, call community EMS.

Patient History

Review for clues to cause of hyperchloremia. Consider the following conditions:

- Acidotic states, including diabetic ketoacidosis, renal acidosis, shock, starvation, and poisoning; contact the poison control center if the agent is unknown to the medical team: 1-800-222-1222
- Acute or chronic metabolic process should be determined, including the potential for renal failure and hypoventilation
- Chronic health problems may contribute, including Cushing's syndrome, diabetes, and other endocrine diseases
- Iatrogenic intervention, including overdoses of sodium chloride, potassium chloride, or ammonium chloride
- Trauma patients should be assessed for brain injury, which could cause chloride retention

Laboratory Assessment and Actions

Values >107 mEq/L reflect hyperchloremia that may need correction. Anticipate treatment for hyperchloremia with symptoms or critical values <115 mEq/L.

If acidosis is present, then:

- Anticipate frequent blood and urine measures of chloride levels, based on frequency and effect of interventions.
- Anticipate frequent blood measures of key electrolytes and ABG measures to determine pH throughout course of therapy. Hypokalemia is a common complication.
- Anticipate arterial blood draw for blood pH measures:
  - If results show metabolic acidosis, pH <7.35, HCO_3 >22, prepare for possible alkalizing treatments.
  - ABG sampling is typically restricted to qualified nurses, respiratory therapists, and physicians.
- Anticipate blood specimen collection for salicylate, ethanol, methanol, and ethylene glycol levels. If the clinical laboratory cannot process alcohol specimens, the medical team may calculate the osmolar gap. A gap of >10 may point to presence of alcohol toxicity (see Chapter 6 for osmolar gap calculation).
- Calculate anion gap (see Chapter 6 for calculation):
  - Elevated ion gap indicates high ion gap acidosis.
  - Normal ion gap indicates hyperchloremia acidosis.
- Anticipate orders for hemodialysis if alcohol toxicity, salicylate poisoning, or renal failure is the cause.

- Anticipate orders for administration of IV bicarbonate. *Note:* Bicarbonate administration is controversial with high anion gap acidosis and may result in increased mortality. See Box 3B–2 for more information (see Chapter 6 for calculation).

Systems Assessment and Actions

If laboratory test results are pending but hyperchloremia is suspected, proceed with a systems assessment. Immediately consult the medical team at the onset or worsening of any of the symptoms that are listed in the following section.

Box 3B–2 Critical Care Medications: Bicarbonate

Sodium bicarbonate is used in critical situations, such as rapid response and code situations. Follow American Heart Association guidelines for advanced cardiac life support for dosage and administration.

The medical team will calculate necessary bicarbonate dose based on the Kaissirer-Bleich equation for desired level of serum bicarbonate and patient's body weight. Safeguards include multiple small-volume IV bags and volume control administration sets for intermittent administration:

- Dose: 2–5 mEq/kg over 4–8 hours
- Onset: Immediate
- Peak: Rapid
- Duration: Unknown

There is a high risk for extravasation with bicarbonate. The medical team should be consulted for any irritation or infiltration of the IV catheter. Anticipate halting infusion and orders for injection of lidocaine or hyaluronidase at the site of infiltration. IV sodium bicarbonate is incompatible with many medications and should be infused separately from any other IV solutions or medications unless compatibility is confirmed in consultation with a pharmacist.

Read the package insert and administration directions thoroughly. Bicarbonate has metabolic contraindications for kidney failure, abdominal pain from an unknown source, hypocalcemia, and respiratory or metabolic alkalosis (low carbon dioxide).

- Caution in use with diabetic ketoacidosis as it may induce cerebral edema and cerebrospinal fluid acidosis.
- Caution with Y-site infusions, as many incompatibilities exist. Do not infuse with Ringer's lactate, Ringer's solution, or Ionosol.
- Caution must be exercised for unintended shift of other electrolytes and/or shift to acidotic state.

Neuro-Musculo-Skeletal

If decreased level of consciousness or weakness is assessed, then:

- Anticipate frequent measures of neurological status using the Glasgow Coma Scale.
- Maintain safety measures including keeping the bed low and call bell in reach.
- Continually reevaluate the patient's ability to follow instructions.
- Consult the medical team to discuss need for one-on-one supervision.
- Assist with transfer, ambulation, and all activities of daily living.

If ethanol withdrawal occurs, observe for agitation and injury to self or others. Anticipate orders for oral or IV medications to help manage withdraw symptoms.

CV

If hypovolemia is causing high concentration of chloride, anticipate orders for IV fluid administration, and watch carefully for signs of hypochloremia and other electrolyte shifts from overhydration.

Respiratory

Perform respiratory assessment for rate, rhythm, and use of accessory muscles. If initial breathing is rapid but shallow, then:

- Be aware that, with a decline of the patient's status, breathing may become slower and deeper.
- Anticipate overexertion leading to respiratory arrest.
- Immediately consult the medical or rapid response team for advanced airway management.
- Keep respiratory support equipment available (ambu-bag, oral airway, suction, and oxygen).
- Measure oxygen saturation, and anticipate orders for supplemental oxygen.
- Raise head of bed to facilitate airway clearance.

> **ALERT**
>
> There is controversy whether to infuse hypotonic saline, isotonic NSS, bicarbonate, or lactated Ringer's solution for chloride replacement. Consult the medical team before preparing hydrating fluids.

GU

Measure fluid volumes; < 30 mL/hr may point to renal insufficiency. If urine output is low, anticipate repeated urine samples to assess effect of fluid loss on electrolyte imbalance.

Prevention

Teach at-risk populations:

- Signs and symptoms of acidosis
- Signs and symptoms of dehydration
- Appropriate dietary intake
- Caution with routine and emergent IV administration of fluids containing chloride

To advocate for public health, advise people to:

- Keep all poisons away from children and cognitively impaired adults
- Become educated on responsible alcohol intake
- Become educated on signs of suicidal depression and availability of hotlines

 CLINICAL SCENARIO

DIAGNOSIS: HYPERCHLOREMIA AND ACIDOTIC STATE FROM ASPIRIN OVERDOSE

Evelyn Smyth, an active 76-year-old woman with new-onset Alzheimer's dementia, approached her husband with an empty bottle of chewable baby aspirin in hand. Mrs. Smyth appeared much quieter than her normal highly active temperament led her to behave. Mr. Smyth called 911 and was told not to give ipecac syrup or induce vomiting. Emergency medical services (EMS) arrived at the house 10 minutes later. When EMS arrived, Mrs. Smyth was lying on the couch and talking calmly with her husband. Her heart rate was 110/min, her respirations were 30/min and shallow, her blood pressure was 135/76, and she was complaining of ringing in her ears.

Mrs. Smyth was placed on a stretcher, and her husband was asked to travel with her in the ambulance because of her underlying dementia. Mrs. Smyth accepted activated charcoal by mouth, but spit most of it out without swallowing. The EMS provider started a large-bore IV and NSS. Blood glucose by finger stick was 125 mg/dL. Mr. Smyth asked if his wife should be forced to vomit. The paramedic responded that induced vomiting is not recommended, but that, based on salicylate levels and other blood studies, they might pump her stomach after they were at the hospital.

In preparation for Mrs. Smyth's arrival at the emergency department (ED), the ED nurse set up her room with liter bags of NSS, D_5W, venous and arterial blood drawing equipment, and a urinalysis kit. Additional activated charcoal, IV Ativan, bicarbonate ampules, and stock bags of low-dose potassium chloride were ordered from the pharmacy. A central hemodialysis catheter kit and tubing were brought to the ED and Surgery, Nephrology, and the hemodialysis nurse were placed on alert for potential emergent hemodialysis.

Once in the ED, stat venous electrolyte laboratory samples, salicylate levels, and arterial blood gases showed normal levels. Mr. Smyth reported that his wife was alone for only a few minutes as he washed the breakfast dishes, so he suspects her ingestion occurred less than 1 hour prior to arrival at the ED. Based on this history and laboratory values, D_5W, bicarbonate, and potassium are given at a slow IV rate. A second dose of activated charcoal was given in biscuit form, which Mrs. Smyth was happy to eat.

The nurse explained to Mr. and Mrs. Smyth that aspirin poisoning levels will rise over the next 6 hours and that her venous and arterial blood will be drawn with frequency. They were told that nurses will carefully observe Mrs. Smyth for other potential symptoms such as fever, shifts between metabolic acidosis and alkalosis, and neurological or respiratory changes.

1. What unique symptom of salicylate toxicity is Mrs. Smyth reporting?
2. Why is Mrs. Smyth at greater risk for salicylate toxicity than the general population?
3. Given Mrs. Smyth's underlying dementia, what special precautions should the nurse initiate?

Cautions for Special Populations

Pediatrics

The normal ranges of serum levels for pediatric patients (in conventional units and SI units) are:

- Premature: 95–110 mEq/L or mmol/L
- 0–1 month: 98–113 mEq/L or mmol/L
- 2 months–adult: 97–107 mEq/L or mmol/L

Special Cautions

Infants may have diarrhea or vomiting from congenital factors including:

- Pyloric stenosis
- Bartter's syndrome (familial chronic diarrhea)
- Renal tubular disorders
- Cystic fibrosis

Pediatric Dietary Intake

Pediatric dietary intake (FDA/adequate intake) of chloride is:

- 0–6 months: 0.18 g/day
- 7–12 months: 0.57 g/day
- 1–3 years: 1.5 g/day
- 4–8 years: 1.9 g/day

Healthy breastfed infants should meet dietary requirements through normal human milk intake.

Geriatric

The geriatric dietary intake (FDA/adequate intake) of chloride is:
- 51–70 years: 2 g/day
- 70 years: 1.8 g/day

Seniors with poor access to fresh foods may consume excess chloride in prepared or canned goods. Dehydration is more common in seniors due to decreased thirst sensors. Low fluid volumes may result in increased serum chloride levels.

Review Questions

1. What is the most common compound in the body that contains chloride?
2. Which ions are compared when evaluating an anion gap?
3. What assessment findings should alert the nurse to chloride losses?
4. Which genetic disorder is associated with chloride loss?
5. Which IV fluid is associated with iatrogenic hypochloremia?
6. Which electrolyte imbalance is associated with decreased chloride reabsorption or vomiting?

3C Magnesium

Magnesium

M agnesium (Mg$^+$) is an alkaline metal, highly soluble in water. In humans, it is the fourth most abundant element, with the average adult holding 24 g in tissues and fluids.

Magnesium is the second most abundant cation (positively charged ion) in intracellular fluid (ICF). Despite this prevalence, only about one-third of the body's magnesium is held in ICF. About half of the body's magnesium is combined with calcium and phosphorus to form bone structures. The balance is stored intracellularly in tissues, with about 27% in muscles and about 1% in the blood. Approximately two-thirds of serum magnesium exists in a free ionized form, and about one-third is bound to albumin. Orders for laboratory testing may be used to measure overall serum magnesium or to measure free ionized magnesium.

Researchers are examining the link between low magnesium states and chronic illnesses such as asthma, cardiovascular (CV) disease, fibromyalgia, and diabetes. They are also examining the relationship between low magnesium levels, energy production, and irregular heart rates. The U.S. Food and Drug Administration (FDA) has been adjusting upward the recommended daily intake (RDI) for magnesium, based on research on the negative health effects of low magnesium states.

Functions

In the human body, magnesium helps to form bone structure, maintain heart rhythm, facilitate nervous and muscle system functioning, and balance electrolytes. It also promotes enzymatic activity, contributes to nucleic acid chemistry, stimulates the immune system, and can be prescribed as a medicinal supplement.

Helps Form Bone Structure

Magnesium is used in formation of bones and teeth. Magnesium is embedded in the skeletal structure, and it coats the bones with a layer that is easily mobilized during periods of dietary magnesium deficiency. Magnesium is essential for the production of parathyroid hormone (PTH). Low PTH levels may induce hypocalcemia and hyperphosphatemia. PTH requires magnesium to release calcium and phosphorus into the blood.

Maintains Heart Rhythm

Magnesium functions as a neuromuscular transmitter in the heart. Low magnesium levels have recently been shown to contribute to higher rates of irregular heartbeats. According to the FDA, people who live in areas where tap water contains more magnesium stores have shown lower risk of heart disease.

Facilitates Nervous and Muscle System Functioning

Magnesium assists in the active transport of potassium and calcium across cell membranes, allowing for normal function of nerves and muscles, especially those involved in cardiac excitatory pathways. It also functions as a neuromuscular transmitter in the central nervous system and as an assistive transmitter to acetylcholine. Without proper serum magnesium levels, muscles are unable to relax.

Balances Electrolytes

Magnesium regulates absorption of key electrolytes, including calcium, phosphorus, potassium, and sodium. Decreased magnesium depresses potassium reabsorption by the kidneys to the extent that potassium levels cannot be restored until magnesium levels return to normal. Serum calcium levels decrease with low magnesium, and calcium's normal actions may be blocked.

Promotes Enzymatic Activity

Enzymes that use or create adenosine triphosphate (ATP) require magnesium. ATP is usually found bound to magnesium as MgATP. Enzymes that activate carbohydrate metabolism and protein and lipid utilization require magnesium. Magnesium is essential for blood clotting.

Contributes to Nucleic Acid Chemistry

Enzymes that stimulate the production of DNA, RNA, lipids, carbohydrates, and the antioxidant glutathione require magnesium. Magnesium is part of the structure of chromosomes and cellular membranes.

Stimulates Immune System

Magnesium works with calcium in interstitial fluid to stimulate the migration of immune active cells to sites of infection.

Supplements and Medicates the Body

In addition to acting as a dietary supplement, magnesium has several uses as a medication. Because magnesium binds with other elements, magnesium supplements are bound with chloride, oxide, gluconate, and citrate. Common magnesium-based medications include:

- **Antacids.** Milk of Magnesia (magnesium hydroxide) is a commonly prescribed antacid. Maalox, another common antacid, is a combination of magnesium hydroxide and aluminum hydroxide.
- **Laxatives.** Magnesium citrate is prescribed as a laxative. Epsom salts (magnesium sulfate) can be prescribed as an ionic laxative.
- **Stabilizers.** Intravenous magnesium is used to stabilize nerve and blood vessel overexcitation, even when magnesium is in balance. It is also used to enhance smooth muscle relaxation, which is needed with asthma- and pregnancy-associated eclampsia.
- **Antiseptics.** Magnesium is prepared as a compound with borate, sulfate, and salicylate.
- **Sedatives.** Magnesium is bound to bromide as a sedative.
- **Anti-inflammatory medications.** One of the most commonly used magnesium-based products is Epsom salts, which are used as both an ionic laxative and as a bath; in a bath, the magnesium is absorbed through the skin in order to decrease inflammation.

Intake

In healthy patients, magnesium intake is through dietary sources and is absorbed through the small intestine. High levels of zinc can interfere with dietary absorption of magnesium, whereas protein and vitamin D intake may allow for more absorption. The jejunum and the ileum are the primary sites of absorption.

Dietary Intake

The body absorbs 25%–65% of dietary magnesium. Adequate magnesium intake for:

- Women 19–30 years: 310 mg/day
- Men 19–30 years: 400 mg/day
- Women over 31 years: 320 mg/day
- Men over 31 years: 420 mg/day

Dietary sources of magnesium include nuts, seeds, whole grains, milk, shellfish, soy flour, and leafy green vegetables. Coffee, tea, and cocoa are also common dietary sources.

Intravenous Infusion

Magnesium sulfate can be administered intravenously if required. However, this must be done with extreme caution. See cautions in the section on hypomagnesemia.

Regulation

Gastrointestinal (GI) absorption and renal mechanisms regulate magnesium levels in the body. When serum magnesium is low, the GI tract absorbs more from dietary sources. In hypermagnesemia, less dietary magnesium is absorbed. Magnesium is partially regulated by renal excretion. In hypermagnesemia, hypercalcemia, or PTH stimulation, less magnesium is reabsorbed by the nephron's loop of Henle. Loop diuretics decrease magnesium reaborption. Low serum magnesium levels stimulate retention by the renal system.

Loss

Excess magnesium from dietary sources is excreted from the kidneys. However, patients taking magnesium supplements, antacids, or laxatives may eliminate unabsorbed magnesium through stool. Hypermagnesemia can occur when renal function is compromised, especially with patients taking oral preparations as laxatives or antacids. Abnormal loss occurs most commonly with patients who are experiencing GI losses, such as diarrhea.

Laboratory Measures

Because less than 1% of magnesium is held in the serum, urine magnesium levels indicate low magnesium prior to when a drop in serum levels becomes apparent. Clinical symptoms of hypomagnesemia may occur before low levels are revealed by blood tests. Note that:
- Normal serum range (adult): 1.32–2.14 mEq/L or 1.6–2.6 mg/dL
- Normal urine range (adult): 73.2–122 mg/24 hr

Serum Specimen Collection

Serum is collected by phlebotomy in a red- or tiger-top tube. Standard phlebotomy procedure requires avoiding blood drawing from a limb with a preexisting intravenous access. To avoid processing errors, ensure that the specimen is delivered to the laboratory according to institutional guidelines.

Urine

Urine measures are typically done to evaluate if low magnesium levels are related to GI losses or renal problems. The medical team will calculate the fractional excretion of magnesium (FEMg) using serum and urine values. A FEMg of < 4% indicates GI losses; an FEMg of > 4% indicates renal losses (see Chapter 6 for calculation). Patients with low stores of magnesium conserve it through the kidneys, and urinary excretion will be low. Magnesium is typically measured using a clean 24-hour collection method with a preservative, but it may be collected as a random specimen. If a urine specimen is required, then assess the patient's ability to perform a clean catch or 24-hour collection, and educate the patient on the process (see Chapter 6 for detailed instructions).

Hypomagnesemia

Hypomagnesemia occurs when the body has too little serum magnesium.

Laboratory Values
- Serum magnesium < 1.32 mEq/L

Basic Concepts

Overall body hypomagnesemia may exist even when serum magnesium levels are within normal ranges. Hypomagnesemia often occurs with hypokalemia and hypocalcemia. Magnesium must be replaced before potassium can be used. This imbalance contributes to associated cardiac problems.

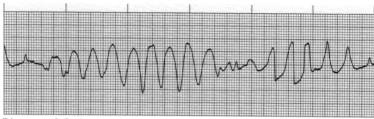

Figure 3C-1: Torsade de pointes.

 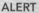
Etiology

Hypomagnesemia can be caused by several factors. A key concern may be distinguishing whether the primary problem is GI, renal, or related to another disorder. Urine measures of magnesium losses are helpful in evaluating the source of low serum levels.

Common causes include:

- Alcoholism, especially with accompanying poor nutritional intake and increased urination
- Acute cellular destruction, such as in burns, myocardial infarction, and sepsis
- GI or psychological problems that effect absorption in the jejunum or ileum, such as anorexia, bulimia, diarrhea, Crohn's disease, ulcerative colitis, celiac disease, fistula-related losses, and malabsorption
- Endocrine problems, including high aldosterone, high antidiuretic hormone, high thyroid hormones, or diabetes mellitus, especially with ketoacidosis, which results in increased urine losses
- Low PTH levels, which may be a reflection of low magnesium levels, where high PTH levels can also cause hypomagnesemia
- Dietary excesses of sodium or calcium increase urinary losses
- Pregnancy-induced hypertension
- Renal diseases, either glomerulonephritis or pyelonephritis, and tubular acidosis, which can decrease reabsorption

Iatrogenic causes can also induce hypomagnesemia, including:

- Drugs that cause excessive renal losses, including antibiotic aminoglycosides such as gentamicin; antifungals such as amphotericin; chemotherapies such as cisplatin; diuretics such as furosemide, bumetanide, and thiazides; excessive calcium and vitamin D

- Decreased GI absorption from medications such as digitalis and insulin or procedures such as radiation or removal of the portions of the small bowel
- GI losses, which can be caused by nasogastric suctioning and the overuse of laxatives, including prescribed bowel preparations for surgery
- Intravenous (IV) fluids or parenteral nutrition without magnesium as the primary source of nutrition, where glucose may pull magnesium from the serum into newly created cells

Symptoms

- **Neurological:** Nystagmus, lethargy, weakness, hyperirritability, personality changes, confusion, dizziness, hallucinations, seizures, positive Babinski's, Cvostek's, or Trousseau's response
- **CV:** Hypocalcemia, hypokalemia that does not respond to supplementation, low blood pressure, premature ventricular contractions, supraventricular tachycardia and other arrhythmia, especially torsade de pointes ventricular tachycardia; ventricular fibrillation, or a prolonged QT interval
- **Respiratory:** Pulmonary edema, stridor, or airway obstruction
- **GI:** Dysphagia, anorexia, nausea, vomiting, weight loss
- **Genitourinary (GU):** Excess diuresis
- **Musculoskeletal:** Weakness, staggering, muscle spasms, tetany, irritability, contractions
  - Chronic low magnesium may contribute to fractures due to osteomalacia and osteoporosis.
- **Electrolytes:** Low serum potassium, phosphorus, or calcium can indicate low magnesium levels

Assessment and Actions

Fluid, electrolyte, and acid-base imbalances can rapidly cause life-threatening neurological, cardiac, and respiratory compromise, requiring immediate notification of the medical or rapid response team. Consult the medical team if any new onset occurs or if worsening symptoms or vital signs occur that are outside the normal range. If neurological, respiratory, or cardiac compromise occurs, call for assistance from the rapid or urgent response team or, if outside an acute care setting, call community emergency medical services (EMS).

Patient History

Review for clues as to cause. The following conditions may be associated with or cause hypomagnesemia:

- Acute or chronic metabolic processes may result in:
  - GI losses or poor absorption, especially in the small bowel
  - Renal losses or decreased reabsorption
- Chronic health problems, including:
  - Alcoholism, anorexia, bulimia, or other poor nutritional states
  - Chronic GI diseases resulting in poor absorption or excess use of diuretics or laxatives
  - Endocrine problems, such as hyperparathyroidism, elevated aldosterone levels, or uncontrolled diabetes, which causes renal losses
- Iatrogenic causes, such as excess fluids or medications that cause magnesium losses

Laboratory Assessment and Actions

If serum values < 1.32 mEq/L reflect hypomagnesemia, then anticipate the need for correction.

- Anticipate orders for frequent serum magnesium levels based on frequency and effect of interventions.
- Anticipate oral administration of magnesium over several days (initial supplements may increase blood levels only temporarily) until magnesium travels into the cells. Tablets must be chewed to allow for full absorption in the GI tract. Common supplements used to correct hypomagnesemia include:
  - Magnesium chloride
  - Magnesium citrate (also used as a laxative)
  - Magnesium gluconate
  - Magnesium hydroxide (also used as a laxative)
  - Magnesium oxide
- Note that each form of magnesium is contraindicated for patients with anuria and heart block.

COACH CONSULT

Special cautions exist for the pregnant population. Magnesium may be given to treat pregnancy-associated conditions such as preeclampsia, eclampsia, and preterm labor. However, magnesium may be contraindicated during active labor or within 2 hours of delivery. Refer to an obstetric resource to determine appropriate treatment of pregnant patients.

MED INFO ℞

Treatment of deficiency requires 200–400 mg/day, typically provided in three or four divided doses. Children between 6 and 11 years receive 3–6 mg/kg/day.

If symptoms occur, or if hypokalemia is demonstrated with normal or low magnesium blood levels, anticipate orders to treat with IV or intramuscular magnesium sulfate.

- Contraindications are hypocalcemia, anuria, and heart block. Frequently measure vital signs because respiratory depression, muscle weakness, arrhythmia, and hypotension are common adverse reactions. Neurological checks should be completed before, during, and after administration.
- Consult the medical team before initiating or continuing infusions if respirations are < 16, patellar reflex is absent, or urine output is < 30 mL/hour. Flushing and sweating are commonly reported side effects of infusions.
- Anticipate orders to measure serum calcium levels because hypocalcemia can occur during IV administration. Calcium gluconate is typically ordered to be infused concurrently to prevent hypermagnesemia.
- IV solutions should be infused via large-bore IV (16- to 18-gauge) or central line access.
  - Reevaluate patient's condition after 1 g of solution. *Note:* Anticipate orders to draw frequent, rapid blood samples that include potassium and calcium levels.
  - The rate should not be > 1 g/hr or 8 mEq/hr.
    - Adult doses are typically 1 g every 6 hours over 4 hours
    - Follow Advanced Cardiac Life Support protocols for emergency treatment
  - Onset is within minutes.
  - Peak is at the end of the infusion.
  - Duration time is 30 minutes.
  - Do not infuse magnesium concurrently in the same IV line with sodium bicarbonate.

Systems Assessment and Actions

If laboratory results are pending but hypomagnesemia is suspected, proceed with a systems

COACH CONSULT

Milligram, gram, and millequivalent doses can easily be confused. Therefore, all IV or intramuscular magnesium doses should be double-checked with a second licensed professional before administration.

COACH CONSULT

All IV electrolyte solutions should be administered via an IV infusion pump or controller. Additional safeguards include multiple small-volume IV bags and volume control sets for intermittent administration.

assessment. Immediately consult the medical team at the onset or worsening of any of the symptoms that are listed in the following section.

Neuro-Musculo-Skeletal

If muscle cramping, tetany, and/or convulsions are present, institute seizure precautions.

- Antiseizure medications should be readily available.
- Side rails should be padded or the bed should be low to the floor. *Note:* Four rails up may be a restraint in some settings. Follow your institutional restraint policies.
- Oxygen, ambu-bag, and suction equipment should be at the bedside.

If weakness, lethargy, personality changes, confusion, hallucinations, or ambulation problems occur, then:

- Anticipate frequent measures of neurological status using the Glasgow Coma Scale (see Chapter 6).
- Institute fall and safety precautions.
- Evaluate orientation and ability of the patient to use the call bell for help.
- Continually reevaluate the patient's ability to follow instructions.
- Consult the medical team to discuss need for one-on-one supervision.

If chronic bone weakness is suspected or deep tendon reflexes are diminished, then assist with all ambulation and transfers to prevent injury.

CV

If signs of cardiac irritability, bradycardia, or changes in ECG morphology occur, anticipate orders to initiate continuous cardiac monitoring. Consult the medical team to determine lead and alarm settings to best monitor for magnesium changes.

Respiratory

Listen carefully for signs of airway closure because stridor may accompany low levels of magnesium. If signs of airway obstruction are present, inform the medical team, and prepare for placement of emergency airway and ventilation support.

Check for rate and depth of respirations frequently. If respiratory rate is slow or respirations are depressed, then:

- Do not leave the patient unmonitored.
- Stimulate the patient to breathe within a normal rate.
- Raise the head of the bed to assist breathing.
- Anticipate orders for continuous respiratory monitoring.

- Prepare patient for chest x-ray. *Note:* Check for potential pregnancy prior to examinations.
- Keep respiratory support equipment readily available (ambu-bag, suction equipment, oral airway, and oxygen).

GI

If dysphagia is noted, hold all oral intake and consult the medical team.

If vomiting or gastric drainage from interventional intubation or fistulas is present, then:

- Measure and document all intake and output.
- Anticipate volume replacement with magnesium, calcium, and potassium if indicated by laboratory values.
  - Fluid orders are typically based on a milliliter-for-milliliter replacement.
  - Communicate need to all ancillary staff for accurate intake and output measures.
- Administer antiemetics as ordered. *Note:* GI symptoms may not resolve until electrolytes are stable, despite use of antiemetics.

GU

Measure fluid volumes. More than 125 mL/hr without concurrent volume replacement may indicate inappropriate diuresis. If excess diuresis is noted, then:

- Anticipate orders for collection of random urine and 24-hour urine collections (see Chapter 6 for specific directions).
- Collect specimen with caution to avoid contamination with water or soap. If drawing from a catheter, make certain to draw urine from the collection tube rather than the bag because urine in the bag will have started to biologically degrade.

Prevention

Teach at-risk populations:

- Signs and symptoms of hypomagnesemia:
  - Inform patients that low potassium may also indicate low magnesium.
  - Report increased urinary or GI losses to primary care provider.
  - Educate patients on digitalis preparations, on the effects of magnesium on digitalis, and the effects of digitalis on magnesium.
- Appropriate ingestion of vitamin D, vitamin B_6, and selenium depending on age-related recommendations and appropriate exposure to sunlight

- Appropriate magnesium ingestion and provide a list of dietary sources

Regarding public health:

- Teach appropriate use of laxatives to avoid magnesium wasting from overuse.
- Promote appropriate dietary sources of magnesium to communities where magnesium is removed from public water sources.

 CLINICAL SCENARIO

DIAGNOSIS: HYPOMAGNESEMIA FROM ALCOHOLIC ABUSE

Mrs. Daj is a 58-year-old widow on Social Security disability from a work-related back injury. The public transportation police brought her to the hospital after finding her on the subway doubled over with abdominal pain. She was ordered to take nothing by mouth (NPO) and was given 2 mg of subcutaneous morphine; in the emergency department she received an abdominal x-ray and IV dextrose 5% with normal saline for hydration. Mrs. Daj's initial blood laboratory tests showed she had a magnesium level of 1.5 mg/dL, and she therefore received 2 g of magnesium over 8 hours. She was then transferred to a telemetry unit because of mild changes in her ECG.

The next morning, Mrs. Daj appeared angry during the nursing assessment. She said she felt much better, did not want any pain medication, and simply wanted to leave the hospital. The nurse told Mrs Daj that she would ask the medical team to see Mrs. Daj as soon as possible and assigned a trained nursing assistant to provide one-to-one observation.

The nurse explained to the medical team that Mrs. Daj appeared anxious and was exhibiting a personality change. The nurse reviewed Mrs. Daj's medical chart and noted Mrs. Daj gave different answers to the emergency room physician, the nurse, and the admitting medical team regarding her alcohol use. The nurse wondered if Mrs. Daj was experiencing withdrawal. She called the laboratory to ask that Mrs. Daj's routine morning bloodwork be evaluated stat, and she reviewed the ECG telemetry strips. Noting that the QT interval was becoming elongated and that a new U wave appeared, the nurse alerted the medical team that she suspected Mrs. Daj may be experiencing alcohol withdrawal.

By late afternoon, Mrs. Daj's serum laboratory tests were evaluated, and she received another dose of IV magnesium and potassium and calcium supplementation. Vitamins and magnesium were added to her IV fluids. She previously received emergent lorazepam (Ativan) but has now begun receiving oxazepam (Serax). She remained NPO because the medical team was evaluating her for pancreatitis. She was placed on a continuous pulse oximeter, which measures oxygen saturation and respiratory rate and pattern. Mrs. Daj was calmer and fully oriented.

Hypermagnesemia

Hypermagnesemia occurs when the body has too much serum magnesium.

Laboratory Values

- Serum magnesium >2.14 mEq/L

Basic Concepts

Hypermagnesemia is rare in patients with healthy kidney function. The highest-risk population includes patients with kidney insufficiency who also ingest magnesium medications.

Because magnesium has a strong link to potassium and calcium levels, hypocalcemia and hyperkalemia should be suspected whenever hypermagnesemia is present. Hypocalcemia may occur due to suppression of PTH, which relates to high levels of magnesium. High magnesium levels inhibit acetylcholine release at the neuromuscular junction, which decreases the

ALERT

Hypermagnesemia occurs when serum magnesium is >2.14 mEq/L. *Critical* hypermagnesemia occurs when serum magnesium is >4 mEq/L, which can lead to decreased reflexes. A critical serum value of >5 leads to slowing of cardiac conduction, and a critical value of >7 mEq/L can lead to cardiac arrest. Patients with elevated serum levels or clinical symptoms should be placed on a continuous cardiac monitor.

excitability of muscles. Magnesium's capacity to function as a calcium channel blocker inhibits electrical conduction in cardiac muscle, which can lead to asystole.

Etiology

Hypermagnesemia can be caused by:

- Renal insufficiency or failure
- Massive hemolysis, rhabdomyolysis, or burns in which intracellular magnesium is released into serum
- Endocrine states, including hypoadrenalism, hypothyroidism, hypoparathyroidism, or uncorrected diabetic ketoacidosis
- Contamination of food or water with mineral salts

Iatrogenic causes can include:

- Use of "hard" water during hemodialysis
- Tumor lysis syndrome from chemotherapy
- Medications
  - Over ingestion of magnesium as a laxative or antacid can occur; especially dangerous for patients who have depressed renal clearance of magnesium
  - Lithium intoxication, causing decreased urinary excretion

Symptoms

- **Neurological:** Weakness, lethargy, drowsiness, coma
- **CV:** Hypotension, bradycardia, generalized feeling of warmth, ECG changes including widened QRS waves, prolonged PR interval, elevated T waves, asystole, and cardiac arrest
- **Respiratory:** Depressed ventilation, respirations leading to apnea
- **GI:** Nausea, vomiting, diarrhea
- **GU:** Decreased urine output associated with renal insufficiency
- **Musculoskeletal:** Decreased neuromuscular excitability, including depressed deep tendon reflexes

Assessment and Actions

Fluid, electrolyte, and acid-base imbalances can rapidly cause life-threatening neurological, cardiac, and respiratory compromise, requiring immediate notification of the medical or rapid response team. Consult the medical team if any new onset occurs or if worsening symptoms or vital signs occur that are outside the normal range. If neurological, respiratory, or cardiac compromise occurs, call for assistance from the rapid or urgent response team or, if outside an acute care setting, call community EMS.

Patient History

The following conditions may be associated with or cause hypermagnesemia.

- Acute or chronic metabolic processes such as:
  - Inability to excrete magnesium through the renal system
  - Cellular release of magnesium into the vascular space through rhabdomyolysis tumor or red blood cell lysis
- Chronic health problems, as well as endocrine diseases, including:
  - Chronic renal failure
  - Hypoaldrenalism, hypothyroidism, hypoparathyroidism
- Iatrogenic intervention, including:
  - Hemodialysis, using water with excess magnesium
  - Chemotherapy-induced tumor lysis or transfusion-related hemolysis
  - Rapid infusion of IV magnesium

Laboratory Assessment and Actions

Values >2.14 mEq/L reflect hypermagnesemia that may need correction. For values >4 mEq/L or with symptoms of hyporeflexia:

- Anticipate treatment including orders for administration of normal saline or lactated Ringer's fluid boluses to reverse hypotension, dilute serum magnesium levels, and promote magnesium losses through diuresis.
- Anticipate orders for administration of a loop diuretic, such as furosemide (Lasix), if the patient is not hypotensive.

For values >5 mEq/L or with cardiac symptoms, anticipate IV administration of calcium gluconate, continuous cardiac and respiratory monitoring and potential emergency airway support.

For values >8 mEq/L, anticipate orders for hemodialysis. See Chapter 2 for details of hemodialysis administration.

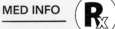

MED INFO

Calcium gluconate is typically ordered at 2–4 mg/kg/hr by IV infusion and is used to counteract the neuromuscular and cardioelectric effects of magnesium.

Systems Assessment and Actions

If laboratory test results are pending but hypermagnesemia is suspected, proceed with a systems assessment. Immediately consult the medical team at the onset or worsening of any of the symptoms that are listed in the following section.

Neuro-Musculo-Skeletal

If the patient displays a decreased level of consciousness or weakness, then perform frequent neurological assessments:

- Anticipate frequent measures of neurological status using the Glasgow Coma Scale.
- Maintain safety measures including keeping the bed low, padded side rails in place, and the call bell in reach.
- Continually reevaluate the patient's ability to follow instructions.
- Consult the medical team to discuss the need for one-on-one supervision.
- If a bilateral strength assessment demonstrates weakness, restrict activity, and institute standard safety measures for all activities of daily living:
  - Keep bed low, side rails up as appropriate, and call bell in reach
  - Assess and reassess patient's ability to follow directions
  - Assist with all ambulation and transfers

CV

- Frequently evaluate the patient for low blood pressure and slow cardiac rate. With any slowing of cardiac rate, anticipate orders for continuous cardiac monitoring to observe for arrhythmia.
- Consult the medical team to determine lead and alarm settings to best monitor for sodium changes.

Respiratory

- With slow or shallow respirations, then:
  - Measure oxygen saturation and anticipate orders for supplemental oxygen.
  - Raise the head of the bed to facilitate breathing.
- Anticipate orders for continuous respiratory monitoring.
- Keep respiratory support equipment readily available (ambu-bag, oral airway, suction equipment, and oxygen).

GI

If nausea, vomiting, or diarrhea occurs, measure and document all intake and output. If volume replacement is required, use caution with concurrent renal insufficiency because fluid overload may ensue.

- Anticipate orders for frequent measures of magnesium, calcium, and potassium because levels may shift with hydration.
  - Fluid orders are typically based on a milliliter-for-milliliter replacement, except in the presence of renal insufficiency.
  - Communicate the need for accurate intake and output measures to all ancillary staff.

- Administer antiemetics as ordered. *Note:* GI symptoms may not resolve until electrolytes are stable, despite use of antiemetics.

GU

- Measure fluid volumes. Less than 30 mL/hr may point to renal insufficiency.
- If renal insufficiency is evident, anticipate orders to administer IV diuretics.
- If severe insufficiency is present, anticipate orders for hemodialysis (see Chapter 2 for hemodialysis precautions).

Prevention

Teach at-risk populations the signs and symptoms of hypermagnesemia, and make certain that all patients with renal insufficiency are aware of which medications contain magnesium and should be avoided.

Health professionals can advocate for public health by ensuring that water with low mineral levels is available for hemodialysis. They can also reinforce Red Cross standards for blood transfusion safety to prevent lysis of red blood cells (see Chapter 2).

 CLINICAL SCENARIO

DIAGNOSIS: HYPERMAGNESEMIA FROM RENAL INSUFFICIENCY

Mr. Anderson has a long history of bipolar disorder treated with lithium. After an episode of strep throat and dosing with cefazolin, Mr. Anderson's primary care provider admits him to the hospital due to decreased urine output and flank pain. Diagnosed with renal insufficiency, Mr. Anderson complains of light-headedness.

The nurse measures Mr. Anderson's blood pressure and finds his systolic level at 85 mm Hg. After consulting with the medical team, chemistry laboratory samples are drawn, and Mr. Anderson's magnesium is found to be 2.75. IV sodium chloride is ordered for a bolus of 250 mL.

Mr. Anderson is transferred to the telemetry unit and is placed on continuous cardiac monitoring; he is also scheduled for blood pressure monitoring every 30 minutes. The nurse finds it difficult to place an IV angiocatheter but is able to start a 22-gauge IV catheter. Mr. Anderson is asked to remain supine in bed. The nurse assigns a nursing assistant to stay with him and contacts the nursing supervisor to ask for an assistant to be assigned for one-to-one supervision.

Continued

Mr. Anderson's systolic pressure after normal saline infusion is 95. Lasix 40 mg IV is ordered and given slowly over 5 minutes. Two hours later, Mr. Anderson has diuresed 200 mL, and the magnesium levels that were sent for laboratory evaluation show a return to normal levels of 2 mEq/L. IV normal saline is ordered for 125 mL/hr. After the first hour, the nurse is able to place an 18-gauge IV catheter. The nursing assistant is instructed to encourage Mr. Anderson to void every hour and to report the output to the nurse.

After 2 hours, Mr. Anderson's blood pressure is 110 systolic, and the nurse raises the head of his bed to 30°. He voids between 30–50 mL per hour.

1. Why does the nurse suspect a renal problem for Mr. Anderson?
2. What ECG changes should the nurse look for on the cardiac monitor?
3. Why would the nurse place an 18-gauge IV catheter in addition to the 22-gauge IV catheter?

Cautions for Special Populations

Pediatric
The normal ranges of serum levels for pediatric patients (in conventional and SI units) are:
- Newborn: 1.23–1.81 mEq/L or 0.62–0.91 mmol/L
- Child: 1.40–1.73 mEq/L or 0.70–0.86 mmol/L

Pediatric Dietary Intake (FDA/Adequate Intake)
Healthy breast-fed infants should meet dietary requirements through normal human milk intake:
- 0–6 months: 30 mg/day
- 7–12 months: 75 mg/day
- 1–3 years: 80 mg/day
- 4–8 years: 130 mg/day
- 9–13 years: 240 mg/day
- 14–18 years—males: 410 mg/day; females: 360 mg/day

Geriatric
According to the FDA, geriatric populations are at high risk for low magnesium intake and excess magnesium loss through the kidneys. This population is also at risk for poor access to magnesium in the diet and the use of magnesium-depleting medications.

Geriatric Dietary Intake (FDA/Adequate Intake)

- For women older than 31 years: 320 mg/day
- For men older than 31 years: 420 mg/day

REVIEW QUESTIONS

1. Where does the body store magnesium for periods of low ingestion?
2. If hypomagnesemia occurs, what effect is seen in the muscles?
3. Which electrolytes are strongly affected by low magnesium?
4. Which common drinks can be a source of magnesium?
5. Why can low body magnesium be masked by normal blood levels?
6. How will low magnesium levels affect urine magnesium?

3D Phosphorus

Phosphorus

Phosphate is the most abundant intracellular negative ion (anion), and it has the chemical symbol PO_4^{3-}. Phosphorus is found in the body in organic and inorganic states.

About 85% of the adult body's 1000 g of inorganic phosphate is bound to calcium in the matrix of bones and teeth. The remainder is found as organic phosphate, which is a structural component in cellular DNA and RNA and in the phospholipid bilayers of cellular membranes. Phosphorus is also a key component of adenosine triphosphate (ATP) and creatinine phosphate, which are the molecules responsible for storing energy in most human cells.

In serum, phosphorus is known as inorganic phosphate. About 10%–15% of serum phosphate is bound to proteins, and 35% forms a complex with other electrolytes, including sodium, calcium, and magnesium. About 55% of phosphate is free in serum.

Serum phosphorus is evaluated in relationship to serum calcium. When phosphorous levels in the blood rise, calcium levels decrease; likewise, when calcium levels rise, phosphorus is excreted. This relationship is due to the feedback cycle of parathyroid hormone (PTH) and calcitriol and the binding of calcium by phosphorus (see the following section on regulation).

Functions

Phosphorus provides structural support to bones and teeth, participates in cellular functions, and delivers oxygen to body tissues. It also helps to maintain the pH of body fluids.

Provides Structural Support to Bones and Teeth

In all, 85% of phosphorus provides structural support to bones and teeth in a matrix with calcium, where it is constantly involved in a cycle of release (resorption) from and deposition into bones. See Chapter 3A for more details on bone minerals.

Participates in Cellular Functions
Phosphorus is an element of the phospholipid bilayer of cellular membranes and is a key component of RNA and DNA. As an element of ATP, phosphorus functions in cellular energy storage and transfer. In low phosphorous states, cellular membranes can break down, and cellular reproduction and functions are interrupted.

Delivers Oxygen to Body Tissues
Phosphorus, as an element of 2,3-diphosphoglycerate (2,3-DPG), binds to deoxygenated hemoglobin. This binding encourages the release of oxygen from hemoglobin in red blood cells into body tissues. In low phosphorous states, oxygen remains more closely bound to hemoglobin and is less available for transfer into cells.

Maintains pH of Body Fluids
Phosphorus acts as a buffer, intracellularly and in the tubules of the kidneys, by accepting or donating hydrogen ions (H^+). Intracellularly, phosphate salts are able to accept or donate hydrogen ions. In the renal system, excess phosphates in the tubular fluid can remove excess hydrogen ions and together they are excreted through the body via urine. Decreasing free hydrogen shifts the pH from acidosis toward alkalosis.

Intake

In healthy patients, phosphorous intake through dietary sources is sufficient, and deficiency is rare. However, patients who have decreased absorption or low intake of vitamin D may not have sufficient levels of phosphorus for essential functions. Vitamin D is metabolized into calcitriol, which allows for absorption of phosphorus and calcium from the intestines.

Dietary Intake
Due to differences in bone formation, adequate intakes of phosphorus are significantly different among age groups (see pediatric concerns at the end of this chapter). For adults older than 19 years, recommended adequate intake is 700 mg/day. Adults older than 70 years should not ingest more than 3000 mg/day because of a decreased ability to excrete phosphorus from the kidneys.

Dietary sources include almost all foods, with adults normally consuming about 1 g/day. Phosophorus-rich foods are similar to calcium-rich foods; some examples include dairy products, seafood, nuts, seeds, and vegetables such as okra, broccoli, and kale. In addition to calcium-rich foods, oats, wheat, and meats are also key dietary sources for phosphorus.

Intravenous Infusion

Intravenous (IV) repletion of low phosphorous levels is not always ordered because much of the body's phosphorus resides intracellularly. If IV phosphorus is ordered, patients are monitored for rebound hyperphosphatemia and hypocalcemia. Sodium phosphate and potassium phosphate are not compatible with Ringer's lactate, dextrose 10%, or dextrose 10% with 0.9% saline. Because phosphorus is not compatible with certain calcium salts, consult the pharmacy to check for interactions with other IV fluids.

Phosphorus should be administered through a dedicated central line, but it may be infused over 4 or more hours through a large-bore IV line. Standard concentration for peripheral infusion of sodium phosphate or potassium phosphate is 15 mmol/250 mL and 15 mmol/100 mL for central-line infusion. It must always be administered via IV controller pump and may never be given as a direct IV push.

COACH CONSULT

Supplements of phosphorus are rarely prescribed because of the dietary availability in most types of foods. However, patients with high calcium levels may receive phosphorus to prevent calcium oxalate stones. Although this is a use approved by the U.S. Food and Drug Administration (FDA), the National Institutes of Health warn that phosphorus supplementation can be dangerous if the stones are composed of magnesium, ammonium, or phosphate.

Regulation

Phosphorous absorption is proportional to ingestion. Like calcium, phosphorous absorption in the small intestine depends on calcitriol, which is the active form of vitamin D. PTH is released when serum calcium is low because it stimulates conversion of vitamin D to calcitriol in the kidneys. This conversion increases intestinal absorption of calcium and phosphorus and the movement of phosphorus and calcium from bones into serum. In addition, PTH stimulates renal excretion of phosphorus while decreasing excretion of calcium, thereby keeping calcium in the bloodstream and getting rid of excess phosphorus. The feedback cycle is completed when high serum phosphorus halts conversion of vitamin D to calcitriol.

Other hormones that affect phosphorous regulation include thyroid hormone and growth hormone, both of which increase the reabsorption of phosphorus in the kidneys. Not all of the hormones that regulate phosphorus are fully understood. Phosphate-regulating factors are hormones that are being studied for their effect on phosphorous bone formation and resorption and renal excretion and reabsorption.

Loss

Phosphorus is added to the body through bone deposits until about age 30, when bone loss begins to occur. Renal excretion is about 200 mg/day, bile excretion accounts for an additional 200 mg/day, and sweat accounts for about 25 mg/day.

High-sodium and high-protein foods increase phosphorous excretion. Caffeine has a negative impact on phosphorous absorption and increases phosphorous excretion. Alcohol reduces both the absorption of phosphorus and the activation of vitamin D in the intestines.

Laboratory Measures

Serum levels are drawn to assess for phosphorus in the blood, which measures only free phosphorus and does not reflect phosphorous levels in bones and teeth or the phosphorus bound to proteins and other electrolytes. Therefore, serum levels may be normal even in the presence of severe depletion of phosphorus from the bones with chronic malabsorption states. In this case, a careful history and clinical assessment should be conducted and discussed with the medical team to look for signs of chronic bone demineralization. The normal serum range for an adult is 2.5–4.5 mg/dL.

Serum Specimen Collection

Serum phosphorus is collected by phlebotomy in a red- or tiger-top tube but may also be drawn in a green-top, heparinized tube. Standard phlebotomy procedure requires avoiding drawing blood from the same arm that has IV access. Hemolyzed blood cells add organic phosphates to serum phosphate, which will return a falsely high result. Note that hemolysis can be caused by tourniquets that are too tight or that are left on too long, by blood that is withdrawn through a syringe instead of a Vacutainer, or by a specimen that is not processed quickly enough after being drawn. To avoid processing errors, ensure that the specimen is delivered according to your laboratory's guidelines.

Urine Phosphorus

Urine may be collected at random using a clean-catch or catheter-obtained specimen, or it may be collected over 24 hours, requiring a hydrochloride fixative (see Chapter 6 for collection method). Urine phosphorous levels depend on dietary intake. High-sodium diets can cause excessive excretion of phosphorus, just as alcohol, pumpkin seeds, and corticosteroids can increase urinary excretion of phosphorus.

Normal adult urine phosphorus range is 0.4–1.3 g over 24 hours. Elevated excretion in the presence of high levels of phosphorus in the blood indicates excess ingestion of phosphorus or cellular lysis, whereas decreased excretion with hyperphosphatemia indicates renal impairment or hypoparathroidism.

Hypophosphatemia

Hypophosphatemia occurs when the body has a phosphorous deficit.

Laboratory Values
- Serum phosphorus < 2.5 mg/dL

Basic Concepts

Hypophosphatemia rarely requires supplementation and is typically seen only in very low nutrition or absorption states. Interventions to correct low phosphorus can cause dangerous electrolytes shifts, and therefore phosphorus's close relationship with magnesium and calcium requires evaluation of these two electrolytes as well.

ALERT

Hypophosphatemia occurs with a serum phosphorus of <2.5 mg/dL. *Critical* hypophosphatemia occurs with serum phosphorus <1 mg/dL.

Etiology

Hypophosphatemia can be caused by:
- Alkalosis, which is one of the most common states that moves phosphate into cells.
  - Alkalosis is especially observed with hyperventilation.
- High energy demand states, where insulin stimulates phosphorus to move into cells. High-energy demand states may be associated with:
  - Recovery from diabetic ketoacidosis
  - Alcohol withdrawal, with a preexisting poor phosphorous absorption

- Cancers, such as acute leukemia and certain lymphomas that consume phosphorus
- Dietary insufficiency or gastrointestinal (GI) disturbances that decrease absorption of phosphorus or vitamin D, including alcohol abuse, starvation, and anorexia
- Vitamin D deficiency or metabolic impairment from lack of exposure to ultraviolet light (including sunlight), poor dietary absorption, or hepatic cirrhosis
- PTH excesses, which cause increased renal excretion of phosphate
- Iatrogenic losses, including:
  - Surgical removal of portions of the stomach or small intestines
  - Renal transplant causing increased urinary excretion
  - Refeeding with high calories but low phosphorus, where metabolism demands deplete serum phosphorus
  - Medications, including:
    - Antacids with aluminum, calcium, or magnesium, which bind phosphorus into unabsorbable compounds
    - Bile acid sequestrants, including cholestyramine and colestipol, which decrease GI absorption
    - Proximal diuretics, which decrease sodium reabsorption and increase phosphorous excretion
    - Laxatives without phosphorous additives
    - Sucralfate, which is a sucrose-sulfate-aluminum medication that is taken before meals

Symptoms

Symptoms of hypophosphatemia include:

- **Neurological:** Anxiety, irritability, numbness, tingling, ascending motor paralysis
- **Cardiovascular (CV):** Fatigue, anemia, low cardiac output, increased infections related to white blood cell dysfunction, hemolytic anemia related to unstable cell membranes, ventricular dysrhythmias
- **Respiratory:** Irregular breathing rhythm, shallow breaths from muscle weakness

- **GI:** Anorexia, difficulty swallowing
- **Musculoskeletal:** Bone pain, soft or fragile bones, stiff joints, muscle weakness, rhabdomyolysis from unstable cell membranes

Assessment and Actions

Fluid, electrolyte, and acid-base imbalances can rapidly cause life-threatening neurological, cardiac, and respiratory compromise, requiring immediate notification of the medical or rapid response team. Consult the medical team if any new onset occurs or if worsening symptoms or vital signs occur that are outside the normal range. If neurological, respiratory, or cardiac compromise occurs, call for assistance from the rapid or urgent response team or, if outside an acute care setting, call community emergency medical services (EMS).

Patient History

The following conditions may be associated with or cause hypophosphatemia:

- Acute or chronic metabolic processes, which may result in alkalotic states, excess renal excretion, impaired GI absorption, low albumin levels, hypomagnesemia, or vitamin D deficiency
- Chronic health problems, including:
  - Anemia
  - Respiratory diseases
  - Neuromuscular disease
  - GI diseases relating to poor albumin or vitamin D absorption, including anorexia, Crohn's disease, pancreatitis, or gastric or intestinal obstruction
  - Liver failure

Laboratory Assessment and Actions

Serum phosphorus < 2.5 mg/dL reflects hypophosphatemia that may need correction. If symptoms are present or critical values of serum phosphorus < 1 mg/dL, immediately consult the medical team and:

- Anticipate orders for frequent blood calcium, magnesium, potassium, and phosphorous levels, based on frequency and effect of interventions
- Anticipate orders for frequent assessment of blood urea nitrogen (BUN) and creatinine to track renal function
- Anticipate orders for oral administration of potassium phosphate as mono-basic potassium phosphate (K-phos) 1 g or potassium phosphate (neutra-phos) 1.45 g times a day as a supplement;

supplements should not be taken with milk to prevent milk-alkali syndrome; phosphorous supplementation is contraindicated with hypocalcemia and is prescribed in divided doses because absorption decreases in the presence of high doses

If oral administration is not effective and phosphorous deficiency is critical, immediately consult the medical team and:

- Anticipate orders for IV administration of phosphorus:
  - Discuss any abnormal chemistry levels with the medical team before IV administration of phosphate.
  - Observe for signs and symptoms of hypocalcemia because IV phosphorus can lower serum calcium to critical levels.
  - IV phosphorous solutions should be infused into a large or central vein.
  - Check compatibility, because phosphate is incompatible with many medications. D_5W, 0.45% NaCl, and 0.9% NaCl are acceptable for dilution. Lactated Ringer's, dextrose 10%, and dextrose 10% with normal saline are not compatible with phosphorus and should not be hung into the same IV line or mixed with phosphorus.
  - If potassium phosphate is ordered, then check serum potassium levels before administration to prevent hyperkalemia.
  - To prevent incorrect dosing, check that the prescription is written in both mmol and mg (1 mmol of phosphorus = 31 mg).

  Anticipate orders to draw laboratory samples for creatinine, calcium, magnesium, and potassium.
- Anticipate orders for frequent, rapid serum chemistry laboratory samples to be drawn:
  - Onset and peak are immediate.
  - Duration is 0.5–2 hours.

- Dosing is usually required for 48 hours or until underlying causes have been identified and treated.

Systems Assessment and Actions

If laboratory test results are pending but hypophosphatemia is suspected, proceed with a systems assessment. Immediately consult the medical team at the onset or worsening of any of the symptoms that are listed in the following section.

Neurological

If confusion, mood changes, anxiety, memory losses, nerve excitability, paresthesias, or paralysis occurs, then:

- Anticipate frequent measures of neurological status using the Glasgow Coma Scale.
- Maintain safety measures including keeping the bed low, padded side rails in place, and call bell in reach.
- Continually reevaluate the patient's ability to follow instructions.
- Consult the medical team to discuss need for one-on-one supervision.
- Institute safety precautions, and assist with all activities of daily living, transfers, and ambulation.

If mental status changes occur, provide supervision, monitoring patient for intolerance of IV lines or other medically necessary devices. If signs of paralysis occur, anticipate rapid correction of hypophosphatemia and emergency respiratory support.

CV

If fatigue, hypotension, low heart rate, low cardiac output, or electrocardiogram (ECG) changes occur, then:

- Immediately consult the medical team for vital signs outside normal limits.
- Frequently measure oxygen saturation, and cardiac and respiratory vital signs.
- Assist with all activities of daily living and transfers.
- Anticipate orders for laboratory samples to assess for anemia.
- Anticipate orders for continuous cardiac, respiratory, and oxygen saturation monitoring.
- Consult the medical team to determine best monitoring leads and alarm settings for cardiac monitoring to observe for ventricular waveform changes.
- Place the patient on bedrest, and anticipate orders for IV fluid support with phosphorus.

If the immune system is compromised, then maintain universal precautions, and anticipate orders for neutropenic precautions if white blood cell count is low. If clotting times are prolonged, then:

- Prepare for transfusion of blood or clotting products (see Chapter 2).
- Educate the patient and family on bleeding precautions.
- Place the patient on bedrest, and consult the medical team regarding activity restriction.

Respiratory
If laryngeal or bronchial spasms develop, then:

- Immediately consult the medical team for emergency laryngeal airway support.
- Measure oxygen saturation, and anticipate orders for supplemental oxygen and continuous respiratory monitoring.
- Raise head of bed to facilitate airway clearance.
- Keep respiratory support equipment available (ambu-bag, oral airway, suction equipment, and oxygen).

GI
If abdominal spasms or pains occur, hold all oral intake, and consult the medical team about potential for laryngeal spasm.

Musculoskeletal
If cramping, tremors, increased reflexes, Trousseau's or Chvostek's sign (see Fig. 3A-2 in Calcium chapter), or tetany occurs, institute safety precautions listed under neurological symptoms, and immediately consult the medical team.

If bone pain is reported or if low bone density is diagnosed, anticipate support with transfers and activities of daily living, and observe for symptoms of stress fracture.

If muscle pain is reported, then:

- Consult the medical team to assess for rhabdomyolysis, including laboratory assessment for creatinine kinase and myoglobin.
- Anticipate orders for high fluid volume IV administration, frequent laboratory assessments for intracellular electrolytes leaking into vascular space, BUN, and creatinine.
- If adequate kidney function is present, anticipate orders for diuretics and/or bicarbonate administration.

Prevention
Teach at-risk populations:

- Signs and symptoms of hypophosphatemia. Emphasize that they should watch for signs of poor clotting, which include bruising and bleeding; changes in immune function, stress fractures, and nerve irritability or muscle weakness, especially with swallowing and breathing.

- Appropriate phosphorous ingestion, and provide a list of dietary sources.

Regarding public health, the health professional can:

- Inform at-risk clients of sources of vitamin D from their diet and sunlight exposure.
- Remind patients that osteoporosis (weak bones) and osteopenia (low bone mass) are common problems resulting in approximately 1.5 million fractures a year (see Chapter 3A for details). Chronic, low ingestion or absorption of dietary phosphorus can cause these bone changes.
- Teach those who abuse alcohol or have experienced starvation or extreme malnutrition that they are at special risk for hypophosphatemia and can have life-threatening phosphorous and calcium shifts when refeeding begins.

 CLINICAL SCENARIO

DIAGNOSIS: MALNUTRITION-INDUCED HYPOPHOSPHATEMIA

Mr. Pettigrew, a 79-year-old widower, is discovered with shallow breathing and extreme weakness by his neighbor after having not been seen in the neighborhood for several days. In the emergency room, he is found to have confusion and a fever of 102°F. He is hydrated with D_5W in 0.45% NaCl and, based on his report of frequent alcohol intake, is given oxazepam (Serax) prophylactically and a daily bag of IV fluids containing thiamine, folic acid, and magnesium. He refuses oral nutrition but agrees to a nasogastric feeding tube. His current weight is down 30 lb from his last admission due to a fall more than a year ago. To prevent refeeding syndrome, his tube feeding is ordered at 20 kcal/kg/day. His phosphorus is 2.3 mg/dL, calcium is 8.5 mg/dL, potassium is 4 mEq/L, and magnesium is 2.2 mEq/L. After a day of feeding, his phosphorus dropped to 1 mg/dL. To stop the decrease, his feedings were cut back, and IV potassium phosphate was ordered every 6 hours for 48 hours, with electrolytes measured every 2 hours during and after each 6-hour infusion. After IV repletion of the phosphorus, oral phosphorus was started and maintained until Mr. Pettigrew was able to take in normal oral nutrition.

1. How does alcohol ingestion affect phosphorous levels?
2. Why are patients with a history of alcohol abuse additionally at risk for low phosphorous levels?
3. Why do special precautions concerning hypophosphatemia have to be observed when delivering foods to Mr. Pettigrew?

Hyperphosphatemia

Hyperphosphatemia occurs when the body has an excess of phosphorus.

Laboratory Values
- Serum phosphorus >4.5 mg/dL

Basic Concepts
Hyperphosphatemia is more common than hypophosphatemia and is typically associated with renal disease. Hyperphosphatemia can cause calcification of organs, especially the kidneys; cardiac valves, blood vessels, and muscles. Plaques in the arteries can lead to high blood pressure, tissue necrosis, and heart failure.

Etiology
Hyperphosphatemia can be caused by:
- Acidosis, causing shifting of phosphate out of cells
- Kidney disease, with functions at or below 50% of normal
- Cellular injuries from burns, trauma, crushing, shock, heat illnesses, hemolysis, ischemic bowel, extensive exercise, rhabdomyolysis, tumor lysis, insulin deficiency, or acute acidosis
- Endocrine disorders, hypoparathyroidism, pseudohypoparathyroidism
- Iatrogenic causes including:
  - Immobilization, leading to bone loss
  - Medications including:
- Amphotericin B
- Glucocorticoid withdrawal
- Overinfusion or ingestion of phosphorus
- Milk-alkali syndrome inhibiting PTH from antacids ingested with milk
- Phosphorus-containing enemas
- Vitamin D toxicity

Symptoms

Symptoms of hyperphosphatemia include:

- **Neurological:** Cataracts, change in mental status, delirium, lethargy, apathy, paresthesias, headache, convulsions, seizures, coma, calcium phosphorus deposits in the eyes, yellow conjunctivae of the eyes
- **Respiratory:** Hypocalcemia-related bronchial or laryngeal spasms may occur
- **CV:** Hypotension, prolonged QT interval on ECG, hypocalcemia, hypomagnesemia, dehydration, metabolic acidosis, chronic arteriole calcification caused necrosis
- **GI:** Tongue coating, foul breath, constipation, anorexia, nausea, reflux, elevated pancreatic enzymes, calcifications, vomiting of phosphorescent materials or blood
- **Genitourinary (GU):** Oliguria, calcifications
- **Musculoskeletal**: Weakness, cramping, tetany, foot and leg swelling, calcium phosphorus deposits in the joints

COACH CONSULT

When renal failure causes the glomerular filtration rate to drop below 30, patients will usually be placed on a low phosphorus diet and phosphate binders. Phosphate binders are based on the patient's phosphorous levels.

COACH CONSULT

Some symptoms of hyperphosphatemia are symptoms of hypocalcemia because both imbalances can be caused by high serum phosphorous levels. Examples of these symptoms include muscle delirium, cramping, tetany, seizures, Chvostek's sign, and Trousseau's sign (see Fig. 3A-2 in the Calcium chapter).

Assessment and Actions

Fluid, electrolyte, and acid-base imbalances can rapidly cause life-threatening neurological, cardiac, and respiratory compromise, requiring immediate notification of the medical or rapid response team. Consult the medical team if any new onset occurs or if worsening symptoms or vital signs occur that are outside the normal range. If neurological, respiratory, or cardiac compromise occurs, then call for assistance from the rapid or urgent response team or, if outside an acute care setting, call community EMS.

Patient History

Review for clues as to cause. The following conditions may be associated with or cause hypophosphatemia:

- Acute or chronic metabolic processes, such as:
  - Acidosis from respiratory or metabolic sources
  - Burns, heat disorders

- Cancer, including leukemia, lymphoma, and bone cancer, with or without chemotherapy-induced bone lysis
- Diabetes acidosis
- Immobilization leading to bone loss
- Ischemic bowel
- Chronic health problems, including:
  - Kidney disease
  - Parathyroid tumors associated with acromegaly or cancers
  - Endocrine diseases such as hypoparathyroidism, thyrotoxicosis, pseudohypoparathyroidism
- Iatrogenic interventions, including:
  - Phosphate therapy, supplements, or enemas
  - Glucocorticoid withdrawal or deficiency
  - Milk-alkali syndrome
  - Vitamin D intoxication

Laboratory Assessment and Actions

Serum >4.5 mg/dL reflects hyperphosphatemia that may need correction. Immediately consult the medical team, and anticipate treatment with symptoms if critical values of serum phosphorus >5 mg/dL.

- Anticipate orders for frequent serum laboratory measures of electrolytes throughout therapy. If serum calcium is low, anticipate measures to correct calcium (see Hypocalcemia section of Chapter 3A).
- Instruct patients to restrict foods that are high in phosphorus.
- Anticipate orders for oral phosphate binders. They bind phosphorus in the GI tract, causing it to be excreted in stool; therefore, oral phosphate binders must be taken with food to bind dietary phosphates. Phosphate binders are also used along with gastric lavage for overingestion or phosphorous poisoning. Examples of phosphate binders include:
  - Aluminum hydroxide (Amphojel). Note that binders with aluminum can put the patient at risk for aluminum toxicity, especially in the presence of renal insufficiency. Aluminum hydroxide is also used to treat stomach acid problems. One to six tablets are prescribed with each meal.
  - Calcium carbonate (Oscal), calcium citrate, and calcium acetate (Phoslo). These binders offset concurrent hypocalcemia, but they may also cause calcification of soft tissues. Oral doses are 250–1500 mg with meals.

- Lanthanum carbonate (Fosrenol) 250–500 mg or sevelamer (Renagel) in doses of two to four capsules with each meal. These are given when aluminum and calcium must be avoided.

With critical levels or if oral binders are not effective, immediately consult the medical team, and anticipate orders for renal dialysis if other measures have not been effective in removing phosphate from the blood.

Systems Assessment and Actions

If laboratory test results are pending but hyperphosphatemia is suspected, proceed with a systems assessment. Immediately consult the medical team at the onset or worsening of any of the symptoms that are listed in the following section.

Neuro-Musculo-Skeletal

For decreased level of consciousness and weakness:
- Anticipate frequent measures of neurological status using the Glasgow Coma Scale.
- Maintain safety measures including keeping the bed low, padded side rails in place, and the call bell in reach.
- Continually reevaluate the patient's ability to follow instructions.
- Consult the medical team to discuss need for one-on-one supervision.
- Institute safety precautions, and assist with all activities of daily living, transfers, and ambulation.

If lethargy, hypotension, convulsions, or seizure occurs, then:
- Immediately consult the medical or rapid response team, provide continuous observation of the patient, and act to protect the patient's airway.
- Institute safety precautions, and assist with all activities of daily living, transfers, and ambulation.

If mental status changes occur, then provide close supervision, monitoring patient for intolerance of IV lines or other medically necessary devices.

Respiratory

If hypocalcemia-related respiratory symptoms of bronchospasm or laryngeal spasm occur, then:
- Immediately contact the medical or rapid response team.
- Provide continuous observation of the patient.
- Measure oxygen saturation, and anticipate orders for supplemental oxygen and continuous respiratory monitoring.
- Raise the head of the bed to facilitate airway clearance.

- Keep respiratory support equipment available (ambu-bag, oral airway, suction equipment, and oxygen).
- Anticipate measures to correct calcium imbalance as discussed in Hypocalcemia section of Chapter 3A.

CV

If ECG changes or hypotension are noted, then:

- Immediately consult the medical team, and discuss the best leads to assess for arrhythmia and prolonged QT interval.
- Anticipate orders for continuous ECG monitoring.
- Place the patient on bedrest, and communicate hypotension to medical team.
- Provide supervision and support for all activities of daily living.
- Anticipate orders for IV fluid administration with electrolyte replacement.

GI

If anorexia, nausea, or constipation occurs, then:

- Hold all oral intake.
- Consult the medical team for antiemetic therapies. Note that antiemetic medications may not be effective until underlying electrolyte imbalance is corrected.
- Consult the medical team for orders to support lower bowel motility. Avoid laxatives or enemas containing phosphorus.

GU

If oliguria is measured, then:

- Measure fluid volumes. Note that < 30 mL/hr may point to renal insufficiency and should be reported to the medical team.
- Instruct all ancillary staff on the need for accurate measurement and documentation of intake and output.
- Anticipate orders for BUN and creatinine laboratory measures.

Prevention

Teach at-risk populations:

- Signs and symptoms of hyperphosphatemia
- Appropriate dietary restriction of phosphorus and necessity of taking phosphorus-binding medications

To advocate for public health, inform patients that:

- High levels of phosphates in soft drinks and snack foods have caused concern for people with low dietary calcium. High-serum phosphorus can lead to high PTH levels, leading to decrease of calcium and phosphorus in the bone.

- Phosphorous poisoning used to be commonplace when people made their own matches. Today, phosphorus is commonly used in fertilizers, detergents, military applications (including nerve gas), and chemical manufacturing. People who work with phosphorus are at high risk for burns, jawbone tissue death necrosis, and smoking stool syndrome, where accidentally ingested white phosphorus still contains incendiary characteristics. Treatment of phosphorous burns can be dangerous because exposure to phosphorus that remains exposed on the patient can cause burns to health-care providers.
- Industrial phosphorus and use of phosphorus-containing household detergents have been linked to the death of natural river and lake flora, which is why many detergents are now made without phosphorus.
- Past beliefs that taking medications with antacids can suppress GI ulceration have proved false, because the combination can

 CLINICAL SCENARIO

DIAGNOSIS: HYPERPHOSPHATEMIA ASSOCIATED WITH END-STAGE RENAL DISEASE

Mrs. Ryan has had kidney disease for 10 years and requires hemodialysis. Her physician has prescribed the phosphate binder sevelamer, but Mrs. Ryan's insurance company will not pay for it. Instead, she is taking calcium acetate.

After taking the calcium acetate, several of her blood laboratory samples show she has hypercalcemia. In addition to renal dysfunction, Mrs. Ryan also has hypertension, anemia, and congestive heart failure, for which she has had several hospitalizations. She complains that the phosphate binders give her nausea and that she does not take them consistently. The nurse explains that high levels of phosphorus can contribute to her nausea and other GI symptoms, along with her muscle cramping and weakness. Mrs. Ryan states that she finds it difficult to manage all of her medications and the frequency of her dialysis, but she agrees to attempt to continue with her phosphate binders to help keep her symptoms at bay.

1. Mrs. Ryan has both high calcium and high phosphorus. What is the normal relationship between calcium and phosphorus?
2. Mrs. Ryan complains of difficulty attending her dialysis sessions regularly. The nurse informs Mrs. Ryan of her elevated blood calcium levels. What precautions should the nurse discuss with Mrs. Ryan?
3. Mrs. Ryan has discussed her difficulty with taking phosphate-binding medications. Based on Mrs. Ryan's history, what other medications should the nurse discuss with the patient?

cause milk-alkali syndrome. Teach appropriate management of GI acid production.

Cautions for Special Populations

Pediatric

The normal ranges of serum levels for pediatric patients after early infancy are higher because of the formation of bones during normal childhood growth. The normal ranges of phosphorous serum levels in pediatric patients are:

- 0–5 days: 4.6–8.0 mg/dL
- 1–3 years: 3.9–6.5 mg/dL
- 4–6 years: 4.0–5.4 mg/dl
- 7–11 years: 3.7–5.6 mg/dL
- 12–13 years: 3.3–5.4 mg/dL
- 14–5 years: 2.9–5.4 mg/dL
- 16–19 years: 2.8–4.6 mg/dL

Pediatric Dietary Intake (FDA/Adequate Intake)

Healthy breastfed infants should meet dietary requirements through normal human milk intake. Cow milk is dangerous for neonates due to the high phosphorous content. Dietary phosphorous requirements are:

- 0–6 months: 100 mg/day
- 7–12 months: 275 mg/day
- 1–3 years: 460 mg/day
- 4–8 years: 500 mg/day
- 9–18 years: 1300 mg/day

Geriatrics

Geriatric dietary intake (FDA/adequate intake) of phosphorus for age 51 + years is 1200 mg/day.

1. Name three to five locations in the human body where phosphorus is in abundance.
2. Which two hormones are primarily responsible for the regulation of the relationship between calcium and phosphorus?
3. When serum phosphorous levels are low, what happens to the oxygen molecules that are bound to hemoglobin?
4. Which key vitamin is essential for the intestinal absorption of phosphorus?
5. Which two common components of beverages can decrease the body's phosphorous levels?
6. Which two tests can be employed to evaluate for hyperphosphatemia and hypocalcemia?

3E Potassium

Potassium

Potassium (K+) is the primary intracellular, positively charged ion (cation) in the body. Approximately 98% of the body's potassium, which is about 3500 mEq, is held within cells in intracellular fluid (ICF); minimal amounts of potassium, approximately 3.5–5 mEq/L, is extracellular. This ratio of intracellular to extracellular concentration helps create a cellular chemical electrical membrane potential, and it is why the body is particularly sensitive to abnormal ranges of extracellular potassium.

The difference in intracellular and extracellular potassium concentration is maintained by a sodium potassium pump in the cellular membrane. Sodium is actively transported out of cells, and potassium is transported into cells with an adenosine triphosphate (ATP) pump.

Functions

Potassium transmits nerve impulses, activates enzymes, and promotes acid-base equilibrium.

Transmission of Nerve Impulses, Cardiac and Skeletal Muscle Contraction

Potassium and sodium are exchanged through active and passive channels to create the depolarization and repolarization of the cellular membranes that allow for transmission of nerve impulses, resulting in cardiac and skeletal muscle contraction (Fig. 3E-1). These polarization changes allow for the transmission of energy across the cellular membrane and the function of these cells. Without the constant pumping of potassium and sodium by ATP pumps, these cells and their organs would not function.

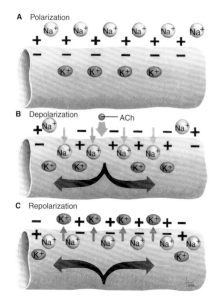

FIGURE 3E-1: Polarization, depolarization, and repolarization in muscle tissue.

Activates Enzymes

Adenosine triphosphate-ases (ATP-ases) are enzymes that catalyze the ATP/adenosine diphosphage (ADP) cycle of energy reaction and release. These enzymes are essential for importation of components of cell metabolism and exportation of waste to outside the cell. ATP-ases are activated in the presence of potassium and sodium. For instance, the gastric hydrogen potassium ATP-ase in the stomach's parietal cells is actually a proton pump responsible for acidification of the stomach fluid.

Pyruvate kinase, an enzyme involved in glycolysis and used for carbohydrate metabolism, is also activated by potassium. Other potassium-dependent enzymes catalyze similarly essential functions and are inhibited in low potassium states.

Promotes Acid-Base Equilibrium

Potassium exchanges with hydrogen on a cellular level as part of the metabolic buffer system. With a pH decrease by 0.1, serum potassium increases by 0.6 mEq/L.

Intake

In healthy patients, potassium intake is through dietary sources. However, many patients admitted to acute care facilities may require oral supplementation or intravenous (IV) infusion.

Dietary Intake

Adequate intake for healthy people over 9 years old is 4.7 g/day. Infants and children younger than 9 years require less potassium per day. More information about potassium and age considerations is at the end of this chapter.

Dietary sources of potassium include apricots, avocado, banana, beans, celery, chocolate, citrus fruits, coffee, cucumbers, dates, dried fruits, kiwi, lima beans, milk, molasses, nuts, peaches, peanut butter, peas, fried potatoes, tomatoes, veal, and yams.

IV Infusion

The kidneys excrete potassium even in the absence of dietary intake. For this reason, if a patient is placed on nothing-by-mouth (NPO) orders or is having any difficulty with ingesting a normal amount of potassium through dietary sources, then hydrating IV fluids will likely be ordered with potassium added. Typically, 20 mEq of potassium is added to a liter of hydrating fluids. Because safety precautions require that potassium be pre-mixed or added by a pharmacist, standard mixtures for hydration are prepared at 20 mEq/L and 40 mEq/L and should always be delivered by IV pump. Potassium diluted at higher concentrations is reserved for electrolyte replacement and must be delivered with precautions, as discussed in the following section on Hypokalemia.

Regulation

Normal regulation of potassium occurs with excretion by the kidney. In a state of low potassium, the kidney excretes less potassium than normal; likewise, in a state of high potassium, the kidney excretes more potassium than normal. An average 70-kg person typically ingests about 70 mEq of potassium per day and excretes the same amount. However, in high potassium states, as long as the kidneys are functioning well, a 70-kg person may excrete up to 700 mEq a day in excess potassium. In low potassium states, the body still excretes about 10–15 mEq per day, which requires that at least this amount must be ingested to avoid hypokalemia.

Potassium regulation by the kidneys is also affected by aldosterone and sodium levels. High potassium levels stimulate excretion of aldosterone.

Aldosterone activates sodium-potassium pumps in the kidney's collecting tubule membrane, which results in potassium losses. High levels of sodium in serum stimulate a higher rate of sodium-potassium exchange in the kidney tubule, also resulting in potassium losses. Increased sodium can also occur during periods of osmotic diuresis, for instance, during diabetic ketoacidosis.

Loss

About 80%–90% of potassium is excreted through urine, with minimal loss from stool and sweat. Abnormal retention occurs most commonly with patients who have renal failure. Although stool losses are normally about 7 mEq/day, this loss can increase when renal excretion is compromised or with states of excess loss of stool, such as diarrhea.

Under normal conditions, a person loses about 2 mEq of potassium a day through sweat. In settings of high sweat loss, however, a person can lose almost 100 mEq per day, averaging 5 mEq/L (to compare, average calcium loss is 1 mEq/L, magnesium 0.8 mEq/L, and chloride 30 mEq/L); the potential for losing such high amounts of potassium puts athletes, patients with uncontrolled fever, and people who exert themselves in hot climates at risk for hypokalemia. Those who are at risk for these losses should be cautious to rehydrate with drinks that contain potassium.

Athletes should consult with trainers and sports medicine specialists when planning for endurance activities because personal characteristics and type of activity can greatly affect losses. People starting exercise regimes or planning recreational or work activities in hot climates should make certain to rehydrate with solutions containing electrolytes and water. The Institute of Medicine recommends solutions that contain 20–30 mEq/L of sodium, 2–5 mEq/L potassium, and 5%–10% carbohydrate. The American College of Sports Medicine's guidelines recommend drinks with about 5%–10% carbohydrates as glucose or sucrose; higher amounts can induce nausea or cramping. Rehydration at the rate of about 1 quart per hour should be offered every 15–20 minutes during strenuous exercise, but this recommendation depends on intensity and duration of exercise and weather conditions.

People who have acclimatized to hot environments may lose less sodium and chloride than those who are newly experiencing them.

Laboratory Measures

Serum levels are drawn to assess for potassium in most inpatient environments as well as frequently during outpatient assessments. In critical care and emergency environments, they may be drawn daily or even hourly, depending on the status of the patient and response to treatment.

The normal potassium serum range for adults is 3.5–5 mEq/L.

Serum Specimen Collection

Serum is collected by phlebotomy in a red-, tiger-top, or green-top heparin tube. Standard phlebotomy procedure requires avoiding blood drawing from the same arm with IV access.

For most accurate results, avoid hand pumping because it can cause hemolysis. Hemolysis and high platelet counts can cause falsely elevated potassium counts. High white blood cell counts of more than 100,000 or an insulin injection right before specimen collection can cause falsely low potassium serum levels. Conditions that affect overall electrolyte balance, such as over- or underhydration, can interfere with obtaining accurate test results.

To avoid processing errors, ensure that the specimen is delivered according to your laboratory's guidelines.

Potassium Urine

Urine can be collected as a timed or random specimen (see Chapter 6 for methods of clean-catch and 24-hour collections). The normal potassium urine range for adults is 26–123 mEq/24 hours.

Urine excretion typically follows serum levels proportionately, whereby low serum levels result in low urine levels, and high serum levels result in high urine levels. When blood is alkalotic, more potassium is excreted in order to allow for the retention of hydrogen ions, thus shifting the pH back toward neutral. With acidotic blood, more hydrogen ions are excreted, and more potassium is retained.

Elevated urine levels of potassium occur with Cushing's syndrome, diabetic ketoacidosis, high aldosterone levels, and cell destruction. A key symptom of bulimia is elevated urine potassium related to frequent vomiting. Decreased levels are associated with low aldosterone levels, nutritional deficiency, and renal failure.

Hypokalemia

Hypokalemia occurs when the body has a potassium deficit.

Laboratory Values
Serum potassium < 3.5 mEq/L

> **ALERT**
>
> Although serum potassium laboratory values of <4 mEq/L are not strictly defined as hypokalemia levels, for patients with cardiac instability this level or below usually requires treatment.

Basic Concepts

Low potassium levels may be true low levels due to loss or lack of ingestion, or they may be only a reflection of potassium leaving the extracellular compartment and flowing into cells. The latter case is called *redistribution hypokalemia*, and it can occur in the presence of alkalosis or high aldosterone levels. A person with redistribution hypokalemia does in fact have sufficient whole body potassium; the potassium is just being used by cells at a higher rate.

In alkalotic states, potassium moves into cells when hydrogen moves out of cells. For each increase of 0.1 in pH, serum potassium drops about 0.3 mEq/L. A stress response causing sympathetic nervous system stimulation or the use of beta-sympathomimetic drugs can force potassium into cells.

Genetic diseases can be associated with high or low potassium levels, causing periods of paralysis lasting from hours to days. Some of these genetic diseases include familial hypokalemic periodic paralysis and familial thyrotoxic periodic paralysis. These diseases are characterized by high or low blood potassium levels that may return to normal between attacks. Treatment for these genetic diseases is focused on correcting serum potassium levels. Thyrotoxic periodic paralysis has symptoms similar to those of hypokalemic flaccid paralysis, but—unlike hypokalemic flaccid paralysis, in which the treatment focuses on correcting hypokalemia—its treatment centers on thyroid management. Paralysis that involves airway or swallowing requires emergency medical attention for airway support and assessment for potential lethal arrhythmia.

Etiology

Hypokalemia can be caused by:

- Alkalosis, in which potassium moves into cells as hydrogen moves out of cells
- Cushing's disease (hyperaldosteronism), in which aldosterone increases excretion
- Dietary intake or absorption deficiency related to alcoholism, anorexia, or pica (where non-nutrients such as clay are substituted for nutrient foods), especially related to low magnesium ingestion or absorption
- Crohn's disease, low meat or vegetable diet content

- Familial periodic hypokalemic paralysis
- Gastrointestinal (GI) loss: diarrhea, fistula, nasogastric suction, vomiting
- Leukemia
- Renal diseases including tubular acidosis and syndromes such as Bartter's, Cushing's, Fanconi's, and Liddle's
- Sweating in excessive amounts
- Thyrotoxicosis, which increases renal excretion (may be associated with familial thyrotoxic periodic paralysis)
- Iatrogenic losses, including medications such as:
  - Acetazolamide
  - Acetylsalicylic acid
  - Albuterol
  - Aldosterone
  - Ammonium chloride
  - Amphotericin B
  - Bicarbonate
  - Bisacodyl
  - Captopril
  - Cisplatin
  - Dexamethasone
  - Digoxin
  - Diuretics (those taking non-potassium-sparing diuretics are at high risk for hypokalemia)
  - Hydrocortisone
  - Insulin excess
  - Licorice root
  - Penicillin
  - Phosphates
  - Theophylline toxicity

Pseudohypokalemia is a state in which there is enough potassium in the body, but the potassium is diluted by excess fluids. Pseudohypokalemia may occur during:

- Congestive heart failure
- Infusion of IV fluids with no electrolytes
- Overhydration/water intoxication

Symptoms

- **Neurological:** Decreased reflexes, fatigue, lethargy, paresthesias, paralysis, psychosis, delirium, hallucinations, depression

- **Cardiovascular (CV):** Palpitations, rapid or slow heart rates, irregular heart rates, ECG changes (Figure 3E-2), depressed T wave, U wave, ventricular arrhythmias, weak pulse, low blood pressure
- **Respiratory:** Respiratory failure
- **GI:** Thirst, anorexia, vomiting, constipation, ileus
- **Genitourinary:** Polyuria, nocturia
- **Musculoskeletal:** Skeletal or abdominal muscle cramps, weakness, decreased reflexes

Assessment and Actions

Fluid, electrolyte, and acid-base imbalances can rapidly cause life-threatening neurological, cardiac, and respiratory compromise, requiring immediate notification of the medical or rapid response team. Consult the medical team if any new onset occurs or if worsening symptoms or vital signs occur that are outside the normal range. If neurological, respiratory, or cardiac compromise occurs, then call for assistance from the rapid or urgent response team or, if outside an acute care setting, then call community emergency medical services (EMS).

Patient History

Review for clues as to cause. The following conditions may be associated with or cause hypokalemia:

- Acute or chronic metabolic processes, which may result in alkalotic states
- Gastric loss of potassium
- Increased aldosterone levels or thyroid levels, increasing renal excretion

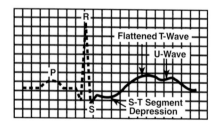

FIGURE 3E-2: Hypokalemia ECG tracing.

- Excessive loss of sweat
- Chronic health problems, such as:
  - Congestive heart failure
  - Cushing's disease
  - Crohn's disease
  - Renal tubular acidosis (hypokalemic)
  - Thyrotoxicosis
- Excess ingestion or infusion of fluids or competitive medications, including diuretics, corticosteroids, aminoglycosides, albuterol, aldosterone, ammonium chloride, amphotericin B, bicarbonate, digoxin, insulin, penicillin, and phosphates
- Teas, herbal preparations, and candies containing licorice that are ingested in large amounts

Laboratory Assessment and Actions

Potassium values < 3.5 mEq/L reflect hypokalemia that may need correction. Patients with cardiac instability may require replacement at 4 mEq/L or below. Anticipate treatment for hypokalemia with symptoms or values < 3.5 mEq/L:

- Anticipate frequent blood potassium, chloride, magnesium, blood urea nitrogen (BUN), creatinine, and urine potassium levels, based on frequency and effect of interventions.
  - Patients with low magnesium levels may not be able to absorb oral potassium.
  - Hypochloremia can be induced if potassium is replaced without sufficient chloride replacement.
  - Decreased renal function can place patients receiving potassium at high risk for hyperkalemia arrhythmias.
  - Continue to monitor potassium levels after replacement because potassium may travel into cells if whole body potassium stores are low.
- Anticipate orders for arterial blood gas measures if the source of hypokalemia is suspected to be related to alkalosis.
- Anticipate orders for continuous cardiac monitoring.
- Anticipate oral administration of potassium:
  - Oral potassium is available in several forms, including potassium acetate, potassium bicarbonate, potassium

COACH CONSULT

Digoxin levels should be measured for patients taking digoxin when hypokalemia is present. Hypokalemia can increase digitalis arrhythmias.

chloride, potassium citrate, potassium gluconate, and combinations of two or more of these forms.

- In most cases, potassium chloride is prescribed, and other forms are used with hyperchloremic acidosis.
- Each form has different levels of potassium and cannot be interchanged with other forms. Therefore, dosing should always be by milliequivilants, not by milligrams.
- Potassium acetate is 10.2 mEq/g, potassium bicarbonate is 10 mEq/g, potassium chloride is 13.4 mEq/g, and potassium gluconate is 4.3 mEq/g.
- Potassium can be given prophylactically at 20–40 mEq/day or for treating hypokalemia at 40–100 mEq/day. Potassium doses >20 mEq will typically be ordered as divided doses.

  - Onset of oral preparations is unknown, peak is 1–2 hours, and duration is unknown.
  - Caution should be used with patients suffering from cardiac or renal disease or upper GI problems and for those taking potassium-sparing diuretics, angiotensin II receptor antagonists, and angiotensin-converting enzyme (ACE) inhibitors. Wax matrix forms of the drug, such as K-Dur, should be used with caution for patients also taking anticholinergics because the combination can lead to GI lesions.
  - Patients with nausea or vomiting may not tolerate drinking fluids until electrolytes have been corrected. In these cases, IV fluids must be introduced to reverse fluid and electrolyte losses before introducing oral fluids.

- Anticipate IV administration containing potassium if oral administration is not effective.
  - Potassium chloride arrives to the nursing unit diluted in normal saline, dextrose solution, or lactated Ringer's solution.

COACH CONSULT

All IV electrolyte solutions should be administered via an intravenous infusion pump or controller. Additional safeguards include multiple small-volume IV bags and volume control sets for intermittent administration.

ALERT

Potassium is never given by IV push or as a bolus drug because both types of administration can be fatal. For this reason, potassium should never be drawn up from a vial or mixed on a nursing unit. Potassium vials are marked as high-alert medications, typically either with black caps or black stripes.

Due to the high-alert nature of this drug, potassium should not be mixed on the nursing unit. Instead, it should be prepared by a pharmacist, or pre-mixed solutions should be used. These solutions should be infused via large-bore IV (18- to 16-gauge) or central line access. Concentrations for peripheral lines should not be >40 mEq/L, with a rate not faster than 10 mEq/hr through a peripheral line for adults. Rates of 20 mEq/hr may be approved for central line infusion as long as the patient is on continuous cardiac monitoring.

- Potassium acetate can cause aluminum toxicity for patients with renal problems.
- Reevaluate patient's condition after 20 mEq of solution. Frequent, rapid serum laboratory samples should be drawn.
- Rate should not be >10 mEq/hr through a peripheral line or 20 mEq/L through a central line, for patients receiving continuous cardiac monitoring.
- Onset is within minutes.
- Peak is at the end of the infusion.

COACH CONSULT

Periodic hypokalemic paralysis and periodic hyperkalemic paralysis are chronic genetic illnesses. They are not true hyper- or hypokalemia but rather incorrect distributions between intracellular and extracellular potassium.

Systems Assessment and Actions

If laboratory test results are pending but hypokalemia is suspected, proceed with a systems assessment. Immediately consult the medical team at the onset or worsening of any of the symptoms that are listed in the following section.

Neuro-Musculo-Skeletal

If fatigue, lethargy, parathesias, or signs of paralysis are present, then:

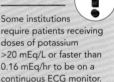

ALERT

Some institutions require patients receiving doses of potassium >20 mEq/L or faster than 0.16 mEq/hr to be on a continuous ECG monitor.

- Anticipate frequent measures of neurological status using the Glasgow Coma Scale.
- Maintain safety measures including keeping the bed low, padded side rails in place, and the call bell within reach.
- Continually reevaluate the patient's ability to follow instructions.
- Consult the medical team to discuss need for one-on-one supervision.
- Institute safety precautions, and assist with all activities of daily living, transfers, and ambulation.

If lethargy or paralysis is severe, anticipate rapid correction of hypokalemia and respiratory support.

If delirium, hallucinations, or other mental status changes occur, provide close supervision, monitoring the patient for intolerance of IV lines or other medically necessary devices.

CV

If ECG changes or cardiac symptoms develop, anticipate orders for continuous cardiac monitoring, and consult the medical team to determine the best monitoring leads and alarm settings for cardiac monitoring to observe for T-wave and U-wave changes.

If hypotension or low pulse develops, place patient on bedrest, and anticipate orders for IV fluid support with potassium.

Respiratory

If respiratory insufficiency develops, then:

- Measure oxygen saturation, and anticipate orders for supplemental oxygen and continuous respiratory monitoring.
- Raise the head of the bed to facilitate airway clearance.
- Keep respiratory support equipment available (ambu-bag, suction, oral airway, suction equipment, and oxygen).

GI

If thirst occurs, anticipate orders for fluid replacement with potassium in solution to prevent increasing hypokalemia.

If signs of constipation occur, carefully assess bowel sounds for signs of ileus, including hyperactive and hypoactive bowel sounds:

- Caution should be exercised to limit laxatives that may cause further loss of potassium.
- Anticipate orders for NPO status until decreased bowel motility is resolved.

If nausea or vomiting is present, then:

- Anticipate administration of antiemetics as ordered.
- Communicate the need to all ancillary staff for accurate intake and output measures. GI symptoms may not resolve until electrolytes are stable, despite use of antiemetics.
- Protect the patient from aspiration by keeping the head of the bed at 30°.
- Keep suction equipment available.

GU

If excess urine loss is observed, then:

- Carefully measure fluid volumes. More than 125 mL/hr without concurrent volume replacement may point to inappropriate diuresis.

- Anticipate repeated urine samples to assess effect of fluid loss on electrolyte imbalance. Collect specimen with caution to avoid contamination with water or soap. If drawing from a catheter, draw the urine from the collection tube rather than the collection bag, because the bag is where the urine will start to biologically degrade.

Prevention

Teach at-risk populations:

- Signs and symptoms of hypokalemia, and provide a list of dietary sources.
- Appropriate potassium ingestion, which is about 4.7 g/day for adults.

Patients with a new diuretic prescription should be taught about potassium losses and how to manage urine losses, potassium supplementation, and dietary potassium.

When promoting public health, recall that endurance athletes are at high risk for hypokalemia and should hydrate with fluids that contain

---

 CLINICAL SCENARIO

DIAGNOSIS: HYPOKALEMIA FROM DIURETIC USE

Mr. Sarandon was recently admitted to the hospital with a non–ST-segment elevation myocardial infarction. At 72 years old, this is his first hospital admission and first serious illness. He is very upset with the idea that he will have to make dietary and lifestyle changes and participate in cardiac rehabilitation. The nurse who observes him arguing with his wife about the seriousness of his illness makes sure to provide the couple with Mr. Sarandon's dietary and medication counseling as well as referral to a post–myocardial infarction support group. Mr. Sarandon's new medications include the diuretic furosemide with a potassium supplement of 10 mEq.

At Mr. Sarandon's 3-month follow-up visit with his cardiologist, he reports episodes of nausea and occasional lightheadedness. His laboratory values demonstrate a mild hypokalemia at 3.4 mEq/L. His wife reports that he is inconsistent with eating fruits and vegetables, and she worries that he is not getting enough potassium in his diet. He reports that his blood pressure readings are typically in the range of 120/60, so the physician keeps his diuretic at the same dose but raises his potassium to 20 mEq/day. Mr. Sarandon will also have weekly blood chemistry laboratory samples drawn to monitor for hypokalemia or hyperkalemia. The nurse spends time at this visit assessing and reinforcing teaching and diet planning with Mr. and Mrs. Sarandon.

Continued

1. In addition to nausea and lightheadedness, what other symptoms should Mr. Sarandon be aware of for signs of hypokalemia?
2. Along with samples for potassium levels, which other electrolytes will the medical team be concerned with?
3. What should Mr. Sarandon be instructed to monitor at home, in addition to his blood pressure?

potassium as well as water in a balance based on their estimated sweat loss with exercise. Sports event organizers should provide a balance of electrolyte fluids and water.

Hyperkalemia

Hyperkalemia occurs when the body has an excess of potassium, which can lead rapidly to lethal dysrhythmia.

Laboratory Values
Serum potassium >5 mEq/L

ALERT

Hyperkalemia occurs when serum potassium is >5 mEq. *Critical* hyperkalemia occurs when potassium serum levels are >6.5 mEq/L. High values of potassium can lead to life-threatening arrhythmias.

Basic Concepts
Hyperkalemia is often categorized based on the severity of effect on the heart. Mild is 5.5–6 mEq/L; moderate is 6.1–7 mEq/L; and 7.0 mEq and above is severe or urgent. At 8 mEq/L, cells can no longer repolarize, and asystole occurs. Although hyperkalemia occurs less frequently than hypokalemia, the percentage of death from untreated severe hyperkalemia can be in the range of 67%. Insulin causes potassium to move into cells, putting diabetic patients with low insulin at risk for hyperkalemia. Caution must be used during blood collection because the destruction of blood cells can release potassium into serum and show an erroneous reading of hyperkalemia.

Etiology
Hyperkalemia can be caused by:
- Acidosis, including diabetic ketoacidosis, when potassium leaves cells in exchange for hydrogen ions

- Low aldosterone states from Addison's disease or hypoaldosteronism, causing decreased excretion
- Renal insufficiency or failure; nephritis caused by infections, lupus, or renal transplant rejection, whereby excretion is decreased
- Cellular damage from asthma-related inflammation, burns, red blood cell lysis, leukocytosis, muscle necrosis, rhabdomyolysis, tumor necrosis, or trauma
- Dietary excesses from citrus, bananas, tomatoes, and hidden sources such as salt substitutes
- Insulin deficiency, causing potassium to shift out of cells
- Renal insufficiency, interstitial nephritis, renal obstruction (including from sickle cell disease), or dehydration, whereby excretion is decreased

Iatrogenic causes are common and should be carefully observed, including:

Overinfusion or overingestion of potassium

- Use of salt substitutes containing potassium with low-salt diets
- High-protein diets
- Medications:
  - Any drug that impairs renal function, including aminoglycosides, antibiotics, nonsteroidal anti-inflammatory drugs (NSAIDs), ACE inhibitors, angiotensin receptor blockers
  - Beta blockers shifting potassium out of cells
  - Dexamethasone
  - Digitalis toxicity
  - Diuretics, potassium-sparing
  - Enalapril
  - Mannitol
  - Methicillin
  - Metoprolol, propranolol
  - Succinylcholine

Psuedohyperkalemia occurs when fluid volumes are low. When fluid volumes are low, potassium is more concentrated. Symptoms of pseudohyperkalemia occur with dehydration states.

COACH CONSULT

Hyperkalemia is often not diagnosed by symptoms because symptoms can be vague. Instead, it is more common to suspect hyperkalemia due to the patient's underlying clinical condition or to changes in ECG; hyperkalemia can also be suspected when identified during routine laboratory assessment. Patients with chronically elevated potassium, such as renal patients, may not show symptoms until potassium levels have reached critical levels.

Symptoms

- **Neurological:** Irritability, speech problems, weakness, fatigue, parasthesias, paralysis, tingling lips or fingers
- **CV:** Palpitations, pauses, bradycardia, ECG changes (Fig. 3E-3) of peaked tented T waves, elevated ST segments, prolonged QT waves, widened QRS complexes, diminished to absent P waves, slow heart rates, ventricular arrhythmias, asystole
- **Respiratory:** Hypoventilation
- **GI:** Diarrhea, abdominal cramps
- **GU:** Decreased urine
- **Musculoskeletal:** Paralysis, decreased deep tendon reflexes, weakness

Assessment and Actions

Fluid, electrolyte, and acid-base imbalances can rapidly cause life-threatening neurological, cardiac, and respiratory compromise, requiring immediate notification of the medical or rapid response team. Consult the medical team if any new onset occurs or if worsening symptoms or vital signs occur that are outside the normal range. If neurological, respiratory, or cardiac compromise occurs, call for assistance from the rapid or urgent response team or, if outside an acute care setting, call community EMS.

Patient History

Review for clues to causes of hyperkalemia. The following conditions may be associated with or cause it:

- Acute or chronic metabolic process such as:
  - Acidotic state
  - Dehydration
  - Diabetic ketoacidosis, renal acidosis, shock, starvation

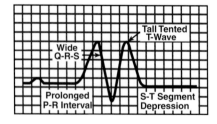

FIGURE 3E-3: Hyperkalemia ECG tracing.

- Cellular damage related to burns, trauma, inflammation, compartment syndrome, or internal hemorrhage
- Infection or sickle cell–induced interstitial nephritis
- Chronic health problems including endocrine diseases may contribute, including:
  - Addison's disease or hypoaldosteronism
  - Diabetes
  - Hyperkalemic familial periodic paralysis
  - Renal insufficiency, especially chronic failure requiring dialysis
- Iatrogenic intervention may be causative, including:
  - Analgesic, antibiotic, diuretic or NSAID-induced interstitial nephritis
  - Medication-induced insufficiency, including potassium insufficiency from digoxin
  - Overingestion of potassium supplementation
  - Tumor lysis from chemotherapy

Laboratory Assessment and Actions

Values >5 mEq/L reflect hyperkalemia that may need correction. Anticipate treatment for hyperkalemia with symptoms or critical values >6.5 mEq/L. Common precautions include frequent blood and urine measures of potassium and key electrolyte levels, and BUN and creatinine based on frequency and effect of interventions.

If the patient has a history of diabetes, then:
- Anticipate frequent blood sugar assessment by finger stick or blood draw or both.
- Anticipate frequent consultation with medical team to manage hyperkalemia with insulin and, potentially, glucose administration. If insulin is ordered intravenously, it should be delivered via programmable pump controller. Only regular insulin is delivered intravenously. If insulin is ordered subcutaneously, keep in mind the onset, peak, and duration of the type of insulin that is ordered, and measure blood sugars to monitor effect of insulins.

If acidosis is suspected, then:
- Anticipate orders for arterial blood gas measures.
- Anticipate consultation with medical team for administration of sodium bicarbonate. IV bicarbonate should be administered via programmable pump controller. It needs to be delivered through a dedicated IV line. If it is ordered as a drip, check

with a pharmacy resource before piggybacking any other medication into the line because sodium bicarbonate is not compatible with most other medications.

- If the patient has a history of taking digoxin, then:
  - Anticipate orders to evaluate serum digoxin level.
  - Observe for signs and symptoms of digoxin toxicity, including slow or irregular pulse, nausea, blurred vision or yellow halos seen around objects. Discuss levels with medical team, and anticipate orders for continuous ECG monitoring.

If arrhythmias are present, then:

- Anticipate consultation with the medical team for administration of IV calcium, unless the patient is receiving digoxin (see Chapter 3A for details on calcium administration). IV administration of calcium may cause hypotension and bradycardia.
- Anticipate orders for IV dextrose and insulin together to push potassium back into cells. Typical doses are 1–2 amps of $D_{50}W$ (25 g of dextrose/amp) and 5–10 units of regular insulin.

If potassium levels are not critical, anticipate orders for oral or rectal administration of polystyrene exchange resin (Kayexalate). Note that:

- 1 g will exchange for 1 mEq of potassium in the intestines. Exchange will begin at 2–12 hours of onset and have a duration of 6–24 hours, with no known peak. Because of the duration of action, patients should be assessed for ongoing signs and symptoms of rebound hypokalemia.
- Typical dose is 15 g four times a day, up to 40 g four times a day. Observe for signs of digoxin toxicity in patients taking digoxin and other electrolyte imbalances related to loss of GI fluids.
- The goal for therapy will be a decrease in serum potassium levels and evidence of one to two watery stools. Sorbitol may be included in the preparation of sodium polystyrene or prescribed concurrently to prevent constipation.
- Rectal preparations are given by retention enema. After instillation and retention for a typical period of 30–60 minutes, anticipate orders for colon irrigation with 1–2 L of nonsodium solution to clear polystyrene and potassium.

If renal failure is the cause of hyperkalemia, then:

- Anticipate orders for hemodialysis (see Chapter 2 for more information on hemodialysis).
- Anticipate a potential sudden shift to lethal dysrhythmia for patients with chronic kidney disease because they may be able to tolerate higher levels of potassium without symptoms for a longer time than patients with acute disease.
- Consult the medical team regarding need for continuous cardiac monitoring and best leads and settings to monitor ECG changes.

Systems Assessment and Actions

If laboratory test results are pending but hyperkalemia is suspected, proceed with a systems assessment. Immediately consult the medical team at the onset or worsening of any of the symptoms that are listed in the following section.

Neuro-Musculo-Skeletal

If weakness, fatigue, or paralysis occurs, then:

- Anticipate frequent measures of neurological status using the Glasgow Coma Scale.
- Maintain safety measures including keeping the bed low, padded side rails in place, and call bell within reach.
- Continually reevaluate the patient's ability to follow instructions.
- Consult the medical team to discuss the need for one-on-one supervision.

If strength assessment demonstrates weakness, then:

- Restrict activity, and institute standard safety measures for all activities of daily living.
- Assist with all transfers and ambulation.

CV

Subtle changes in potassium levels may cause lethal arrhythmias. If rhythm changes or palpitations occur, then:

- Anticipate orders for continuous cardiac monitoring.
- Anticipate communication with the medical team regarding any changes in the ECG tracing that might indicate worsening cardiac status.
- Consult the medical team to determine the best monitoring leads and alarm settings to observe for T-wave and ST-wave changes.

If hypovolemia is causing high concentration of potassium, then:

- Anticipate order for IV fluid administration.
- Watch for signs of hypokalemia and other electrolyte shift from overhydration.

Respiratory

Check for rate and depth of respirations. If deep, shallow, rapid, slow, or irregular breathing or shortness of breath is present, then:

- Measure oxygen saturation, and anticipate orders for supplemental oxygen and continuous respiratory monitoring.
- Raise the head of the bed to facilitate airway clearance.
- Keep respiratory support equipment available (ambu-bag, oral airway, suction equipment, and oxygen).
- Observe for any signs of vocal or airway paralysis.
- Anticipate orders for airway support.

If respiratory rate is slow or respirations are depressed, then:

- Do not leave the patient unmonitored.
- Stimulate the patient to breathe within a normal rate.

GI

If abdominal cramping or diarrhea is present, then:

- Anticipate orders for stool assessment of potential source of diarrhea, including occult blood, bacteria, or parasite.
- Assess the patient for chronic malabsorption disease, food intolerance, and potential ileus.
- Provide hydration with and add electrolytes based on laboratory values, and anticipate orders for medications to slow or stop diarrhea *unless* ileus is suspected. Antidiarrheal medications will aggravate ileus.
- Anticipate orders for volume replacement. Fluid orders are typically based on milliliter-for-milliliter replacement.
- Communicate the need to all ancillary staff for accurate intake and output measures.

GU

If urine output is low, anticipate orders for collection of random urine and 24-hour urine collections (see appendix for specific directions). Measure fluid volumes, and note that < 30 mL/hr may point to renal insufficiency.

If renal insufficiency is evident, anticipate administration of IV diuretics with frequent monitoring for elevations in BUN and creatinine. Communicate the need to all ancillary staff for accurate intake and output measures.

If severe insufficiency is present, anticipate hemodialysis. Collect the specimen with caution to avoid contamination with water or soap. If drawing from a catheter, make certain to draw urine from the collection tube rather than the collection bag, because the bag is where the urine will start to biologically degrade.

Prevention

Teach at-risk populations the signs and symptoms of hyperkalemia. Also teach:

- Appropriate dietary intake: < 50 mEq of potassium/day for those at risk of hyperkalemia
- High-potassium foods to avoid and ways to decrease potassium in foods, such as rinsing peeled potatoes before eating
- Food choices that are low in potassium, which include applesauce, asparagus, blackberries, green or yellow beans, cauliflower, cucumbers, corn, grapes, and tangerines

To promote public health:

- Ensure that water with low mineral levels is available for hemodialysis.
- Reinforce Red Cross standards for blood transfusion safety to prevent lysis of red blood cells.
- Counsel patients to prevent extension of renal disease by managing high blood pressure and diabetes.

 CLINICAL SCENARIO

DIAGNOSIS: HYPERKALEMIA FROM LACK OF COMPLIANCE RELATED TO CHRONIC RENAL FAILURE

Mrs. Hapman is a 75-year-old patient with chronic diabetes and hypertension who has recently descended into dialysis-dependent renal failure after an infection that required high doses of antibiotics. During the beginning of her treatment with dialysis, she is hospitalized for implantation of a short-term central catheter and establishment of an arteriovenous fistula. After her hospital stay, she begins outpatient dialysis at a freestanding community center.

Three times a week, Mrs. Hapman's daughter drives her and picks her up from the center for her 3 hours of treatment. At the center, Mrs. Hapman receives counseling from nurses, social workers, and a dietitian on medications, lifestyle, and dietary modifications to manage her disease. She then requires re-hospitalization for removal of the short-term catheter after her fistula has matured.

After the resumption of her regular dialysis treatments, the nurse notes that Mrs. Hapman's potassium and phosphorous levels are consistently higher than goal. After discussion with Mrs. Hapman, the nurse learns that Mrs. Hapman is depressed and states that she has no interest in limiting her diet and does not want to take her phosphorous binders when she is eating in public. The nurse calls a team meeting and plans for a discussion with Mrs. Hapman and her daughter for decision making around the long-term management of her disease and treatment options, including monitoring of symptoms of electrolyte imbalance, fluid management, and transplantation.

Continued

CLINICAL SCENARIO—cont'd

1. In addition to fatigue, parasthesias, and abdominal discomfort, what other symptoms of hyperkalemia should Mrs. Hapman and her daughter become familiar with?
2. Why are patients with renal disease at risk for high levels of potassium?
3. What foods should the nurse caution Mrs. Hapman about?

Cautions for Special Populations

Pediatrics

The normal ranges of potassium serum levels for pediatric patients are:
- Newborn: 3.7–5.9 mEq/L
- Infant: 4.1–5.3 mEq/L
- Child: 3.4–4.7 mEq/L

Pediatric Dietary Intake (USDA/Adequate Intake)

Pediatric dietary intake (USDA/adequate intake) of potassium is:
- 1–3 years: 3 g/day
- 4–8 years: 3.8 g/day

Healthy breastfed infants should meet dietary requirements through normal human milk intake.

Geriatrics

The Geriatric Dietary Intake (FDA/adequate intake) for adults 50+ years of age is 4.7 g/day. Intake is the same for adults age 14 years and older as it is for seniors.

Review Questions

1. Why should IV potassium never be given as a bolus injection?
2. If a patient presents with or develops dehydration under the nurse's care, how should standing orders for a daily dose of potassium be managed?

3F **Sodium**

Sodium

I n nature, sodium does not appear in an unbound, elemental form. Because sodium is highly soluble in water, most sodium appears in seawater as a sodium chloride compound. Sodium also commonly occurs as sodium bicarbonate, known as *soda,* and as sodium borate, called *borax.*

In the body, sodium is the major positively charged ion (cation) in extracellular fluid (ECF), normally 135–145 mEq/L. For a 70-kg (154-lb) person this is about a total of 50 g. Minimal amounts of sodium, approximately 12 mEq/L, are found intracellularly.

Sodium distribution is closely linked to ECF balance, so it is essential to know the patient's hydration status when determining the cause and care for low sodium states in the blood (hyponatremia) or high sodium states in the blood (hypernatremia). Some problems are directly related to sodium regulation, whereas others stem from fluid regulation. Over- or undercorrection of abnormal sodium levels can cause significant problems that are similar to the problems caused by the underlying fluid imbalance.

Functions

Sodium has many functions in the body. For example, it creates most of the osmotic pressure of ECF, which helps to regulate blood pressure; it influences renal excretion of water; and it participates in acid-base balance. Sodium also regulates chloride levels, initiates neuromuscular reactions, and creates an electrostatic charge in opposition to potassium.

Creates Most of the Osmotic Pressure of ECF

Sodium cations combine with the anions chloride and bicarbonate to create most of the osmolality in ECF, thus maintaining blood pressure. When sodium is pumped out of cells by the sodium-potassium pump, water tends to follow sodium out of the cell.

Influences Renal Excretion of Water

As blood flows through the kidneys, molecules and electrolytes are filtered out into the kidneys' filtration system due to normal blood pressure. This fluid is called *renal filtrate,* and it consists of amino acids, glucose, urea, uric acid, and electrolytes. The kidneys are able to reabsorb many of these substances back into the bloodstream. This reabsorption is based on physiological need for these substances. Reabsorption of sodium is regulated by the renal excretion of the hormone renin and requires active transport. Renin stimulates the production of the hormones angiotension II and aldosterone, which regulate how much sodium is reabsorbed. Water follows sodium back into the interstitial space because of the osmotic pressure that sodium exerts over water.

Participates in Acid-Base Balance

In the kidney, sodium and hydrogen are exchanged between tubular fluid in the lumen of the proximal-collecting tubule in a process called Na^+-H^+ counter transport. A sodium ion is transported into cells, and a hydrogen ion is exchanged from the cell and into the renal filtrate. This exchange lowers the number of hydrogen ions in the cell, thus decreasing the cell's acidity.

Regulates Chloride Levels

When sodium ions move from renal tubules into the bloodstream, the blood becomes more positively charged. This positive charge allows chloride and bicarbonate, which are negatively charged, to follow sodium out of the renal filtrate and into the blood.

Once sodium and chloride are released from the renal tubules into the bloodstream, they rely on each other to reach their next destination. Sodium is actively transported into the proximal tubule, and chloride is actively transported into the ascending tubule. Therefore, if sodium is needed in the ascending tubule, it can follow the actively transported chloride to the ascending tubule. Likewise, if chloride is needed in the proximal tubule, it can follow actively transported sodium to that destination.

Initiates Neuromuscular Reactions

Proteins in the cellular membrane form channels that allow for sodium transport across the cellular membrane. In neurological and muscle cells, action potentials are linked to sodium transport through the channels and the change of the electric gradient of the cell. Cells that are regulated by voltage-gated sodium channels include central and peripheral neurons, heart and skeletal muscles, adrenal gland cells, and kidney cells. See Figure 3F-1 for activity of sodium at the neurological synapse.

Creates an Electrostatic Charge in Opposition to Potassium

Sodium and potassium create an electrostatic charge on nerve and muscle tissue that transmits signals for contraction. The sodium-potassium pump, Na^+/K^+ ATPase, which helps return cells to a resting charge, was discovered in 1950 by scientists who later won the Nobel Prize in chemistry. This enzyme pumps two potassium ions out of a cell in exchange for three sodium ions pumped into the cell.

Intake

In healthy patients, sodium intake is through dietary sources. However, patients who are admitted to acute-care facilities may occasionally require sodium supplementation through intravenous (IV) infusion in the form of sodium chloride or saline. Although low concentrations of sodium

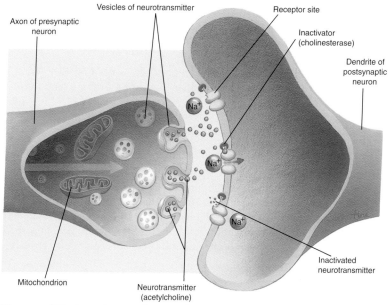

Figure 3F-1: Sodium at the neurological synapse.

solution, like 0.45% and 0.9% saline, are prescribed for routine hydration and fluid balance, higher concentrations, such as 3% saline, are only given during low-sodium states in emergency situations. When these higher concentrations are required, special precautions are essential and are detailed in the later section on hyponatremia.

Dietary Intake

One teaspoon of table salt (NaCl) (or 5 mL) contains about 2.3 grams of sodium. Adequate intake for people 9–50 years old is 1.5 g/day, according to the United States Department of Agriculture. However, the American Heart Association cautions that patients with high blood pressure need less than 1.5 mg/day, or about half a teaspoon. Proper sodium intake for infants and geriatric patients is at the end of this chapter.

Dietary sources include table salt, baking soda (sodium bicarbonate), monosodium glutamate, and salted, pickled, or canned foods. Patients with lower sodium requirements are encouraged to read food labels to identify hidden sources of sodium because it is used to prepare many foods.

IV Infusion

Sodium chloride is commonly used for hydration in the form of hypotonic, half-normal saline solution or 0.45% sodium chloride; 0.45% saline may also be ordered as treatment for hyperosmolar hyperglycemic nonketotic syndrome.

Isotonic, normal saline, which is 0.9% saline, is used for ECF volume expansion or fluid maintenance, to flush or prime IV tubing, and to treat metabolic alkalosis.

Hypertonic saline of 3% or 5% is only used with extreme caution and is usually restricted to critical care or emergency settings. See cautions in the section on hyponatremia.

Irrigation Solutions

Normal or half-normal saline solutions are used to irrigate wounds or flush tubes, including nasogastric tubes, Foley catheters, and gastric tubes. Most institutions require physician orders or standing orders for irrigation with any solution. Although irrigation solutions are not meant to be absorbed, unintended absorption can occur and sodium levels can rise as a result.

Regulation

Sodium levels in serum are regulated along with osmolarity by thirst and baroreceptor mechanisms, hormone secretion, and renal excretion. When osmoreceptors in the hypothalamus sense that osmolarity has risen above normal levels because of elevated sodium levels or other particles, they stimulate the release of antidiuretic hormone (ADH). The kidneys, stimulated by ADH, reabsorb water, making urine more concentrated and serum less concentrated. This change in osmolarity also stimulates thirst, causing increases in free water ingestion, if water is available.

Aldosterone is also involved in sodium regulation. When low serum volume stimulates the renin-angiotension-aldosterone cascade—which is the hormone system that regulates fluid and blood pressure balance—the kidneys absorb sodium, and free water reabsorption follows sodium. Kidneys also respond to hypovolemic and hypervolemic states by excreting or retaining sodium and free water in response to hormonal stimulation.

Loss

About 90%–95% of sodium is excreted through urine, with less than 5% lost from stool with normal intake levels. Sodium loss from sweat is 0.025–8.7 g/day; the amount of sweat lost depends on intake, rate of sweating, and heat. Sodium concentration in sweat decreases with decreased available dietary sodium. In healthy individuals, sodium loss is equivalent to sodium intake.

Laboratory Measures

Serum levels are drawn to assess for sodium levels during routine chemistry evaluations as part of a basic metabolic panel, called chem 7. Normal serum sodium range is 135–145 mEq/L.

COACH CONSULT

Atrial natriuretic peptide is secreted in response to hypervolemia, which stimulates several changes in the kidneys, including inhibiting renin and aldosterone secretion, decreasing sodium reabsorption, and increasing glomeruler filtration rate by stimulating dilation and constriction of glomerular vessels.

Serum Specimen Collection
Serum is collected by phlebotomy in a red- or tiger-top tube. Standard phlebotomy procedure requires avoiding drawing blood from the same arm that has IV access. It is particularly important to avoid contamination of the specimen by infused or instilled NaCl. To avoid processing errors, ensure that the specimen is delivered according to your laboratory's guidelines.

Hyponatremia

Hyponatremia occurs when the body does not have enough sodium.

Laboratory Values
- Serum sodium < 135 mEq/L

Basic Concepts

Low sodium levels may be true low levels due to loss or lack of ingestion/infusion, or they may be only a reflection of hemoconcentration. Extracellular hyponatremia can be caused by high levels of solutes, such as mannitol or sorbitol, that pull fluid into the vascular space; extracellular hyponatremia can also be caused by patients who ingest water while they are receiving hypotonic IV solutions, because water ingestion dilutes sodium levels. Intracellular hyponatremia can be caused if fluid is pulled into cells. In clinical settings, intracellular hyponatremia cannot be measured, so serum hyponatremia must be evaluated along with an understanding of the patient's overall fluid balance.

Hyponatremia causes symptoms when low levels of sodium in ECF cause an osmotic shift of fluid intracellularly. Brain cells cannot accommodate the influx of fluid because of the restriction of the skull. Swelling of brain cells causes pressure in the brain that impairs neurological function. For this reason, critical symptoms associated with hyponatremia are typically neurological. Slow shifts toward hyponatremia can typically be accommodated by brain cells, but acute shifts can cause coma or death. Shifts of chronic hyponatremia can stimulate seizures and are associated with cerebral pontine

🗣 NURSE TO NURSE TIP

Hyponatremia can be chronic or acute. *Chronic* is defined by long-standing hyponatremia of more than 48 hours, and it is associated with sodium levels 120–125 mEq/L. Patients with long-standing hyponatremia can typically tolerate low sodium with less cerebral edema than patients with acute or less than 48 hours of low sodium. *Acute* is defined by low sodium states occurring over less than 48 hours. Those with acute hyponatremia may suffer death from brainstem herniation and compression of the mid-brain. Those with chronic hyponatremia may suffer death from status epilecticus or cerebral pontine myelinolysis/demyelination at sodium levels less than 120 mEq/L. However, chronic hyponatremia must be reversed slowly to prevent CPM during return of sodium levels to normal.

myeinolysis (CPM), in which brain nerve cells lose their protective myeline covering. Acute hyponatremia is defined as less than 48 hours in duration, and chronic shifts are defined as occurring over more than 48 hours.

Etiology

There are four types of hyponatremia: hypervolemic, euvolemic, hypo-volemic, and pseudohyponatremia.

Hypervolemic Hyponatremia

Hypervolemic hyponatremia is caused when excess fluid dilutes sodium concentration. Excess ingestion of fluids and excess fluid retention are two possible reasons for hypervolemic hyponatremia. Examples of patients who experience hyponatremia because of excess ingestion of fluids include:

- Endurance athletes, such as marathon or triathlon runners, who lose sodium through sweat and replenish with water instead of electrolyte fluids
- Fad dieters, who may consume excess water and restrict salt intake
- Patients with psychiatric or developmental delay–associated psychogenic polydipsia, who drink dangerously excessive amounts of water
- Heavy beer drinkers with malnutrition
- Recreational drug users of the substance MDMA, also known as ecstasy

Examples of states that cause excess fluid retention include:

- Congestive heart failure (CHF)
- Liver disease
- Low protein states
- Renal insufficiency or failure or nephrotic syndrome
- Syndrome of inappropriate antidiuretic hormone (SIADH); SIADH can also cause euvolemic hyponatremia

Euvolemic Hyponatremia

Euvolemic hyponatremia is caused when normal fluid volumes contain low sodium; this state can also be described as "low sodium osmolarity in ECF." Chronic health conditions and iatrogenic losses are the usual causes of euvolemic hyponatremia. Examples of chronic health conditions that cause low sodium osmolarity in ECF are:

- Cancers, including nasopharyngeal, gastrointestinal (GI), ureter, prostate, or uterus
- Addison's disease
- Hypothyroidism

- GI diseases
- Infections of the central nervous system
- Lung diseases, such as asthma, pneumonia, tuberculosis, or pulmonary abscess
- Trauma

Examples of iatrogenic losses that could cause euvolemic hyponatremia are those associated with:

- Surgical patients treated with hypotonic solutions
- Patients receiving irrigation fluids for wounds or gastric lavage

Hypovolemic Hyponatremia

Hypovolemic hyponatremia is present when sodium and fluids are lost together, causing low overall body sodium and normal to low sodium osmolarity in fluid. This can be associated with acute or chronic problems and with iatrogenic causes. Examples of patients with acute or chronic problems include:

- Those with cerebral salt-wasting syndrome (CSWS) secondary to traumatic brain injury, subarachnoid hemorrhage, or intracranial surgery
- Patients with a fever
- Women who are lactating
- GI patients with acute or chronic vomiting or diarrhea
- Athletes who lose sodium and water through sweat and do not replace either
- Travelers unaccustomed to hot weather, humidity, or high altitudes who lose sodium and water
- People living in poverty who lose sweat during excessive heat exposure and do not have access to clean water

Examples of patients with iatrogenic causes include:

- Patients on "nothing by mouth" status with insufficient fluid and sodium replacement
- Patients taking diuretics and low-salt diet, causing water and salt losses
- Patients held on an inappropriate fluid restriction

Pseudohyponatremia

Pseudohyponatremia is a state in which sodium and fluid are near normal but fluid has shifted intravascularly. It commonly occurs:

- In patients with massive hyperlipidemia, hyperproteinemia, or hyperglycemia, which causes intravascular fluid retention
- In patients who are receiving glucose infusions, which pulls fluids into the vascular space

Medications associated with low sodium states include:

- Amphotericin B
- Bicarbonate
- Diuretics
- Fluoxetine
- Cathartics or laxatives
- Nicardipine
- Theophylline

Symptoms

Symptoms include:

- **Neurological:** Confusion, headache, irritability, lethargy, seizures, decreased consciousness, coma related to brain swelling, pupil changes to dilation, fixed nonreactive state, decorticate or decerebrate posturing, respiratory arrest, or lethal hypertension
- **Cardiovascular (CV):** Symptoms may point either to hypovolemia or hypervolemia; hypovolemia correlates with tachycardia, decreased skin turgor, dry or cracked tongue, or hypotension; hypervolemia correlates with peripheral or lung edema, moist cough or shortness of breath, jugular venous distention, ascites, or rapid weight gain
- **Respiratory:** Respiratory depression
- **GI:** Anorexia, nausea, vomiting related to brain swelling
- **Genitourinary (GU):** Increased or decreased urinary losses depending on hypervolemic or hypovolemic state
- **Musculoskeletal:** Muscle weakness, spasms, cramping, or pain associated with rhabdomyolysis

AGE-RELATED IMPLICATIONS

Small children can become easily dehydrated and lose sodium much faster than adults. Consult a healthcare provider when fever, diarrhea, or vomiting occurs.

ALERT

Hyponatremia symptoms may be related to acute brain swelling. Chronic hyponatremia may be asymptomatic until sodium drops to as low as 110 mEq/L. Patients with acute hyponatremia typically develop neurological symptoms at levels at or near 120 mEq/L.

Assessment and Actions

Fluid, electrolyte, and acid-base imbalances can rapidly cause life-threatening neurological, cardiac, and respiratory compromise, requiring immediate notification of the medical or rapid response team. Consult the medical team if any new onset occurs or if worsening symptoms or vital signs occur that are outside the normal range. If neurological, respiratory, or cardiac compromise occurs, call for assistance from the rapid or urgent response team or, if outside an acute care setting, call community emergency medical services (EMS).

Patient History

Review for clues as to cause. The following conditions may be associated with or cause hyponatremia:

- Acute or chronic metabolic processes may result in hyponatremia including CSWS, diarrhea, eosinophilia, high potassium states, hyperlipidemia, hyperproteinemia, infections, lactation, low blood pressure, lymphocytosis, SIADH, vomiting, excessive sweating from fever or exercise, or lack of renal excretion of water
- Chronic health problems may be associated with hyponatremia, including:
  - Endocrine problems, such as Addison's disease, adrenal insufficiency, hypothyroidism, SIADH
  - Cancers such as nasopharyngeal, GI, uterine, or prostate
  - Chronic heart failure
  - Chronic lung diseases such as asthma or tuberculosis
  - Chronic renal failure
  - Hepatic disease
- Excess ingestion or infusion of low-sodium fluids or competitive medications may result in low sodium levels related to or including:
  - Recent athletic contest or exertion with excessive heat
  - History of mental illness or developmental delay with polydipsia
  - IV fluid infusion with low-sodium osmolarity
  - Recent ingestion of excessive amounts of beer or the drug MDMA (ecstasy)
- Other iatrogenic causes may include:
  - Concurrent fluid and sodium restriction
  - Diuretic use with a sodium restriction
  - Administration of competitive medications
  - Inappropriate restriction of fluids

Laboratory Assessment and Actions

Sodium values <135 mEq/L reflect hyponatremia that may need correction. Anticipate more aggressive, emergent treatment for hyponatremia with symptoms or critical values of < 120 mEq/L because, at this level, hyponatremia can cause brainstem herniation. If sodium levels are < 120 mEq/L, then:

- Anticipate orders for frequent blood sodium levels, based on frequency and effect of interventions.
- Anticipate orders for oral administration of electrolyte replacement if sodium levels are not critical and neurological symptoms are absent or mild.
  - Electrolyte solutions are the most common form of replacement in noncritical situations.
  - Tablets may be ordered to be mixed in a specific ratio of water. Electrolyte tablets typically contain sodium together with potassium, dextrose, and other electrolytes.

MED INFO

Dosing of salt tablets is typically 1–2 g three times per day.

  - Oral sodium is easily absorbed, but the rate of onset, peak, and duration are unknown.
  - If hyponatremia occurs at the same time as low fluid states, anticipate orders to cautiously replace sodium and fluids together.
  - If patients with nausea or vomiting cannot tolerate drinking fluids until electrolytes have been corrected, then IV fluids must be introduced to reverse fluid and electrolytes losses before introducing oral fluids or medications.
- Anticipate orders to administer fluids slowly so that sodium levels are increased from 120–125 mEq/L at a rate of 0.5 mEq/L/hr or 12 mEq/L/day, then gradually increased over 48 hours to normal levels.

ALERT

IV infusion of hypertonic saline is indicated only in extreme cases of hyponatremia and is done slowly and carefully because it can cause CPM. See Box 3F–1 for more details.

- Anticipate orders for continuous oxygen therapy to prevent hypoxia related to potential for CPM.
- Anticipate orders for IV administration containing **isotonic** sodium (0.9% saline) if oral administration is not effective; 1 L of normal, isotonic saline contains 150 mEq of sodium. Although there is less risk of venous irritation from isotonic solutions, it is still essential to observe for signs of

Box 3F–1 **Hypertonic Saline**

Administration of hypertonic saline (3% or 5% saline) may be ordered in emergency or critical care settings where a patient can be closely monitored. Hypertonic saline administration requires special safeguards to prevent CPM (destruction of the myelin sheath of the brain's pons), which is associated with chronic hypernatremia and reversal of chronic hyponatremia.

When hypertonic saline is ordered, anticipate orders for concurrent administration of supplemental oxygen to diminish potential for CPM response; 3% and 5% saline are ordered in low doses of no more than 100-mL bags and must be administered with an IV pump controller; 100 mL of 3% saline contains 50 mEq of sodium; 100 mL of 5% saline contains 83.3 mEq. Rate of infusion should not exceed 1 mEq/kg/hr. For a 70-kg (154-lb) patient, this infusion rate would be no faster than 140 mL/hr of 3% saline or 84 mL/hr of 5% saline. Hypertonic saline requires IV administration via large-bore IV or central line to prevent infiltration.

irritation or leaking at the insertion site to prevent infiltration, especially when high volumes are administered over a short period. See Box 3F–2 for tips regarding isotonic saline infusion.

If critical levels of <120 mEq/L are measured or neurological symptoms are present, then:

- Anticipate orders for transfer of patient to a critical care environment for continuous neurological, respiratory, and cardiac monitoring.
- Initiate safety and seizure precautions including keeping the bed in low position and padded side rails.

Box 3F–2 **Isotonic Saline: Infusion Tips**

When isotonic saline is used to treat low sodium, smaller-gauge IV lines can be used because the rate of infusion should not be greater than 1 mEq/kg/hr. Normal saline is 154 mEq/L, so for a 70-kg (154-lb) patient, this infusion rate would be no more than 454 mL/hr.

Some institutions require that all IV solutions be administered via control pump. However, other institutions have policies that allow for infusion of isotonic or hypotonic saline solution using straight tubing with a control mechanism, such as a roller clamp. Check institutional policies for limits on rate, volume, and tonicity of saline solutions that may be administered without a pump.

Due to the dangers associated with too rapid sodium administration, a programmable pump should be used when correcting low sodium levels.

- Discuss the need for one-on-one continuous observation with the medical team.
- Place emergency respiratory equipment at the bedside, including an ambu-bag, oral airway, and suction equipment.
- Anticipate orders for continuous cardiac monitoring and discuss with the medical team preferred leads and alarm setting for monitoring of sodium-related electrocardiogram changes.
- Anticipate orders for radiological studies to rule out CSWS induced by tumor, hematoma, cerebral lesion, or other causes of confusion.
- Anticipate orders for slow, continuously monitored infusion of hypertonic 3% saline solution.
- Anticipate orders for frequent laboratory draws to assess for raise in sodium levels. An increase of 4–6 mEq/L is typically sufficient to reverse neurological symptoms.

If hypervolemia is the source of low sodium, anticipate conservative treatment of fluid restriction orders. If fluid restriction is ineffective, anticipate the use of Vaprisol (conivaptan) because an arginine vasopressin antagonist is used to increase urine output of free water with little output of sodium.

If high-volume hyponatremia is related to chronic etiology, such as heart failure, liver cirrhosis, or SIADH, anticipate orders for administration of oral Samsca (tolvaptan), which is a selective vasopressin receptor antagonist.

If fasting glucose levels are >99 mg/dL in adults, then:

- Anticipate orders for frequent laboratory studies of glucose, including blood finger stick assessment.
- Anticipate orders to correct glucose levels with subcutaneous regular or aspart insulin.
- Anticipate a sodium increase of 1.6 mEq/L with each decrease of blood glucose by 100 mg/dL.

MED INFO Rx

For arginine vasopressin antagonists like Vaprisol, it is typical for a 20-mg loading dose to be ordered intravenously over 30 minutes, followed by a continuous infusion of 20 mg over 24 hours, then 20 mg/day for 24–72 hours. Doses of up to 40 mg/day may be ordered.

MED INFO Rx

Orders for selective vasopressin receptor antagonists (e.g., Samsca [tolvaptan]) are typically 15 mg PO for initial dosing, with increases to 30 mg after 24 hours and up to 60 mg after 48 hours if necessary. Although this drug is administered orally, it must be started and monitored for effect in a hospital setting to observe for CPM and other effects of sudden increase of sodium levels.

Rebound hypernatremia may occur with treatment of hyponatremia. If reversal of low sodium is too rapid or if neurological symptoms of high sodium develop during administration of IV saline, then:

- Anticipate orders to reverse sodium levels with the administration of hypotonic sodium (0.45% saline) or desmopression. *Note:* Hypotonic saline (0.45%) is not used to treat low sodium and may cause sodium levels to drop further, especially in pediatric populations.
- Anticipate that desmopression DDAVP (an analogue of vasopressin) or vasopressin—antidiuretic hormone that enhances reabsorption of water by the kidneys—may be administered to reverse sodium levels that rise too quickly. (See the section of this chapter on hypernatremia.)

These actions are necessary because serum glucose is measured as part of a chemistry panel to evaluate if hyperglycemia is causing ECF retention and dilution of serum sodium. Serum glucose is collected in a red- or tiger-top tube. For each 100 mg/dL in glucose above normal, sodium levels fall by 1.6 mEq/L.

If urine osmolality levels are >100 mOsm/L, anticipate serum osmolality assessment to help distinguish causes of hyponatremia. This is because urine osmolality levels >100 mOsm/L point to SIADH. The normal serum osmolality range for children and adults is 275–295 mOsm/kg. Low serum osmolality points to hypervolemic causes of low blood sodium, and high serum osmolality points to hypovolemic causes. Serum osmolality samples are also collected in a red- or tiger-top tube.

CLINICAL COACH

SIADH must be distinguished from CSWS. Although both sets of patients present with low sodium, patients with CSWS have dehydration with hypovolemia, and patients with SIADH are typically normal to hypervolemic. Urine sodium with CSWS typically is >100 mEq/L, and in SIADH it is typically >20 mEq/L and <100 mEq/L.

If dehydration is the suspected cause of hyponatremia, the nurse should assess endocrine function and make sure that:

- Thyroid-stimulating hormone and free thyroxine are checked to rule out hypothyroidism
- Cortisol levels are checked for adrenal function, especially if the patient was recently treated with oral steroids

With dehydration states, most electrolytes are concentrated in urine. Sodium, however, is retained by the kidneys as a mechanism to retain water with osmotic pressures that are dependent on sodium. During dehydration states, urine sodium measures are low, but they can be used to assess for causes of dehydration.

- Normal sodium urine levels for adults are 25–50 mmol/L; < 10 mmol/L from a random specimen points to depletion of sodium from outside the kidneys; 10–20 mmol/L points to losses caused by diuretics or GI losses; 20–40 mmol/L points to renal or adrenal causes such as Addison's disease or hypothyroidism; SIADH can produce levels > 20 mmol/L up to > 40 mmol/L; levels > 40 mmol/L may point to acute tubular necrosis, as kidneys are not able to reabsorb sodium.
- Urine sodium is used with serum sodium, serum creatinine, and urine creatinine to estimate whether low urine output is due to dehydration or to kidney dysfunction. This calculation is called the fractional excretion of sodium (see formula in Chapter 6).

Systems Assessment and Actions

If laboratory test values are pending but hyponatremia is suspected, proceed with a systems assessment. Immediately consult the medical team at the onset or worsening of any of the symptoms listed in the following section.

Neuro-Musculo-Skeletal

If serum sodium is < 120 mEq/L or neurological symptoms develop, including lethargy, apathy, decreased consciousness, or seizure activity, then:

- Anticipate frequent measures of neurological status using the Glasgow Coma Scale.
- Anticipate institution of seizure precautions.
- Maintain safety measures including keeping the bed low, padded side rails in place, and the call bell in reach.
- Continually reevaluate the patient's ability to follow instructions.
- Consult the medical team to discuss the need for one-on-one supervision.
- Anticipate orders for antiseizure medications.
- Anticipate orders for radiological examinations to evaluate for brain or brainstem swelling and potential causes in addition to hyponatremia. Check for potential pregnancy before the examination.
- Anticipate orders for hyperventilation with signs of increased intracranial pressure.

CV

If symptoms of moderate dehydration exist, such as dry mucous membranes, tachycardia, decreased skin turgor, thirst, cool extremities, or decreased urine output with a decrease in body weight of <9%, antici-pate orders for oral or slow rehydration with isotonic, 0.9% saline solution.

If symptoms of dehydration or cardiac arrhythmia exist, including neurological changes, weak pulse, sunken eyes, absent tears, skin recoil >2 seconds, prolonged capillary refill, mottled extremities and a weight loss of >9% body weight, then:

- Anticipate orders for IV rehydration with extreme caution and continuous observation.
- Anticipate orders for continuous cardiac monitoring.
- Consult the medical team to determine lead and alarm settings to best monitor for sodium changes.

If symptoms of hypervolemia exist, including pulmonary rales/crackles, S3 cardiac gallop, jugular venous distention, peripheral edema, or ascites, anticipate orders for diuretic by IV infusion (see Chapter 2 for diuresis precautions). Initiate intake and output measures and daily weights to eval-uate for fluid losses or gains.

Respiratory

Check for rate and depth of respirations. If deep, shallow, rapid, slow, or irregular breathing or shortness of breath is present, then:

- Measure oxygen saturation, and anticipate orders for supplemen-tal oxygen.
- Raise the head of the bed to facilitate airway clearance.
- Prepare the patient for chest x-ray to assess for pneumonia, CHF, or pulmonary edema or effusion. Check for pregnancy prior to examination.
- Keep respiratory support equipment available (ambu-bag, oral airway, suction equipment, and oxygen).

GI

If vomiting, volume of suction, or gastric drainage from interventional intubation or fistulas is present, then:

- Measure and document all intake and output.
- Anticipate volume replacement:
  - Fluid orders are typically based on a milliliter-for-milliliter replacement.
  - Communicate need for accurate intake and output measures to all ancillary staff.
- Administer antiemetics as ordered; GI symptoms may not resolve until electrolytes are stable, despite use of antiemetics.

GU

Measure fluid volumes; >125 mL/hr without concurrent volume replacement may indicate inappropriate diuresis; <30 mL/hr may indicate dehydration or renal dysfunction. Anticipate repeated urine samples to assess effect of fluid loss on electrolyte imbalance. Collect specimen with caution to avoid contamination with water or soap. If drawing from a catheter, make certain to draw urine from the collection tube rather than the collection bag, because the bag is where the urine will start to biologically degrade.

Prevention

To prevent hyponatremia, teach at-risk populations:

- The signs and symptoms of hyponatremia
- Appropriate sodium ingestion, and provide a list of dietary sources, including hidden sources
- Appropriate fluid ingestion at 2.7 L/day for nonlactating, nonpregnant, healthy female adults and 3.7 L/day for healthy adult males
- Signs, symptoms, and management of fluid retention, including edema, shortness of breath, and weight gain; daily weights should be measured at the same time of day, on the same scale, with the same amount of clothing (see the hypervolemia section of Chapter 2).

Regarding public health, health professionals can:

- Teach sporting event organizers and athletes that the International Marathon Medical Directors Association publishes guidelines for electrolyte and fluid planning for treatment and events, based on expected energy expenditure. The Institute of Medicine guidelines suggest adequate intake for individuals engaged in recommended levels of physical activity in temperate climates to be 1.5 g/day for healthy males or females 9–50 years of age (less for older than 50 years)
- Educate emergency room personnel to observe for recent ingestion of the recreational drug MDMA (ecstasy) and beer because both are associated with hyponatremia. Beer drinkers with accompanying malnutrition are at risk for dilution of sodium. Recreational drug

AGE-RELATED IMPLICATIONS

Pediatric patients are at higher risk for hyponatremia related to ingestion of inappropriate water. Educate families to replenish fluids lost to vomiting or dehydration with electrolyte solutions instead of free water, and advise caregivers not to dilute infant formula in an effort to stretch nutrition.

DIAGNOSIS: HYPONATREMIA FROM DIABETES AND RENAL INSUFFICIENCY

Mr. Jones is a 35-year-old obese male with a history of poorly controlled diabetes mellitus (hemoglobin HA_{1C}= 18%; renal insufficiency, glomerular filtration rate = 20), and he was recently transferred from the intensive care unit to a medical/surgical unit after being treated for an admission diagnosis of diabetic ketoacidosis (DKA). Mr. Jones is found standing at the bathroom sink ladling handfuls of water into his mouth, stating, "I just need something to drink." On assessment, Mr. Jones is no longer oriented to location or time.

The nurse calls for assistance. After returning Mr. Jones safely to his bed, the nurse obtains vital signs, measures Mr. Jones' Glasgow Coma Scale, and assigns the nursing assistant to take Mr. Jones' capillary blood glucose. The nursing assistant is instructed to stay with Mr. Jones, ensuring that he has no more water intake and that he remains safely in bed.

Mr. Jones' blood glucose is 227. While the nurse awaits laboratory test results to determine probable treatment options, the patient's primary problem is safety. Although the patient has a history of DKA, a blood sugar of 227 makes this diagnosis unlikely. Both DKA and acute hyponatremia can lead to seizures, brainstem herniation, and death. The nurse needs to be alert for other signs of clinical neurological deterioration. Mr. Jones currently has a GCS rating of 14.

1. Based on Mr. Jones' presentation, the nurse suspects that he has hyponatremia. Which IV fluid is anticipated for correction?
2. Based on Mr. Jones' renal history, what symptoms should the nurse consider when infusing ordered fluids?
3. Which objective scales can help the nurse measure Mr. Jones' neurological status?

use stimulates SIADH due to sweating and water ingestion associated with the use of ecstasy.

Hypernatremia

Hypernatremia occurs when the body has too much sodium.

Laboratory Values
- Serum sodium >145 mEq/L

Basic Concepts
Hypernatremia is rare, but it has an accompanying high mortality rate. Cellular changes begin to

occur after 1 hour of high sodium levels, leading to intracranial hemorrhage. Patients with an intact thirst stimulus and access to water can drink sufficient amounts of water, even during states of high undiluted urine production, such as diabetes. High sodium levels may be true high levels due to excess ingestion, or they may be only a reflection of hemoconcentration.

Etiology

High sodium levels may be related to excessive intake, excessive renal retention, or loss of fluids with no accompanying loss of sodium. Increased sodium ingestion is related to diet patterns or limited access to low sodium foods. Increased renal retention/resorption of sodium occurs with azotemia, Cushing's syndrome, and hyperaldosteronism. Hemoconcentration may be related to free water losses from:

- Burns
- Dehydration states, especially when water is not easily accessible
- Fever states in which water is lost in excess of sodium losses
- GI losses from diarrhea, drains, fistula, suction, or vomiting
- Lack of thirst stimulus, often related to aging or hypothalamus lesion
- Urination in excess amounts or unconcentrated urine related to uncontrolled diabetes mellitus, diabetes insipidus, lack of antidiuretic hormone, or kidneys that are resistant to vasopressin

In addition, iatrogenic causes should be carefully considered, including:

- Overinfusion of sodium from hypertonic or isotonic infusions
- Tube feeding with insufficient free water in the regimen
- Medications, including:
  - Anabolic steroids and corticosteroids
  - Angiotension
  - Bicarbonate
  - Carbenoxolone
  - Cisplatin
  - Gamma globulin
  - Mannitol

Euvolemic hypernatremia occurs when fluid is lost from intercellular or interstitial spaces instead of from the vascular space. This is related to central diabetes insipidus or nephrogenic diabetes insipidus. Euvolemic hypernatremia is associated with brain injuries, tumors, vascular or congenital problems, pregnancy, sickle cell anemia, amyloidosis, sarcoidosis, and renal tubular acidosis.

Symptoms

Symptoms include:

- **Neurological:** Lethargy, change in mental status, restlessness, seizures, coma
- **CV:** Poor skin turgor, cracked lips or tongue, low blood pressure, tachycardia
- **Respiratory:** Hyperventilation
- **GI:** Anorexia, nausea, intense thirst, swollen tongue, vomiting
- **GU:** Urine volumes of up to 20 L/day
- **Musculoskeletal:** Weakness, tremors, twitching, hyperreflexia, ataxia

Assessment and Actions

Fluid, electrolyte, and acid-base imbalances can rapidly cause life-threatening neurological, cardiac, and respiratory compromise, requiring immediate notification of the medical or rapid response team. Consult the medical team if any new onset occurs or if worsening symptoms or vital signs occur that are outside the normal range. If neurological, respiratory, or cardiac compromise occurs, call for assistance from the rapid or urgent response team or, if outside an acute care setting, call community EMS.

Patient History

Review for clues as to the cause of hypernatremia. The following conditions may be associated with or cause hypernatremia:

- Acute or chronic metabolic process such as azotemia, dehydration, diarrhea or other
- GI losses, fever, hemoconcentration, lack of thirst stimulus
- Chronic health problems, including endocrine diseases, may contribute, including:
  - Amyloidosis
  - Congenital vascular disorders
  - Chronic kidney disease
  - Endocrine problems, such as Cushing's syndrome, diabetes mellitus, diabetes insipidus, hyperaldosteronism
  - Sarcoidosis
  - Sickle cell anemia
- Iatrogenic intervention may be causative, including:
  - Overinfusion of sodium from IV or tube feeding sources
  - Amphotericin B
  - Bicarbonate administration

- Carbenoxolone
- Cisplatin
- Colchicines
- Furosemide and osmotic diuretics
- Gentamicin
- IV dyes
- Lithium
- Mannitol
- Steroids

Laboratory Assessment and Actions

Serum sodium values >145 mEq/L reflect hypernatremia that may need correction. Anticipate treatment for hypernatremia with symptoms or critical values >160 mEq/L.

If laboratory values of hypernatremia exist:

- Anticipate orders for laboratory measures of electrolytes every 1–2 hours during treatment, then after each liter of fluid or every 4 hours.
- Anticipate close monitoring of intake and output and daily weights.
- Anticipate orders for central nervous system scans to rule out vascular changes.
- Confirm absence of pregnancy before any radiological exams.

If hypernatremia is mild (without critical symptoms), then it may be treated by sodium restriction and oral free water.

If hypernatremia and low fluid volumes are causing symptoms, then:

ALERT

Any treatment of hypernatremia requires extreme caution. When high sodium is treated, water leaving the vascular compartment will return to cells and may cause swelling of brain cells as well as intracranial hemorrhage. Slow, cautious return to normal levels is required to allow cells to return gradually to equilibrium. Goals for correction should be no faster than 1 mEq/L/hr.

- Anticipate consultation with medical team to calculate fluid losses based on total body water and insensible losses.
- Anticipate order to replace fluids gradually over a 48-hour period.
- Anticipate order to replace fluid with IV isotonic, 0.9% normal saline. These fluids stay in the vascular space, whereas hypotonic saline causes intercellular swelling because free water passes into cells.

If symptoms of hypernatremia are not related to low fluid volumes or if hemodynamics have been corrected, anticipate orders to reduce sodium levels with IV infusion with hypotonic 0.45% saline or $D_5W/0.45\%$ (dextrose 5% in half-normal saline).

If elevated sodium occurs with high fluid volumes, anticipate orders for IV infusion of diuretics along with D_5W.

If high sodium and hypervolemia are associated with renal insufficiency or renal failure, anticipate orders for hemodialysis (see the section on hypervolemia in Chapter 2).

If high sodium is related to diabetes insipidus, anticipate consulting the medical team to identify the cause of diabetes insipidus. The nurse should also:

- Anticipate orders to treat central diabetes insipidus with desmopressin by the oral, subcutaneous injection, or nasal spray route to increase reabsorption of water by the kidneys. To prevent dehydration, oral fluid replacement may be ordered at 2.5 L/day or more until the loss is under control.
- Anticipate orders to treat renal diabetes insipidus with salt restrictions and diuretics of the thiazide class.

Systems Assessment and Actions

If laboratory test results are pending but hypernatremia is suspected, proceed with a systems assessment. Immediately consult the medical team at the onset or worsening of any of the symptoms that are listed in the following section.

Neuro-Musculo-Skeletal

Perform frequent neurological assessments for decreased level of consciousness and weakness. Record point scale using the Glasgow Coma Scale (see Chapter 6).

If a bilateral strength assessment demonstrates weakness, restrict activity, and institute standard safety measures for all activities of daily living: bed low, side rails up as appropriate, and call bell in reach. Assess and reassess the patient's ability to follow directions.

CV

If hypovolemia is causing high concentration of sodium, then:

- Prepare for IV fluid administration of hypotonic sodium.
- Watch carefully for signs of rebound hyponatremia and other electrolyte shifts from overhydration.

Respiratory

Check for rate and depth of respirations. If deep, shallow, rapid, or irregular breathing or shortness of breath is present, then:

- Place emergency respiratory equipment at the bedside, including ambu-bag, oral airway, and suction equipment.

- Measure oxygen saturation, and anticipate orders for supplemental oxygen.
- Raise the head of the bed to facilitate airway clearance.

GU
- Measure fluid volumes; < 30 mL/hr may indicate renal insufficiency
- Anticipate repeated urine samples to assess effect of fluid loss on electrolyte imbalance

Prevention

To prevent hypernatremia, teach at-risk populations:
- Signs and symptoms of hypernatremia
- Appropriate sodium ingestion (approximately 1/2 teaspoon per day for adults) and provide a list of dietary sources, including hidden sources; sodium bicarbonate may be a hidden source and should not be prescribed for those at risk for hypernatremia
- Appropriate fluid ingestion at 2.7 L/day for nonlactating, nonpregnant healthy female adults and 3.7 L/day for healthy adult males
- Appropriate dietary intake based on health concerns and medications

Regarding public health:
- Teach new parents that hypernatremia may be associated with poor feeding, especially with premature or low-birthweight infants. Poor feeding is an indication to call the medical team for assessment and support to prevent electrolyte shifts and dehydration.
- Teach caregivers of vulnerable populations to ensure water is accessible and that they are drinking the water that is provided. Monitor disabled people, poorly mobile seniors, and young children to ensure they have sufficient access to water during periods of illness that include fever or GI losses.

 CLINICAL SCENARIO

DIAGNOSIS: HYPERNATREMIA FROM HYPERTHERMIA

Mr. Odam, 76 years old, has a history of mild dementia and mild CHF, with symptoms of dehydration including decreased skin turgor, low blood pressure, and dry mouth and throat. He has been brought to the emergency room by his daughter, who found him in a closed third-story room when she arrived home. Although air conditioning was available, Mr. Odam had not turned it on.

Continued

His skin was dry and hot, and his clothes showed signs of sweating. Although he had clear signs of dehydration, the nurse was uncertain about his sodium status until his tests indicated sodium of 155 mEq/L. His daughter also noted that she had given him his Lasix that morning. She explained to the nurse that, although he did have mild dementia, the change of mental status he was demonstrating on arrival at the emergency department showed an unusual level of confusion.

Once the nurse's suspicions of hypernatremia are confirmed by blood test results, Mr. Odam is started on an isotonic saline drip of 0.9% at 100 mL/hr. Fluid loss calculations have resulted in orders for 5 L over 48 hours at 100 mL/hr.

After a slow infusion of 500 mL, Mr. Odam begins to show less confusion. At 800 mL, he is able to make urine, and after 1000 mL, a second blood test result showed sodium at 148 mEq/L. His samples are measured every 2 hours, then every 4 hours during his treatment. This rate is less than 1 mEq/hr correction, but Mr. Odam has already begun to show improvement in his neurological and cardiovascular symptoms. The nurse consults social work service to discuss alternative care options for Mr. Odam during the day, which is when he is normally home alone. The medical team has scheduled Mr. Odam for a full neurological work-up to rule out any acute or chronic conditions that may be affecting his underlying dementia.

1. When Mr. Odam arrives at the emergency department, his veins are flat and difficult to access. Will the nurse be able to infuse normal saline through a small-gauge IV line?
2. List two factors that placed Mr. Odam at special risk for dehydration and hypernatremia?
3. When providing hydration to Mr. Odam, what symptoms should the nurse be aware of in relationship to his CHF?

Cautions for Special Populations

Pediatrics

The normal ranges of sodium serum levels for pediatric patients are:
- Newborn: 133–146 mEq/L
- Infant: 133–144 mEq/L
- Child is same as adult: 135–145 mEq/L

Healthy breastfed infants should meet U.S. Food and Drug Administration (FDA) dietary requirements through normal human milk intake:
- 0–6 months: 0.12 g/day
- 7–12 months: 0.08 g/day

- 1–3 years: 1 g/day
- 4–8 years: 1.2 g/day
- 9–18 years: 1.5 g/day

Geriatrics

Geriatric dietary intake of sodium is (FDA/adequate intake):
- 51–70 years: 1.3 g/day
- 70 years: 1.2 g/day

Review Questions

1. Low sodium can be associated with excess free water. Which populations are at risk for this type of hyponatremia?
2. What is the danger from too rapid infusion of sodium?
3. Why is 0.45% hypotonic saline not used to correct low sodium levels?
4. Why is slow, cautious correction of hypernatremia at a rate of 1 mEq/L/hr necessary?
5. What are some hidden sources of sodium in the diet?
6. What pattern is a key symptom of diabetes insipidus?

3G Minerals

Essential Minerals and Elements

I n addition to the effects of electrolytes, certain minerals and elements also have an effect on a patient's health and well-being. Examples of essential minerals include: boron, chromium, copper, fluoride, iodine, iron, manganese, molybdenum, selenium, and zinc. Each of these elements is discussed in this chapter.

The impact of these elements on acute and chronic health status is understood to some extent, but it is also under intense study by health and nutritional researchers. This chapter provides a general overview of minerals and elements as related to the current studies listed in the References section at the end of this book.

Even though the full effect of under- or overingestion of these minerals is not fully understood, nutritional pharmacists formulate medically prescribed nutritional supplements and parenteral nutrition to provide for the United States Department of Agriculture (USDA) adequate daily intake (ADI) values; ADI values for the minerals discussed are in Table 3–1. In some cases, the medical team may also prescribe supplements at higher or restricted amounts to account for losses through disease process.

Essential minerals can be lacking in patients with poor diets, inadequate absorption, or chronic illness states. Modified diets, including vegetarian diets, may not be planned adequately to include all essential micronutrients.

The American Dietetic Association recommends education of patients and caregivers to ensure adequate dietary intake. Some foods are bio-fortified with these minerals, and others may also be fortified with substances that promote the absorption of minerals, such as beta-carotene polypeptides.

Table 3–1 USDA ADI Amounts

AGE/SEX	CHROMIUM (mcg/day)		COPPER (mcg/day)	FLUORIDE (mg/day)		IODINE (mcg/day)	IRON (mg/day)		MANGANESE (mg/day)		MOLYBDENUM (mcg/day)	SELENIUM (mcg/day)	ZINC (mg/day)	
	M	F	M & F	M	F	M & F	M	F	M	F	M & F	M & F	M	F
0–6 MO	0.2	0.2	200	0.01	0.01	110	0.27	0.27	0.003	0.003	2	15	2	2
7–12 MO	5.5	5.5	220	0.5	0.5	130	11	11	0.6	0.6	3	20	3	3
1–3 Y	11	11	340	0.7	0.7	90	7	7	1.2	1.2	17	20	3	3
4–8 Y	15	15	440	1	1	90	10	10	1.5	1.5	22	30	5	5
9–13 Y	25	21	700	2	2	120	8	8	1.9	1.6	34	40	8	8
14–18 Y	35	24	890	3	3	150	11	15	2.2	1.6	43	55	11	9
19–30 Y	35	25	900	4	3	150	8	18	2.3	1.8	45	55	11	8
31–50 Y	35	25	900	4	3	150	8	18	2.3	1.8	45	55	11	8
51–70 Y	30	20	900	4	3	150	8	8	2.3	1.8	45	55	11	8
>70 Y	30	20	900	4	3	150	8	8	2.3	1.8	45	55	11	8

MO = months; Y = years; M = male; F = female; M & F = male and female

Source: United States Department of Agriculture, National Library of Agriculture, Food and Nutrition Information Center, Dietary Guidance, Dietary Reference Intakes, DRI tables

Available: http://www.iom.edu/Global/News%20Announcements/~/media/48FAAA2FD9E74D95BBDA2236E7387B49.ash

Nutrition researchers also seek to reduce the presence of food elements that can interfere with absorption of essential micronutrients. For instance, iron can decrease zinc and copper levels, and zinc can reduce iron and copper; fiber additives can compete with calcium absorption. Although these absorption blockers are still being studied, it is important to be aware that highly processed foods may be interfering with absorption when mineral loss is apparent in patients.

Short- and long-term toxicity can be caused by overingestion or overabsorption of minerals from respiratory or integumentary exposures. For example, exposure to copper, iron, and manganese in industrial settings has been linked to greater incidence of Parkinson's disease.

Boron

The periodic table denotes boron by the letter B and the atomic number 5. Boron has a number of industrial uses and is an essential biological element in plants. The National Institutes of Health (NIH) report that boron may have a role in calcium absorption and estrogen metabolism.

Adequate Intake
According to the NIH, investigations of boron in humans have yielded only uncertain scientific evidence for the use of boron as a supplement. Therefore, there is no adequate intake information for boron.

Dietary Sources
Boron is found in avocados, nuts, peanut butter, and prune juice.

Adverse Effects of Inadequate Consumption
Adverse effects are currently unknown.

> **ALERT**
>
> Boron is sometimes used as a traditional remedy for skin or vaginal applications, for cleaning baby pacifiers, and for diaper rash. It has been associated with fatality in infants. If boron exposure is suspected, contact the National Poison Control Center: 1-800-222-1222.

Adverse Effects of Excess Consumption
Excess boron is usually excreted. However, exposure to excess boron on the skin or in the mouth may cause acidosis, abdominal pain, agitation, diarrhea or vomiting of a blue-green color, fever, hypotension, lethargy, rash, seizure, tremors, weakness, and even death. Note that death is more typical among small children or infants. Excess boron may lower insulin levels and interfere with medications that are cleared through the kidney.

Sensitivity
Sensitivity is currently unknown.

Chromium

The periodic table denotes chromium by the symbol Cr and the atomic number 24. Chromium is a tasteless and odorless metal. Chromium at the oxidation state of $+3$, trivalent chromium (chromium III), is required by humans as a trace element, because it is the active ingredient in glucose tolerance factor, a compound that helps insulin bring glucose from blood into cells. Chromium III is found in compounds used to treat diabetes. Several valent forms are used for industrial purposes; chromium VI, or hexavalent chromium, with an oxidation state of VI, is toxic and carcinogenic.

Adequate Intake
Recommended levels are age- and sex-specific (see Table 3–1). Women who are pregnant need 29–30 mcg/day, depending on age. Lactating women need 44–45 mcg/day, depending on age.

Function
Chromium is essential for glucose and lipid metabolism, and it is needed to maintain normal blood glucose levels. Investigation is ongoing for the relationship among chromium, obesity, muscle mass, and muscle strength. Scientists believe that chromium may have a role in lowering low-density lipoproteins. It is also being investigated for a potential role in treating certain types of atypical depression.

COACH CONSULT

Low chromium levels are associated with geriatric patients, extreme athletes, pregnant women, and those whose diets contain large amounts of sugar. Antacids may decrease chromium absorption, and chromium may enhance the effect of some diabetes medication.

Dietary Sources
Cereals, whole grains, meat, poultry, fish, cheese, black pepper, thyme, and brewer's yeast are common sources of chromium.

Adverse Effects of Inadequate Consumption
Chromium deficiency is under investigation for its relationship to diabetes, gestational diabetes, and steroid-induced diabetes.

Adverse Effects of Excess Consumption
For children, the recommended range of chromium consumption is still under investigation because

controversy exists over the full scope of the biological role of chromium, including potential chromosome damage. The Institute of Medicine has not set an upper limit for adults. However, investigators have suggested that high levels of chromium may interfere with insulin's role in glucose transport. It may also cause flushing, itching, or gastrointestinal irritation.

Sensitivity
Sensitivity is currently unknown.

Copper

The periodic table denotes copper with the symbol Cu and the atomic number 29. Copper can inhibit the growth of bacteria, and it has been used on hospital surfaces to stop the transmission of bacteria. Research has proposed positive and negative health effects in diseases such as arthritis, cancer, growth and development disorders, rheumatoid disorders, and psychiatric and neurological conditions. The NIH do not consider these study results as strong evidence.

Copper is used to treat malnutrition under medical supervision at a dose of 20–80 mcg/kg/day.

Copper toxicity has occurred from drinking fluids stored in copper containers. Because of this find, the Environmental Protection Agency regulates the amount of copper in drinking water.

Adequate Intake
USDA recommendations are age-specific (see Table 3–1). Pregnant women need 1000 mcg/day, and lactating women need 1300 mcg/day. Calcium supplementation may decrease available copper.

Function
Copper is used to form enzymes for iron metabolism. It also acts as an antioxidant, is necessary for cellular metabolism, and is used in the production of melanin. Copper is required for the enzymes that regulate bone matrix formation.

Dietary Sources
Foods with copper include avocado, fruits, vegetables, organ meats (kidney and liver), seafood, nuts, wheat bran, cocoa, whole grains, and nonfiltered drinking water.

Adverse Effects of Inadequate Consumption

Copper deficiency can occur with restricted diets. Babies who are not breast-fed and receive only cow's milk–based formula; patients who have malabsorption or cystic fibrosis; and patients on a restricted diet may not receive adequate amounts of copper in their diets. Decreased absorption may occur in the presence of high levels of iron, calcium, and zinc.

Adverse Effects of Excess Consumption

Copper has USDA-recommended upper limits. For children, the range is age-dependent and 1000–3000 mcg/day. For this reason, children should not take adult copper supplements. For teens and adults, the range is 5000–10,000 mcg/day. Too much copper can cause gastrointestinal upset and vomiting, neurological weakness, kidney failure, liver damage, coma, and death.

Sensitivity

Certain patients are at special risk of effects from too much copper. These include patients with Wilson's disease, which is a genetic disorder in which excess copper accumulates in the liver and nerves; patients with Indian childhood cirrhosis (related to cooking in copper pots); and patients with preexisting idiopathic copper toxicosis. Copper deficiency makes patients susceptible to molybdenum toxicity, and excess molybdenum can cause copper deficiency. Zinc and penicillamine are used to bind excess copper.

Fluoride

Fluoride is the reduced form of fluorine, which the periodic table denotes with the symbol F and the atomic number 9. Fluoride is a common component of toothpastes and mouthwashes, and it is used as an additive in municipal water sources.

Adequate Intake

Adequate intake of fluoride is age- and sex-specific (see Table 3–1). Women who are pregnant or lactating need 3 mg/day.

Function

Fluoride stimulates new bone formation, works to create teeth, and prevents production of the bacteria responsible for cavities (also called caries).

Dietary Sources

Tea and ocean fish are common sources of fluoride. Many communities add fluoride to water sources. It is also added to most dental cleansers. It is important to teach children not to swallow or eat toothpaste because doing so can cause ingestion of excess fluoride.

Adverse Effects of Inadequate Consumption
The adverse effects are currently unknown.

Adverse Effects of Excess Consumption
Fluoride has age-dependent USDA-recommended upper limits. For infants and children, this level is 0.7–2.2 mg/day. For males and females age 9 years and older, the upper limit is 10 mg/day. Too much fluoride can cause fluorosis, excessive absorption of fluoride in teeth and bones. Effects can range from slight discoloration to cracking and pitting of teeth and bones and ossification of tendons and ligaments.

Sensitivity
Sensitivity is currently unknown.

Iodine

The periodic table denotes iodine with the symbol I and the atomic number 53. Iodine intake is based on the amount of iodine in the soil. Dietary enrichment is provided through table salt, cattle feed, and dough additives. Iodine itself is not usually prescribed to treat a thyroid deficiency; instead, thyroid hormone in the form of levothyroxine sodium is ordered. Potassium iodine may be prescribed to prevent toxicity from exposure to radioactive iodine. Povidone-iodine, also known as betadine, is a topical agent used to prepare surgical sites, or it is applied to wounds as a disinfectant. Research is ongoing for the use of topical iodine for a variety of skin and mucous membrane applications. Some people are sensitive to these products and may develop a rash or burn.

Adequate Intake
Recommendations are age- and sex-specific (see Table 3–1). Women who are pregnant or lactating need 220–290 mcg/day.

Function
Iodine is a component of thyroid hormones T3 (triiodothyronine) and T4 (thyroxine).

Dietary Sources
Ocean fish, such as bass, cod, haddock, and perch, and the sea vegetable kelp are sources of iodine. Kelp must be used in cautious amounts to avoid

toxicity. Iodine is added to foods and salt in order to guarantee adequate consumption in diets that do not contain fish. Vegetables grown in iodine-rich soils also provide a source of iodine.

Adverse Effects of Inadequate Consumption

Low levels of iodine can cause thyroid dysfunction, such as goiter and neurological dysfunction, during fetal development. Research is also pointing to hearing loss and loss of cognitive function as associated with low levels of iodine.

Dietary deficiencies can be related to soil distribution of iodine. People whose diets are from areas with heavy rainfall or glacial water are at higher risk for deficiency because the water drains the iodine from the soil. Pregnant women from these climates should be cautioned about iodine deficiency because it may lead to severe mental retardation in the fetus. Nursing babies whose mothers have iodine deficiency may develop neurological problems.

Adverse Effects of Excess Consumption

Iodine has age-dependent USDA-recommended upper limits. For infants and children, this level ranges 200–300 mcg/day. For males and females age 9 years and older, the upper limit is 600–1000 mcg/day. Too much iodine can elevate thyroid-stimulating hormone. Symptoms of iodine toxicity include gastrointestinal pain, vomiting, diarrhea, and decreased consciousness descending into coma. Kelp, a type of seaweed used in teas and supplements, contains iodine and has been linked to hypothyroidism.

COACH CONSULT

Potassium iodine is part of the emergency kits that are prepared for toxic exposures to radioactive iodine. Potassium iodine prevents the thyroid gland from absorbing the radioactive isotope. Iodine tablets are used to purify water and are sold in camping stores or in areas with poor water quality.

Chronic overexposure to iodine can cause the preceding symptoms and eye irritation, metallic taste, increased saliva, anorexia, flu-like symptoms, respiratory problems, neurological complaints, irregular heart rhythm, thyroid and parathyroid problems, and decreased immunity.

Iodine toxicity is prescribed based on Poison Control Center protocols and may involve gastric lavage, activated charcoal, milk, cornstarch mixed with water, or flour mixed with water.

Sensitivity

Patients with a history of autoimmune thyroid disease, iodine deficiency, or nodular goiter are at special risk for adverse effects of normal dietary levels of iodine.

Iron

The periodic table denotes iron with the symbol Fe and the atomic number 26. Iron is an essential material for most species and therefore is present in many foods. In humans, the majority of iron is held in red blood cells.

Adequate Intake
Recommended iron intake is age- and sex-specific (see Table 3–1). Women who are pregnant or lactating need 9–27 mg/day.

Function
Iron is found as an element of all human cells, and it is key to the formation of the hemoglobin in red blood cells and the myoglobin of muscle cells. Iron is an essential component of hemoglobin because it carries oxygen in red blood cells. It is also required for the enzymes that regulate bone matrix formation.

Dietary Sources
Iron is available as heme iron and non-heme iron. Fruits, legumes, and vegetables such as raisins, spinach, chard, turnip, and collard are considered non-heme sources, whereas meat and poultry are considered heme sources. Some grain products, such as breakfast cereals, oatmeal, breads, and grits, are fortified with non-heme sources. Non-heme iron from dietary sources is significantly less well absorbed than from heme sources, so the USDA recommends that vegetarians consume twice the daily recommended adequate intake as meat and poultry eaters.

Adverse Effects of Inadequate Consumption
Microcytic hypochromic anemia, gastrointestinal distress, increased risk of infectious disease, decreased intellectual functioning, fatigue related to anemia, and pica, which is the craving and consumption of non-food products like ice or clay, are symptoms of iron deficiency. Low birth weight, premature birth, and reproductive problems are linked to iron deficiency.

Adverse Effects of Excess Consumption
The USDA's recommended upper limit for infants and children is 40 mg/day. For males and females age 9 years and older, the upper limit is 40–45 mg/day. Humans are unable to excrete excess iron, and

ALERT

Hyperkalemia can occur when potassium iodine is taken in combination with amiodarone, ACE-inhibitors, angiotension receptor blockers, or potassium-sparing diuretics. Hypothyroidism or lithium toxicity may be induced by the use of potassium iodine with lithium salts.

therefore their intake of iron is regulated by mechanisms that limit iron absorption. Too much iron can cause gastrointestinal distress, cirrhosis, diabetes, heart failure, and increased skin pigmentation. Excess iron can also accumulate in the liver, heart, and some endocrine glands to the point of causing dysfunction. This inability to excrete excess iron can be genetically linked or can occur as a result of blood disorders. Iron toxicity can occur secondary to excess intake, internal hemorrhage, blood transfusions, or liver dysfunction. Excess iron can be removed by treatment with a chelating medication that binds the iron to stool or urine for excretion or by the technique of repeated withdrawal of blood.

Sensitivity
Sensitivity is currently unknown, but predisposition to iron toxicity hemochromatosis is more common in people with Northern European genetic heritage.

Manganese

The periodic table denotes manganese with the symbol Mn and the atomic number 25. Manganese is abundant, is an essential element for most species, and occurs in most human foods. Toxic levels can accumulate through exposure through food or respiratory sources. It is a component in antioxidant enzymes of the mitochondria, and it activates enzymes that control metabolism of carbohydrates, cholesterol, and amino acids.

Adequate Intake
Recommended intake is age- and sex-specific (see Table 3–1). Women who are pregnant or lactating need 2–2.6 mg/day. Manganese has age-dependent USDA-recommended upper limits. For infants and children, this level ranges 2–3 mg/day. For males and females age 9 years and older, the upper limit is 6–11 mg/day.

Function
Manganese is used in formation of nerves and is required for the enzymes that regulate bone matrix formation.

Dietary Sources
Manganese is available from nuts, legumes, teas, whole grains, and unfiltered drinking water.

Adverse Effects of Inadequate Consumption

Adverse effects include metabolic problems resulting in inappropriate bone and cartilage formation and poor wound healing.

Adverse Effects of Excess Consumption

Too much manganese can cause neurotoxicity. Patients with a history of liver dysfunction are at higher risk for adverse effects of manganese.

Sensitivity

People who consume large amounts of manganese from dietary sources should use caution when drinking manganese-fortified water or when taking any supplements that are also fortified with manganese.

Molybdenum

The periodic table denotes molybdenum with the symbol Mo and the atomic number 42. Molybdenum is used medically for conditions like Wilson's disease, which is a genetic disease that causes the toxic buildup of copper in the organs. Molybdenum is under investigation as a potential antioxidant and for a potential protective effect when used at the same time as some oncology medications.

Adequate Intake

USDA intake guidelines are age- and sex-specific (see Table 3–1). Women who are pregnant or lactating need 50 mcg/day.

Function

Molybdenum acts as a co-factor for enzymes that catabolize sulfur amino acids, purines, and pyridines. It is also involved in cellular energy production, neurological cell development, and kidney function.

Dietary Sources

Nuts, leafy green vegetables, legumes, liver, and grains contain molybdenum. Regional variations of molybdenum in soil influence how much is ingested.

Adverse Effects of Inadequate Consumption

Molybdenum deficiency is rare because the body requires only very small amounts. However, molybdenum deficiency can occur with long-term dependency on intravenous fluids for nutrition or with inadequate levels in total parenteral nutrition and peripheral parenteral nutrition (TPN/PPN).

Adverse Effects of Excess Consumption

Molybdenum has age-dependent USDA-recommended upper limits. For infants, the levels are not established. For children age 1–8 years, the levels range 300–600 mcg/day. For males and females age 9 years and older, the upper limit is 1100–2000 mcg/day. Based on studies in animals, too much molybdenum is theorized to cause adverse effects on reproduction. It can cause fatigue, dizziness, gout symptoms, and decreased white and red blood cell count.

Sensitivity

Copper deficiency makes patients susceptible to molybdenum toxicity. Excess molybdenum can cause copper deficiency.

Selenium

The periodic table denotes selenium with the symbol Se and the atomic number 34. Selenium has been intensely studied for its antioxidant role. In particular, it is believed to play a role for patients undergoing chemotherapy. However, this role is controversial: some oncologists restrict selenium during chemotherapy, and others prescribe it.

Selenium at higher than required levels may have a protective role against some cancers, and research is being conducted into selenium's protective role in antioxidant enzyme activity and the inflammatory response. It is also being studied for a potentially protective role against mercury toxicity from fish and shellfish ingestion.

Selenium is found in soils and water. Patients who live in areas with low soil selenium may be at risk for deficiency. Selenium found naturally in foods grown in selenium-rich soil may have it depleted or removed during processing. Several diseases related to selenium deficiency are named after Keshan, which is a region of China that has low selenium levels in soil and large populations of these diseases.

Adequate Intake

Adequate intake of selenium is age- and sex-specific (see Table 3–1). Women who are pregnant or lactating need 60–70 mcg/day.

Function

Selenium is important for immunity functions because it oxidates free radicals; it is also important in the regulation of thyroid hormone. Selenium may protect from radiation and chemical carcinogens. It is believed to have a supportive role in male fertility and prostate health. It may also assist in antibody formation.

Dietary Sources

Food sources include organ meats; seafood and freshwater fish; grains and brewers' yeast; sunflower seeds, Brazil nuts, and walnuts; and plants grown in selenium-rich soils, including chives, fennel, ginseng, onions, radishes, and shiitake mushrooms.

Adverse Effects of Inadequate Consumption

A decrease in immune system function and hypothyroidism changes leading to Keshan cardiomyopathy disease, Kashin-Beck joint disease, myxedematous endemic cretinism, and cardiomyopathy are linked to low selenium. Lack of selenium is under investigation for a relationship to cancers of the bladder, bowel, mammary glands, ovaries, prostate, skin, and uterus. It also correlates with behavioral problems in children, but this relationship is still being researched. Deficiency can be associated with poor gastrointestinal absorption, long-term dependency on intravenous fluids for nutrition or inadequate levels in TPN/PPN, and high-dose steroid therapy.

Adverse Effects of Excess Consumption

Selenium has age-dependent USDA-recommended upper limits. For infants and children, this level ranges 45–150 mcg/day. For males and females age 9 years and older, the upper limit is 280–400 mcg/day. Too much selenium can cause abdominal problems, including pain, vomiting, and diarrhea; neurological problems, including fatigue, dizziness, hyperreflexia, tremors, and neuropathies; organ problems, including thyroid, renal, and hepatic dysfunction; endocrine problems such as delayed physical development and reduced sperm motility; integumentary problems such as nail and hair loss or brittleness; and immune system deficiencies. Toxicity is associated with respiratory distress, electrocardiogram changes, and death.

Sensitivity

Sensitivity is currently unknown.

Zinc

The periodic table denotes zinc with the symbol Zn and the atomic number 30. Zinc is commonly prescribed for patients with malnutrition and significant wounds, and it is commonly included in sunscreen applications, diaper rash preparations, dandruff shampoos, and toothbrushes. It is under investigation for reduction in the symptoms of the common cold

NURSE-TO-NURSE TIP

Zinc can be delivered by mouth and intravenously as a supplement. Doses must always be delivered in dilution of at least 100-mL volumes. Doses are 2.4–4 mg/day for adults, and they may be higher for patients in highly catabolic states or for patients experiencing high volumes of small-bowel fluid losses, such as through an ileostomy. The dose for full-term babies to children up to 5 years is 100 mcg/kg/day. Premature infants may receive higher doses.

by dietary supplement or nasal application and for treatment in attention deficit hyperactivity disorder.

ALERT !

Intramuscular and direct intravenous (IV) (IV push) zinc administration is contraindicated due to tissue irritation. IV zinc must always be diluted. IV administration without concurrent copper can cause decreased copper levels.

Adequate Intake

Recommendations for intake are age- and sex-specific (see Table 3–1). Women who are pregnant or lactating need 34–40 mg/day. Calcium supplements may interfere with gastrointestinal absorption of zinc.

Function

Zinc is necessary for various enzymes and proteins, including those that regulate bone matrix formation. It is a co-enzyme for RNA and DNA polymerase. Zinc is a component of blood cells, the retina, muscle, bone, skin, and organs such as the kidney, liver, pancreas, and prostate. It is involved in healing wounds, promoting normal growth rates, skin hydration, and the senses of taste and smell.

Dietary Sources

Zinc is provided by red meat, poultry, seafood, grains, beans, nuts, and fortified cereals. Nonmeat sources of zinc are more difficult to absorb, requiring consumption of double the recommended daily allowance when zinc is ingested from only these sources.

Adverse Effects of Inadequate Consumption

Zinc deficiency may be related to endocrine problems such as delayed growth (including delayed development of reproductive organs) and prosthetic hypertrophy; integumentary problems, including skin irritation, hair loss, and parakeratosis; gastrointestinal problems, including anorexia, diarrhea, and enlarged liver; and depression.

Adverse Effects of Excess Consumption

Zinc has age-dependent USDA-recommended upper limits. For infants and children, this level ranges 4–12 mg/day. For males and females age 9 years and older, the upper limit is 8–11 mg/day. Too much zinc can cause copper deficiency, and long-term excess exposure to zinc may have a detrimental effect on the immune system and raise the risk of prostate cancer. Toxicity occurs at concentrations above 200 mcg/dL. Symptoms include increased serum amylase, sweating with low body temperature, decreased mental status, blurred vision, rapid heart rate, pulmonary edema, low urine output, and gastrointestinal symptoms, including diarrhea, vomiting, and jaundice.

Sensitivity

Sensitivity is currently unknown.

4 Acid-Base Balance and Imbalance

CHAPTER 4

Acid-Base Balance and Imbalance

Acids are molecules that can release hydrogen ions. Some fluids in the body are naturally acidic, including urine, gastric secretions, and bile.

Bases are molecules that can accept or bind free hydrogen ions.

Like bases, *alkalis* are molecules that can bind free hydrogen. Chemically, they are a combination of alkaline metals with strong bases, such as sodium (Na^+) combining with hydroxyl (OH^-). Sodium bicarbonate ($NaHCO_3$) is usually discussed as the primary alkali in vascular and extracellular fluid. When the body's pH is in normal range, there are about 20 times more base (alkaline) bicarbonate molecules than acid molecules present in extracellular fluid.

Pancreatic secretions are one example of a body fluid that is naturally basic/alkaline.

Acids and bases/alkalis affect respiratory and metabolic processes. For example, sulfuric, hydrochloric, and phosphoric acid are products of various stages of metabolism. Lactic acid is produced by the incomplete oxidation of glucose, and ketoacids are produced from the incomplete oxidation of fats. These acids are buffered by bicarbonate in extracellular compartments or by proteins inside cells. Bases are also generated by the metabolism of amino acids, but in a typical, meat-dependent U.S. diet, acid production is higher.

COACH CONSULT

The neutral acid-base midpoint in the human body is pH 7.4, with a normal range of pH 7.35–7.45.

Acids and bases also play a role in cellular respiration or gas exchange. For example, the carbon dioxide (CO_2) in tissues combines with water (H_2O) in cells to form H_2CO_3, which is a carbonic acid. However, because acids release hydrogen ions, H_2CO_3 dissociates into HCO_3^- and H^+:

$$CO_2 + H_2O > H_2CO_3 > (H^+) + (HCO_3^-)$$

The resulting free hydrogen increases the body's acidity. To compensate for the acidity, the free hydrogen binds to hemoglobin (Hb) that has released its oxygen (O_2). Hemoglobin—which is a base—then returns to the lungs to "drop off" its excess H^+ and pick up more O_2 for the body to use. If something goes wrong in this balanced acid-base transmission, respiratory acidosis or respiratory alkalosis can occur. More details about these latter two conditions are provided later in the chapter.

The body's acid-base balance is measured by calculating the number of hydrogen ions (H^+) in the body and is expressed as pH. The neutral acid-base midpoint in the human body is pH 7.4, with a normal range of pH 7.35–7.45. Acid and base imbalance is discussed as acidosis when pH is low (<7.35) and alkalosis when pH is high (>7.45). Acidosis, then, is a state where there is an excess of hydrogen ions in the body, and it occurs when there is a deficiency of molecules that can accept hydrogen ions. In turn, alkalosis is a state where there is a deficiency of hydrogen ions, which occurs when there is a deficiency in molecules that can release hydrogen. Figure 4-1 shows the acid-base continuum.

Evaluation and treatment of acidosis and alkalosis are focused on observation for symptoms, interpretation of laboratory values, identification of a source of the imbalance, and correction toward normal range. These imbalances are divided into metabolic and respiratory causes based on whether the dysfunction stems from the lungs or kidneys. Typically, an initial response to pH changes occurs in the respiratory system because it is able to respond more quickly to these changes, whereas the renal system is slower to respond.

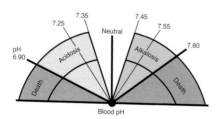

FIGURE 4-1: The pH scale, which ranges 1–14. Normal blood pH is 7.35–7.45.

Intake

Dietary intake affects the pH of body fluids. In a typical U.S. diet, high protein ingestion increases the amount of amino acids in the body, which promotes acid production. In contrast, vegetarians have more bases in their metabolism because of a higher ingestion of organic anions. The pH values of selected body fluids and solutions are in Figure 4-2.

COACH CONSULT

The terms *basic* and *alkalotic* are used interchangeably to refer to a high pH.

Regulation

The respiratory system, the kidneys, intracellular buffer proteins, and other extracellular chemical buffers regulate acid and base levels. In healthy individuals, buffer systems are constantly exchanging excess acids and bases to maintain a balanced pH. Phosphorus can also play a role in regulating body pH.

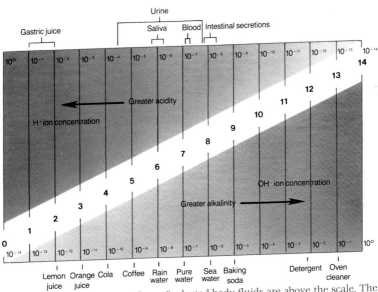

FIGURE 4-2: The pH values of selected body fluids are above the scale. The pH values of selected solutions are below the scale.

Respiratory Buffering

Carbon dioxide (CO_2) is controlled by the respiratory system. In the brain, once carbon dioxide crosses over the blood-brain barrier, it joins with water (H_2O) to form carbonic acid (H_2CO_3). When this molecule breaks down into hydrogen (H^+) and bicarbonate (HCO_3^-), hydrogen stimulates the brain's respiratory center, causing increased ventilation to blow off excess CO_2. This response to acidosis can occur within minutes, but it will not completely buffer a large shift toward acidosis, which could be caused by ingestion of strong acids, destruction of tissues, or other critical metabolic disorders. Other mechanisms that take longer to react must be functioning in order to balance extremely acidic conditions.

Renal Buffering

The kidneys change the acidic or alkaline components of urine in response to pH changes. During acidosis, they can excrete excess hydrogen ions or reabsorb or create bicarbonate molecules. During alkalosis, the kidneys can excrete excess bicarbonate. These processes (Fig. 4-3) continue over many hours until the balance of pH is resolved.

Protein Buffers

Proteins are large molecules that have the ability to act as a base or an acid, releasing or accepting hydrogen ions as necessary. Most protein buffers are inside cells.

Hydrogen can diffuse into cells and be taken up by buffering proteins. When this occurs, potassium (K^+) leaves the cell to make room for the hydrogen, which causes serum hyperkalemia. This shift occurs more markedly with metabolic acidosis than it does with respiratory acidosis.

Extracellular proteins—such as albumin, hemoglobulins, and oxyhemoglobin in the blood—can also act as protein buffers.

Bicarbonate Buffer System

The bicarbonate buffer system is active in the blood and is responsible for about 80% of buffering in extracellular fluid. It responds to both metabolic acidosis and the presence of strong acids, such as hydrochloric acid (HCl), by combining these acids with bicarbonate salts, such as sodium bicarbonate ($NaHCO_3$).

Combining acids with bicarbonate salts forms both a weak acid and neutral salts; for example, combining acid with bicarbonate salts results in carbonic acid (H_2CO_3) and sodium chloride (NaCl). The carbonic acid

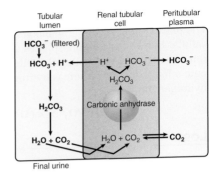

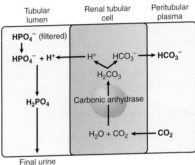

FIGURE 4-3: Kidney exchange. (A) Reabsorption of filtered bicarbonate; (B) Excretion of secreted hydrogen ions combined with phosphate.

then changes to water (H_2O) and carbon dioxide (CO_2). The CO_2 is then exhaled, and the new molecule of NaCl remains in the serum:

$$(H^+) + (HCO_3^-) > H_2CO_3 > CO_2 + H_2O$$

When a strong base is formed (i.e., sodium hydroxide [NaOH]), then a buffering system introduces a weak acid (i.e., carbonic acid [H_2CO_3]) to form both $NaHCO_3$ and H_2O. Carbon dioxide that is taken up by the buffer system is then replaced by carbon dioxide that is retained by the respiratory system. The kidneys can conserve or excrete bicarbonate (HCO_3^-) as required by this buffer system:

$$NaOH + H_2CO_3 > NaHCO_3 + H_2O$$

COACH CONSULT

Chemical reactions occur within the blood to buffer strong acids, such as hydrochloric acid, or strong bases, such as sodium hydroxide. These combinations yield weak acids, such as carbonic acid, and sodium bicarbonate. The other end product for these reactions is water.

Phosphorus

The phosphorous level in the blood is too low to act as an effective extracellular buffer. Instead, phosphates act more effectively as buffers in the renal system and intracellularly. Dihydrogen phosphate ($H_2PO_4^-$) can donate a hydrogen ion, whereas hydrogen phosphate [HPO_4^{2-}] can accept a hydrogen ion:

$$H_2PO_4^- > < (H^+) + (HPO_4^{2-})$$

Loss

Dietary intake and metabolism are responsible for the ingestion and production of acids and bases. Phosphoproteins, sulfur-containing amino acids, and chloride salts are contained in most diets. The metabolism of carbohydrates, fats, and proteins yields lactic acid, ketoacids, sulfuric acid, phosphoric acids, and uric acid. A high-protein diet results in more acids, whereas a vegetarian diet results in more bases. Excess hydrogen and acids are excreted via the kidneys, whereas excess carbon dioxide is lost through lungs. Excess base is lost through the urine and stool.

Laboratory Measures

Levels of pH can be detected through serum and urine laboratory studies.

Blood

Venous and arterial samples are two ways to collect blood gases when testing for acidity or alkalinity. Arterial blood gas samples can be more accurate, but they are difficult to obtain.

Venous Samples

Venous samples can be used to obtain CO_2 and HCO_3^- levels. A venous blood level of CO_2 reflects both free CO_2 and approximately 70% of CO_2 that is in the serum as a component of HCO_3^-. Total venous CO_2 is normally 23–29 mEq/L. Low CO_2 levels indicate alkalosis, and high CO_2 indicate acidosis.

Bicarbonate is used to estimate the overall serum content of buffers, including bicarbonate, protein, and phosphorus buffers. If bases are determined to be in excess, this indicates metabolic alkalosis. Base deficit indicates metabolic acidosis. The normal range of bicarbonate is +/- 3 mEq/L.

Venous samples are also used to calculate the anion gap, which helps health-care professionals estimate the amount of unmeasured serum ions in the blood to determine whether there is an excess of acid in the body.

Anion Gap

Venous samples are used to estimate phosphates, sulfates, organic acids, and proteins in the blood, which are commonly called unmeasured anions. Sodium, which is the most abundant positive serum ion (cation), is compared with the sum of the most abundant negative ions, which are chloride (Cl^-) ions and bicarbonate (HCO_3^-) molecules. The cause of the metabolic acidosis is evaluated using an anion gap measurement. The normal gap ranges 8–16 mEq/L. A gap that is < 8 mEq/L indicates alkalosis, and a gap that is > 16 mEq/L indicates acidosis. Anion gap formulas are in Chapter 6.

Blood Gases

Blood gases are used to evaluate pH and related changes. Normal serum pH is in the range of 7.35–7.45. A pH < 7.35 is considered acidotic, and a pH > 7.45 is considered alkalotic. Blood gases also reflect the cause of an imbalance as respiratory, metabolic, or mixed. This evaluation includes an assessment of how extreme the imbalance is and whether the patient has begun to compensate for the imbalance.

Carbonic acid (H_2CO_3) is difficult to measure in the blood because it only occurs in small amounts. Therefore, it is estimated based on the partial pressure of serum CO_2 in blood gases. CO_2 levels are estimated based on measured (pressure) P_{CO_2}, which is normally 38–42 mm Hg. If the level of CO_2 is > 42 mm Hg, a person is alkalotic; if the level of CO_2 is < 38 mm Hg, the person is acidotic.

When blood gases are ordered, the nurse must assess the patient for arterial perfusion, teach the patient about the process, communicate with respiratory and medical staff, and prepare for immediate transport of samples.

The medical team may order *arterial blood gases* (ABGs) instead of venous blood gases. ABGs refer to blood gases that are drawn from the radial arteries and—if necessary—from the femoral arteries. Most facilities have restrictions on which personnel may obtain a direct arterial serum sample, so refer to your institution's guidelines. General information about ABG withdrawal and interpretation is in Chapter 6. Before communicating ABG orders to the personnel who will perform the draw, the nurse must assess the patient's arterial function. Any decrease in pulses should be reported to the medical team before attempting to obtain blood gases.

ALERT

Blood gases must be placed on ice immediately for transport and must be analyzed very quickly, but at least within 60 minutes of collection.

Urine

The anion gap can be calculated from urine specimens in order to look for renal response to metabolic acidosis. Na^+ and K^+ levels are added together and compared with Cl^- levels. This number estimates ammonium (NH_4^+) excretion:

$$[(Na^+) + (K^+)] - (Cl^-) = NH_4^+$$

Normal ammonium secretion is 20–40 mmol/L.

Respiratory Alkalosis

Respiratory alkalosis occurs when excess carbon dioxide is expelled from the lungs, causing a decrease in circulating hydrogen ions.

Laboratory Values (Arterial)

Arterial laboratory values for respiratory alkalosis can be uncompensated or compensated:

- **Uncompensated:** Arterial PCO_2 < 35 mm Hg; pH > 7.45; HCO_3^- = 18–23 mEq/L
- **Compensated:** Arterial PCO_2 < 35 mm Hg; pH = 7.35–7.45; HCO_3^- < 18 mEq/L

Uncompensated respiratory alkalosis means that the partial pressure of carbon dioxide is decreased, causing the pH to be elevated, thus indicating alkalosis. Note that blood bicarbonate values are within a normal range and have not begun to compensate for decreased levels of the partial pressure of carbon dioxide levels. With *compensated respiratory alkalosis*, the blood bicarbonate levels have decreased to offset the decreased partial pressures of carbon dioxide, causing the pH to return to a normal range.

Basic Concepts

Respiratory dysfunction can result in lower than normal levels of carbon dioxide in the body. This lack is typically caused by increased rate and/or depth of breathing. When alkalosis occurs, there is no automatic respiratory response to attempt to compensate or balance pH; instead, renal compensation occurs by decreasing excretion of hydrogen and decreasing bicarbonate reabsorption. As the body returns to a more normal pH, respiratory rates and depth may return to near normal.

Etiology
Hyperventilation, the main form of respiratory alkalosis, can be linked to:
- Anxiety
- Asthma
- Brain lesions of the respiratory center
- Brain trauma
- Cerebrovascular accident
- Congestive heart failure
- Fever
- High altitudes
- Hyperthyroidism
- Infection
- Interstitial lung disease
- Liver disease
- Pain
- Pneumonia
- Pneumothorax
- Pregnancy
- Pulmonary edema
- Pulmonary embolus
- Sepsis
- Iatrogenic causes, including:
  - Increased mechanical ventilation
  - Salicylate intoxication (wintergreen or aspirin)
    - Initial stimulation of respiratory centers causes alkalosis, then develops into metabolic acidosis

Symptoms
Common symptoms of respiratory alkalosis include:
- **Neurological:** Verbalizing anxiety or pain, agitation, mental status, personality or memory changes; nonverbal pain scale findings, hypervigilance, report of recent brain trauma, fear of "impending doom" with presence of pulmonary embolus
- **Cardiovascular (CV):** Anemia, fever, neck vein distention, peripheral edema, elevated heart rate
- **Respiratory:** Elevated respiratory rate, use of accessory muscles, production of sputum, pain associated with breathing,

decreased breath sounds, absent breath sounds in one or more lung fields, rales/crackles in lung fields, hypoventilation associated with pregnancy related to decreased thoracic-abdominal space
- **Gastrointestinal (GI):** Ascites, jaundice

Assessment and Actions

Management of alkalosis is related to identifying its source and treating it while attempting to correct the imbalance.

Fluid, electrolyte, and acid-base imbalances can rapidly cause life-threatening neurological, cardiac, and respiratory compromise, requiring immediate notification of the medical or rapid response team. Consult the medical team if any new onset occurs or if worsening symptoms or vital signs occur that are outside the normal range. If neurological, respiratory, or cardiac compromise occurs, call for assistance from the rapid or urgent response team or, if outside an acute care setting, call community emergency medical services (EMS).

Patient History

Review for clues as to cause. The following conditions may be associated with or cause respiratory alkalosis:
- Brain injury related to lesions, trauma, stroke, anoxia, or liver disease
- Chronic CV disease, leading to fluid overload in the lungs and decreased oxygen-carrying capacity
- Chronic or acute respiratory disease or dysfunction related to decreased gas exchange, poor ventilatory effort, or trauma to the anatomy of the lung
- Infection by bacterial or viral source
- Iatrogenic causes, including mechanical ventilation or overdosing or poisoning with salicylates

Laboratory Assessment and Actions

If a patient has symptoms or disorder history that points to alkalosis, then:
- Anticipate orders for an arterial blood draw for blood gas evaluation:
  - See the arterial access precautions in Chapter 6.
  - If pH is >7.45, consult the medical team for application of supplemental oxygen.
- Anticipate orders for venous serum sample to measure a complete blood count:
  - If the white blood cell count is >12,000/mm³, which points to infection, or <4000/mm³, pointing to sepsis, then:
    - Discuss results with the medical team.

- Anticipate orders for blood, urine, sputum, and wound cultures to identify potential sources of infection.
- Anticipate orders for antipyretics if fever develops $> 101.5\,°F$ $(38.6\,°C)$.
- Anticipate orders for broad-spectrum antibiotics and fluid replacement if fever develops $> 100.5\,°F$ $(38\,°C)$ or $< 96.8\,°F$ $(36\,°C)$, indicating systemic inflammatory response syndrome (SIRS) or sepsis.
- If hemoglobin is < 12.6 g/dL for adult males or 11.7 g/dL for adult females, or if hematocrit is $< 43\%$ for adult males or 38% for adult females (indicating anemia), then:
  - Discuss results with the medical team.
  - Anticipate measures to reverse anemia as discussed in Chapter 2 in the section on blood administration.
- Anticipate orders to draw a venous serum sample to evaluate electrolyte imbalance and liver imbalance:
  - If calcium, sodium, potassium, or phosphorus is low, anticipate measures discussed in electrolyte chapters for correction of imbalances.
  - If liver enzymes are elevated, anticipate measures to reduce exposure to stressors, such as medications that are metabolized in the liver.
- Anticipate orders for serum specimen salicylate levels:
  - If > 30 mg/dL, discuss with the medical team.
  - If > 40 mg/dL, discuss with the medical team, and observe for symptoms of respiratory alkalosis or metabolic acidosis.
  - If > 100 mg/dL, anticipate immediate alert to medical team and initiation of emergency measures for a life-threatening toxic level:
    - Anticipate communication with the Poison Control Center.
    - In acute episodes, anticipate orders for activated charcoal administration at a normal dose of 1–2 g/kg:
      - Anticipate orders for gastric lavage or whole-bowel irrigation with recent ingestion.
      - Anticipate orders for hemodialysis with high toxicity levels or chronic absorption.
      - Anticipate orders for fluid resuscitation.

COACH CONSULT

A slow reversal of blood alkaline levels may be ordered to allow for increased urinary excretion of salicylates through ion trapping.

- Anticipate orders to assess serum potassium and to replete decreased potassium stores in an effort to support alkalization of urine and excretion of salicylates through the kidneys. Once potassium levels are corrected, then:
  - Anticipate orders for intravenous sodium bicarbonate to increase blood and urine pH.
  - Anticipate orders for repeated potassium levels to ensure that urine remains alkaline throughout treatment.
  - Anticipate emergency measures to prevent rebound acidosis because low pH allows for salicylates to transfer into the brain.
- Anticipate orders to redraw levels with frequency because peak levels do not occur until 4 hours after ingestion.
- Anticipate orders for thyroid levels because increased levels may cause increased ventilation and depletion of carbon dioxide.

Systems Assessment and Actions

If laboratory test results are pending but respiratory alkalosis is suspected, proceed with a systems assessment. Immediately consult the medical team at the onset or worsening of any of the symptoms that are listed in the following section.

Neurological

Perform frequent neurological assessments for decreased level of consciousness, mental status, and personality or memory changes. If mental status changes occur, then:

- Anticipate frequent measures of neurological status using the Glasgow Coma Scale.
- Maintain safety measures, including keeping the bed low, padded side rails in place, and the call bell in reach.
- Continually reevaluate the patient's ability to follow instructions.
- Consult the medical team to discuss need for one-on-one supervision.
- Institute safety precautions, and assist with all activities of daily living, transfers, and ambulation.
- Observe nonverbal and verbal indications of pain or anxiety:
  - An institution-approved, research-normed pain scale or verbal pain scale should be used to assess for pain:
    - Provide comfort measures and a calm environment.
    - If possible, teach or reinforce techniques such as slowing breaths or visualization to decrease pain.
    - Anticipate orders for medicinal pain relief.

- Observe carefully for decrease in respiratory rate and depth.
- An institution-approved, research-normed anxiety scale, a verbal report, or observation of agitation should be used to assess for anxiety:
  - Provide a calm, safe environment and interventions as described for pain.
  - Assign a caregiver to stay with the patient until anxiety has decreased.
  - Reassure the patient that sources of anxiety are being addressed.
  - Anticipate orders for medicinal anxiety relief.
  - Observe carefully for decrease in respiratory rate and depth.
- Immediately contact the medical and rapid response team if the patient reports feeling of impending doom:
  - Anticipate emergent respiratory support for potential pulmonary embolus.
  - Anticipate orders for ventilation perfusion screening or computerized tomography (CT) scan if a pulmonary embolus is suspected.
- If no other source for respiratory alkalosis is determined, anticipate orders for head CT or magnetic resonance imaging (MRI) to rule out brain disorders:
  - Inquire as to potential for pregnancy in premenopausal women.
  - Review results of urine pregnancy tests before sending premenopausal women for radiological studies.
  - Ensure that patients are screened for interfering metal implants and shrapnel before sending them for MRI.

CV

If fever of $>101.5°F$ $(38°C)$ or $<96.8°F$ $(36°C)$ is present and SIRS or sepsis is suspected, then:
- Anticipate orders for blood, sputum, wound, and urine cultures.
- Anticipate orders for administration of broad-spectrum antibiotics and hydrating fluids.
- Anticipate orders for continuous cardiac and blood pressure monitoring. Carefully assess the patient for signs of hypotension associated with capillary permeability from sepsis.

If signs of congestive heart failure are present, then:
- Provide assistance with all activities of daily living to decrease the work of breathing.
- Place the patient in an upright position to support ventilation.

- Discuss with the medical team the need for supplemental oxygen.
- Anticipate orders for diuretic medications.
- Monitor intake and output.
- Anticipate orders for fluid restriction.

If heart rate is elevated >100, discuss with the medical team the need for continuous cardiac monitoring.

Respiratory

If respiratory rate is increased, then:

- Instruct patient on slow deep-breathing techniques.
- Discuss with medical team the option of having patient breathe into a paper bag or a rebreathing mask to retain carbon dioxide.
- Anticipate orders to place patient on continuing pulse oximetry.

If the oxygen levels drop <93%, or if the patient's baseline or respiratory support or mechanical ventilation is required, anticipate reassuring the patient that the support is temporary while the underlying condition is corrected. If the patient is placed on mechanical ventilation, then:

- Explain the necessity for the ventilation support.
- Inform patients who are ordered to receive noninvasive positive pressure ventilation (NIPPV), such as bi-pap or c-pap, the need to wear a tight mask over their face until carbon dioxide levels return to normal or until underlying conditions are corrected.
- Inform patients requiring endotracheal intubation that speech is temporarily inhibited, and provide tools for the patient to communicate, such as a picture board or pencil and paper.
- Anticipate orders to modify tidal volume and respiratory rate, and carefully monitor oxygen saturation, neurological changes, and respiratory effort response to changes in mechanical ventilation.

If sputum is present, then:

- Discuss orders for sputum specimen with the medical team.
- Document color, consistency, and amount of sputum produced.
- Perform oral suctioning, or provide suction catheter and instruction to the patient for self-suctioning.

If nasal, pharyngeal, or tracheal secretions are present, discuss orders with the medical team for sterile suctioning, and follow institutional guidelines to ensure sterility, oxygenation, and airway protection. Use caution, as excessive suctioning can decrease oxygen levels.

If changes in lung sounds occur, then:

- Report diminished, absent, or adventitious lung sounds to the medical team:
  - If rales/crackles are present, anticipate orders for fluid restriction and diuretic therapy.
  - If rhonchi are present, then:
    - Perform oral suctioning, or provide suction catheter and instruction to the patient for self-suctioning.
    - If nasal, pharyngeal, or tracheal secretions are present, discuss orders with the medical team for sterile suctioning, and follow institutional guidelines to ensure sterility, oxygenation, and airway protection. Use caution, as excessive suctioning can decrease oxygen levels.
  - Anticipate orders for antibiotics.
- Anticipate orders for chest x-ray to rule out lung disorders:
  - Inquire as to potential for pregnancy in premenopausal women.
  - Review results of urine pregnancy test before sending premenopausal women for radiological studies.
  - If x-ray test results are inconclusive but symptoms persist, then:
    - Anticipate orders for CT scan or MRI. Review allergies to screen for allergy or sensitivity to radiological dye or seafood.
    - Screen patients for interfering metal implants and shrapnel, and discuss with the medical team before sending patients for MRI.

GI

If abdominal girth is increased, then:

- Help the patient into an upright position to allow for maximum inspiration.
- If inspiration effort persists, anticipate orders to assist the medical team in a sterile, bedside paracentesis or to transfer the patient to interventional radiology for paracentesis.
- If jaundice is present, anticipate orders for ammonia serum sampling.

COACH CONSULT

If ammonia levels are elevated >102 mcg/dL for adult males or >87 mcg/dL for adult females, anticipate orders for low-protein diet and for either (1) intravenous sodium phenylacetate with sodium benzoate or lactulose by mouth or enema or (2) a GI antibiotic, such as neomycin.

Prevention

Staff at inpatient settings should carefully evaluate patients for pain and anxiety associated with hospitalization and treat patients with supportive measures before respiratory problems develop. Patients with chronic respiratory or cardiac problems should be taught to observe themselves carefully for elevated respiratory rate and/or work on breathing as a symptom of abnormal respiration. Families should be taught to observe for mental status changes as a sign of respiratory problems. Adult patients should be taught to carefully read all drug labels and to keep all medications away from children and adults with diminished mental capacity.

 CLINICAL SCENARIO

DIAGNOSIS: RESPIRATORY ALKALOSIS RELATED TO SALICYLATE TOXICITY

Mrs. Aslam arrives at her physician's office complaining of unrelieved headache and diarrhea. She reports having taken aspirin 325 mg four times a day and a pink liquid antidiarrheal medication she purchased over the counter. In addition, she report treating her stuffy nose with menthol aerosol drops that she places in her humidifier at home. Finally, she reports treating her aching bones with a pain rub that she also purchased over the counter.

The nurse notes that her respirations are in the high 20s, her heart rate is 98, and her skin in very dry. The nurse queries Mrs. Aslam if she has also been taking her normal medications. Mrs. Aslam informs the nurse that she did not know that Ecotrin contained aspirin. The nurse learns that Mrs. Aslam took recent doses of the nonprescription aspirin, her normal prescription Ecotrin, and the pink medication before she came to the office today. Although she suspects that Mrs. Aslam's salicylate toxicity is acute, the chronic pattern of ingesting aspirin, inhaling wintergreen salicylates, and applying salicylates to her joints over the past week makes the nurse concerned for a chronic problem. She immediately calls Poison Control and consults with the office nurse practitioner.

On the advice of Poison Control, the nurse calls 911. While awaiting EMS, the nurse and nurse practitioner reassure Mrs. Aslam that she will be fine. They do not attempt to slow her breathing, with the knowledge that maintaining her alkaline blood and urine will be essential to ridding her body of excess salicylates. Instead, they attempt to have Mrs. Aslam consume fluids, and they conduct a thorough physical assessment head to toe.

When the EMS team arrives, they find her heart in sinus rhythm and her oxygen saturation at 99%, and they begin administration of activated charcoal and intravenous fluids under direction of the Poison Control Center and the EMS medical director. The nurse practitioner makes a report to the receiving emergency room physician. Together, the nurse practitioner and the nurse make a plan to contact Mrs. Aslam's family and secure all sources of salicylates in the household. A home-care visit is planned for after discharge. The nurse takes a further step, calling Mrs. Aslam's local pharmacy and—without breeching patient confidentiality—asks that the pharmacist warn patients about purchasing over-the-counter salicylates in combination with prescription salicylates.

1. Why is Mrs. Aslam breathing rapidly?
2. When should the nurse anticipate salicylate blood levels to peak?
3. The nurse conducts a history and physical assessment to rule out other causes of hyperventilation. What are critical concerns?

Respiratory Acidosis

Respiratory acidosis occurs when carbon dioxide is not expelled from the lungs, causing a decrease in circulating bicarbonate.

Laboratory Values (Arterial)
Arterial laboratory values for respiratory acidosis can be uncompensated or compensated:

- **Uncompensated:** Arterial P_{CO_2} >45 mm Hg, pH <7.35, HCO_3^- 18–23 mEq/L
- **Compensated:** Arterial P_{CO_2} >45 mm Hg, pH 7.35–7.45, HCO_3^- >23 meq/L

Uncompensated respiratory acidosis means that the partial pressure of carbon dioxide is increased, causing the pH to be decreased and thus indicating acidosis. Blood bicarbonate values are within a normal range and have not yet begun to compensate for elevated levels of the partial pressure of carbon dioxide. With *compensated respiratory acidosis*, the blood bicarbonate levels have increased, offsetting the increased partial pressure of carbon dioxide, to return the pH to a normal range.

Basic Concepts
Respiratory dysfunction can also result in levels of carbon dioxide that are higher than normal. This high level of carbon dioxide is typically caused

by a decreased rate and/or depth of breathing. As the presence of hydrogen ions increases in the blood, there is an automatic increase in the rate and depth of ventilation, thus reversing the acidosis if the patient's respiratory response center is intact. However, if the respiratory response system is impaired, the patient may not be able to self-correct and will need ventilator support.

Chronic acidosis can occur over months to years and may lead to acute acidosis. If the patient who has chronic acidosis is otherwise in good health, the body's renal buffer systems should be able to compensate for low-level acidosis by increasing hydrogen excretion and increasing reabsorption of bicarbonate. Additionally, the otherwise healthy patient's bicarbonate should increase 3.5 mEq/L for a rise of $Paco_2$ by 10 mm Hg. However, the level of bicarbonate increase lowers substantially in the patient with acute respiratory acidosis: bicarbonate will increase only by 1 mEq/L for each increase in $Paco_2$ of 10 mm Hg.

Etiology

There are many possible causes of respiratory acidosis, including:

- Hypoventilation, or decreased respiratory exchange of carbon dioxide, which can be linked to:
  - Acute lung disease, such as influenza, pulmonary edema, pulmonary embolism, pneumonia, pneumothorax, or respiratory distress syndrome
  - Anemia
  - Brain injury, disease, or infection
  - Trauma to the thoracic cavity
- Chronic cardiac disease leading to pulmonary hypertension, including congenital heart disease, congestive heart failure, or valvular stenosis or prolapse
- Chronic lung disease, including chronic obstructive pulmonary disease (asthma, bronchitis, emphysema), infiltration of lungs with industrial irritants (asbestos, coal dust), interstitial fibrosis, sarcoidosis, or tuberculosis
- Endocrine disease, such as hypothyroidism
- High altitudes
- Neurological diseases, such as amyotrophic lateral sclerosis, Guillain-Barré syndrome, muscular dystrophy, and myasthenia gravis
- Obesity hypoventilation syndrome
- Poisoning with gases like carbon monoxide

COACH CONSULT

In patients with chronic lung disease, chronic acidosis can occur over months to years.

- Thoracic skeletal deformity
- Tumor
- Iatrogenic causes, including:
  - Inhibiting respiratory capacity due to:
    - Abdominal or thoracic surgery or intubation
    - Pain medication
    - Sedatives or sleeping medication
    - Salicylate toxicity in late stage (due to wintergreen or aspirin)
  - Aldosterone bicarbonate
  - Corticosteroids
  - Ethacrynic acid (Edecrin)
  - Isoproterenol
  - Radiological contrast agents

Symptoms
Symptoms of respiratory acidosis include:
- **Neurological:** Mental status, personality or memory changes, fear of impending doom with presence of pulmonary embolus, asterixis, myoclonus, seizures
- **CV:** Anemia, fever, distended neck veins, peripheral edema, dilation of superficial blood vessels, retinal papilledema
- **Respiratory:** Decreased respiratory rate, decreased recoil of respiratory muscles, production of sputum, pain associated with breathing, decreased breath sounds, absent breath sounds in one or more lung fields, rhonchi, wheezing, rales/crackles in lung fields
- **GI:** Ascites

Assessment and Actions
Management of acidosis is related to identifying its source and treating it while attempting to correct the imbalance.

Fluid, electrolyte, and acid-base imbalances can rapidly cause life-threatening neurological, cardiac, and respiratory compromise, requiring immediate notification of the medical or rapid response team. Consult the medical team if any new onset occurs or if worsening symptoms or vital signs occur that are outside the normal range. If neurological, respiratory, or cardiac compromise occurs, call for assistance from the rapid or urgent response team or, if outside an acute care setting, call community EMS.

Patient History

Review for clues as to cause. The following conditions may be associated with or cause respiratory acidosis:

- Brain lesions or trauma leading to hypoventilation
- Chronic or acute respiratory disease or dysfunction leading to decreased ventilation
- Endocrine dysfunction, including hypothyroidism
- Neurological or neuromuscular diseases leading to hypoventilation
- Poisoning with competitive gases
- Chronic thoracic cavity deformity or insufficiency related to obesity
- Iatrogenic causes, including:
  - Surgery
  - Pain and sedative medication
  - Corticosteroids

Laboratory Assessment and Actions

If a patient has symptoms or etiological history that indicates acidosis, anticipate arterial blood draw for blood gas evaluation and venous blood for anion gap assessment (see the arterial blood draw precautions).

If pH is < 7.35, consult the medical team to evaluate anion gap and collaborate for management:

- Anticipate orders for venous serum sample to evaluate electrolyte imbalance. If calcium or potassium is high, anticipate measures discussed in the electrolyte chapter for correction of imbalances.
- Anticipate orders for serum thyroid levels. If TSH, T3 and/or T4 levels are elevated, anticipate orders to support a medical workup for hypothyroidism.
- Anticipate orders for serum and urine drug levels for opiates, barbiturates, and benzodiazepines, and discuss results of screening tests with the medical team:
  - If narcotics are confirmed as a source of respiratory depression, anticipate orders for administration of one or more doses of naloxone (Narcan), with an adult dosing of 0.4–2 mg intravenously, intramuscularly, or subcutaneously every 2–3 minutes to a maximum of 10 mg:
    - Lower doses are required for patients who are opiate-dependent to prevent severe pain response.
    - Observe patients closely for a return to sedation after effects of Naloxone wear off and opiate sedation persists.

- If benzodiazepines are confirmed as a source of respiratory depression, then:
  - Anticipate orders for administration of flumazenil (Romazicon), with an adult dose of 0.2 mg intravenously over 30 seconds, with repeated 0.5-mg doses 1 minute apart, administered over 30 seconds, up to a maximum of 3 mg.
  - Anticipate application of seizure precautions with the use of flumazenil, as reversal of benzodiazepines may precipitate seizure activity.

Systems Assessment and Actions

If laboratory test results are pending but respiratory acidosis is suspected, proceed with a systems assessment. Immediately consult the medical team at the onset or worsening of any of the symptoms that are listed in the following section.

Neurological

Perform frequent neurological assessments for decreased level of consciousness, mental status, and personality or memory changes. If mental status changes occur, then:

- Anticipate frequent measures of neurological status using the Glasgow Coma Scale.
- Maintain safety measures including keeping the bed low, padded side rails in place, and the call bell in reach.
- Continually reevaluate the patient's ability to follow instructions.
- Consult the medical team to discuss need for one-on-one supervision.
- Institute safety precautions, and assist with all activities of daily living, transfers, and ambulation.

Immediately contact the medical and rapid response team if the patient reports feeling of impending doom:

- Anticipate emergent respiratory support for potential pulmonary embolus.
- Anticipate orders for ventilation perfusion screening or CT scan if a pulmonary embolus is suspected.

If neuromuscular disease or insufficiency is suspected, anticipate orders for electromyography testing to analyze potential ventilatory muscle weakness. If weakness is diagnosed, see the following respiratory section for mechanical ventilatory support actions.

If no other source for acidosis is determined, anticipate orders for head CT or MRI to rule out brain disorders:

- Inquire as to potential for pregnancy in premenopausal women.
- Review results of urine pregnancy tests before sending pre-menopausal women for radiological studies.
- Ensure that patients are screened for interfering metal implants or shrapnel before sending them for MRI.

CV

If fever is $>100.5\degree$ F ($38\degree$ C), then:

- Consult the medical team for evaluation of infectious process, such as influenza, pneumonia, or other infectious lung diseases.
- Anticipate orders for antipyretics for temperatures $>101.5\degree$ F ($38.6\degree$ C).

If sputum or rhonchi are present, then:

- Anticipate orders for sputum specimen.
- Perform oral suctioning or provide suction catheter and instruction to patient for self-suctioning.
- If nasal, pharyngeal, or tracheal secretions are present, discuss orders with the medical team for sterile suctioning, and follow institutional guidelines to ensure sterility, oxygenation, and airway protection. Use caution, as excessive suctioning can decrease oxygen levels.

If influenza symptoms such as GI distress or aches are present, then:

- Anticipate orders for a nasal swab culture.
- Anticipate orders for respiratory isolation.
- Anticipate teaching the patient careful hand-washing and hygiene techniques.

If signs of congestive heart failure are present, then:

- Provide assistance with all activities of daily living to decrease the work of breathing.
- Place the patient in an upright position to support ventilation.
- Discuss with the medical team the need for supplemental oxygen.
- Anticipate orders for diuretic medications.
- Monitor intake and output.
- Anticipate orders for fluid restriction.

If the heart rate is elevated >100, discuss with the medical team the need for continuous cardiac monitoring.

Respiratory

If the respiratory rate is decreased or cyanosis is present, then:

- Carefully observe for barrel chest and other symptoms of chronic lung disease, such as clubbing of fingers and pursed lip breathing.
- Anticipate orders to place the patient on continuing pulse oximetry.
- Anticipate orders for supplemental oxygen support:
  - Discuss potential for low-flow oxygen in the presence of COPD, in which oxygen and carbon dioxide exchange is chronically out of ratio and excessive oxygen may destroy a fragile balance.
  - Anticipate drawing repeated blood gases and discussion with the medical team to adjust oxygen to keep Pao_2 60–65 mm Hg.

If oxygen levels drop <93% or below the patient's oxygenation baseline, and/or if respiratory support or mechanical ventilation is required, then:

- Anticipate reassuring the patient that support is temporary while the underlying condition is corrected:
  - If the patient is placed on mechanical ventilation, then explain the necessity for the support.
  - Inform patients who are ordered to receive NIPPV, such as bi-pap or c-pap, the need to wear a tight mask over their face until carbon dioxide levels return to normal or until the underlying conditions are corrected.
  - Inform patients requiring endotracheal intubation that speech is temporarily inhibited, and provide tools for the patient to communicate, such as a picture board or pencil and paper.
  - Anticipate orders to modify tidal volume and respiratory rate, and carefully monitor oxygen saturation, neurological changes, and respiratory effort response to changes in mechanical ventilation.

If sputum is present, then:

- Discuss orders with the medical team for a sputum specimen.
- Document the color, consistency, and amount of the sputum produced.
- Perform oral suctioning, or provide suction catheter and instruction to the patient for self-suctioning.
- If nasal, pharyngeal, or tracheal secretions are present, discuss orders with the medical team for sterile suctioning, and follow

institutional guidelines to ensure sterility, oxygenation, and airway protection. Use caution, as excessive suctioning can decrease oxygen levels.

- If blood is present in sputum, immediately report to the medical team. Anticipate efforts by the medical team to differentiate between tumor, tuberculosis, and pulmonary edema through bedside assessment, cultures, and radiological scans.

If changes in lung sounds occur, then:

- Report diminished, absent, or adventitious lung sounds to the medical team.
- If rales/crackles are present, anticipate orders for fluid restriction and diuretic therapy.

If rhonchi are present, then:

- Perform oral suctioning, or provide suction catheter and instruction to the patient for self-suctioning.
- If nasal, pharyngeal, or tracheal secretions are present, discuss orders with the medical team for sterile suctioning, and follow institutional guidelines to ensure sterility, oxygenation, and airway protection. Use caution, as excessive suctioning can decrease oxygen levels.
- Anticipate orders for antibiotics.

If wheezing is present, then:

- Consult the medical team for potential need for medications to open the airway:
  - Medications may include bronchodilators such as:
    - Beta-agonist albuterol, with adult dosing of 2–4 mg orally three times a day or by inhalation nebulizer 2.5 mg in 1–2.5 mL of normal saline every 4–6 hours.
    - Anticholinergic medications, such as ipratropium bromide (Atrovent) by inhalation, with adult dosing of 250 mcg diluted in 2.5 mL of normal saline every 4–6 hours.
    - Theophylline, used with caution for rebound respiratory alkalosis:
      - Orally in an adult dose of 10 mg/kg/day every 8–12 hours and then on a maintenance dose of 10 mg/kg/day once or twice a day.
      - Intravenously with a loading dose of 5.6 mg/kg over 20 minutes followed by a drip of 0.1–1.1 mg/kg/hr.
      - Theophylline is dosed based on blood levels; for adults, the range is 5–15 mcg/mL.

- Caution should be used with pediatric dosing of these medications because the ratios are different.
- Anticipate orders for chest x-ray to rule out lung disorders:
  - Inquire as to potential for pregnancy in premenopausal women.
  - Review results of urine pregnancy tests before sending premenopausal women for radiological studies.
  - If x-rays are inconclusive but symptoms persist, then:
    - Anticipate orders for CT scan or MRI.
    - Screen patients for interfering metal implants and shrapnel, and discuss with the medical team before sending them for MRI.

GI

If abdominal girth is increased, assist patient in an upright position to allow for maximum inspiration. If inspiration effort persists, anticipate orders to assist the medical team in a sterile bedside paracentesis or to transfer the patient to interventional radiology for paracentesis.

Prevention

Teach adult and child patients to wash their hands and to cover the mouth and nose during flu season. Remind patients with chronic respiratory and cardiac disease to avoid crowds during flu season. Remind patients to wear seat belts, and make certain all passengers are wearing seat belts to avoid thoracic trauma. Advise patients to maintain a carbon monoxide detector in their home, especially if they have an attached garage or an indoor fireplace. Encourage patients with symptoms of sleep apnea to discuss an assessment with their primary care provider and not to drive or operate machinery without sufficient sleep.

 CLINICAL SCENARIO

DIAGNOSIS: RESPIRATORY ACIDOSIS RELATED TO SLEEP APNEA

Mr. Riley had suffered with familial obesity, gastroesophageal reflux disease, and sleep apnea throughout most of his adult life. After extensive counseling, he was advised to undergo elective laparoscopic bariatric gastric bypass surgery to decrease his weight and improve his overall health. His surgery went well, but in the intensive care unit a day later he was noted to be somnolent and then had evolving mental status changes during the day. Narcan was delivered with consideration that a morphine patient-controlled analgesia pump might have been causing decreased respiratory exchange.

Continued

After the Narcan, Mr. Riley's condition improved somewhat. Physicians ordered a CT scan to rule out a potential postsurgical stroke. No anatomical changes were found on the CT scan and, over the next 24 hours, Mr. Riley appeared to be more wakeful. He was transferred to the bariatric surgery unit, where he was encouraged to be active in his care and to increase his supervised ambulation and activities of daily living. During visiting hours, while receiving physical therapy, and during meal times, Mr. Riley was assessed as awake, alert, and oriented. At night, his home c-pap machine was placed for sleeping.

However, on his second morning out of the intensive care unit, the morning shift nurse noted that Mr. Riley did not seem himself. Although he was able to answer orientation questions when being stimulated, he seemed unable to pour the 2-oz portions he was allowed to drink into the small medicine cups he had been provided. Concerned, the nurse measured his oxygen saturation and found it to be 85%. A rapid consultation was made with the physician, oxygen at 4 L was placed, and a blood gas sample was obtained. The sample demonstrated a respiratory acidosis with a pH of 7.32 and a P_{CO_2} of 55 mm Hg. Orders were placed for Mr. Riley to have his c-pap machine in place during the day when no one was present to stimulate him or when he was too sleepy to stay awake. Within 48 hours, his mentation and his respiratory gases returned to normal. The nurse assessed that a combination of postoperative hypoventilation, increased need for sleep, and decreased respiratory exchange related to a longer than typical response to pain medication had resulted in overall decreased gas exchange.

1. What signs should the nurse look for that show a patient is at risk for respiratory acidosis?
2. What common factors can interfere with respiratory function?
3. Why are patients with morbid obesity at risk for respiratory compromise when hospitalized?

Metabolic Alkalosis

Metabolic alkalosis occurs when there is a loss of circulating hydrogen ions or an excess of circulating bicarbonate molecules.

Laboratory Values (Arterial)
Arterial laboratory values for metabolic alkalosis can be uncompensated or compensated:

- **Uncompensated:** HCO_3^- >23 mEq/L; pH >7.45; P_{CO_2} = 35–45 mm Hg
- **Compensated:** HCO_3^- >23 mEq/L; pH = 7.35–7.45; P_{CO_2} >45 mm Hg

Uncompensated metabolic alkalosis means that blood bicarbonate values are increased, causing the pH to be increased, thus indicating alkalosis. Partial pressure of carbon dioxide values is within a normal range and has not yet begun to compensate for elevated levels of blood bicarbonate. With *compensated metabolic alkalosis*, the partial pressure has increased, offsetting the increased blood bicarbonate values, to return the pH to a normal range.

Basic Concepts

Metabolic dysfunction can result in higher than normal levels of bicarbonate in the bloodstream or loss of hydrogen or chloride ions. Loss of chloride in gastric secretions stimulate increased gastric acid secretion and a corresponding increase in serum bicarbonate. Loss of intravascular volume stimulates increased renal sodium reabsorption and, in the absence of chloride, bicarbonate is reabsorbed at the same time. Respiratory response will include slower and shallower breathing in order to retain carbon dioxide. Renal response will be to decrease hydrogen excretion and bicarbonate reabsorption. Renal disturbances can impair response to states of metabolic alkalosis. Metabolic alkalosis can also occur as a compensatory response to respiratory acidosis.

Etiology

There are many possible causes of metabolic alkalosis, including:
- Anoxia
- Hyperaldosteronism or stimulation of the renal renin-angiotensin-aldosterone system
- Low chloride ingestion or excessive loss from kidneys or GI losses
- Low potassium ingestion or excessive loss of potassium
- Gastric loss of hydrogen ions from bulimia or vomiting
- Ingestion of large amounts of licorice (or medical glycyrrhiza) or oral tobacco
- Shock

ELECTROLYTE ALKALOSIS

Electrolyte alkalosis is a subtype of metabolic alkalosis and indicates treatment associated with correcting electrolyte imbalance: Hypochloremic alkalosis is linked to low chloride levels (see Hypochloremia in Chapter 3B). Hypokalemic alkalosis is linked to low potassium levels (see Hypokalemia in Chapter 3E).

ALERT

Seizures, coma, and lethal dysrhythmias may occur at or above pH 7.55.

- Iatrogenic causes, including:
  - Blood transfusion with citrate preservative
  - Calcium carbonate ingestion
  - Corticosteroid use
  - Diuretic induced hydrogen, potassium, and sodium ion losses
  - Gastric suctioning or surgery
  - Magnesium-containing antacids
  - Milk alkali syndrome (milk ingestion with calcium-containing antacids)
  - Ringer's lactate infusion
  - Sodium bicarbonate ingestion or infusion, especially as an antacid
  - Total or partial parenteral nutrition with acetate or lactate

Symptoms

Metabolic alkalosis is often asymptomatic, except for symptoms of volume depletion. Concurrent hypokalemia or hypocalcemia may cause similar symptoms.

- **Neurological**: Confusion, change in mental status, weakness, seizures, and coma
- **CV:** Dysrhythmias may occur at or above pH 7.55:
  - Hypervolemia with non-chloride–associated alkalosis
  - Hypovolemia with chloride-associated alkalosis
- **Respiratory:** Slow, shallow breathing leading to failure
- **GI:** Vomiting causing decreased potassium and chloride, hepatic encephalopathy
- **Genitourinary (GU):** Polyuria
- **Musculoskeletal:** Increased reflexes, spasms, tetany

Assessment and Actions

Management of alkalosis is related to identifying the source of alkalosis and treating it while attempting to correct the imbalance.

Fluid, electrolyte, and acid-base imbalances can rapidly cause life-threatening neurological, cardiac, and respiratory compromise, requiring immediate notification of the medical or rapid response team. Consult the medical team if any new onset occurs or if worsening symptoms or vital signs occur that are outside the normal range. If neurological, respiratory, or cardiac compromise occurs, then call for assistance from the rapid or urgent response team or, if outside an acute care setting, then call community EMS.

Patient History

Review for clues to etiology. The following conditions may be associated with or cause metabolic alkalosis:

- Respiratory compromise, trauma, CV arrest, and other conditions causing anoxia, respiratory acidosis (compensatory response), or shock
- GI illness associated with vomiting, diarrhea, suctioning, or fistulas, causing either chloride, hydrogen, and/or potassium losses or the inability to ingest chloride or potassium from dietary sources
- Electrolyte imbalance resulting in low chloride or low potassium levels
- Conditions requiring medical intervention with blood transfusion, diuretics, parenteral nutrition, steroids, Ringer's lactate, or alkaline medications, such as antacids

Laboratory Assessment and Actions

If the patient has signs and a disease history that indicate alkalosis, anticipate orders for an arterial blood draw for blood gas evaluation and potassium levels. If pH is >7.45, then:

- Carefully monitor respiratory rate and depth.
- Anticipate efforts to decrease ventilation rate and depth:
  - If mechanical ventilation is in place, anticipate orders for reduced tidal volume or rate.
  - If patients are breathing on their own, provide a quiet environment and reassurance, and teach patients to slow breathing through relaxation techniques.

If pH is >7.55, then:

- Anticipate emergent hemodialysis to prevent cardiac arrhythmias, encephalopathy, coma, or death.
- Nephrologists may order intravenous infusion of hydrochloric acid solutions in continually monitored critical care environments.
- See Chapter 2 for precautions regarding hemodialysis.

If potassium is <3.5 mEq/L, then:

- Anticipate collaboration with medical team for orders of intravenous or oral potassium administration (see the hypokalemia section in Chapter 3E for a description of and details regarding the procedure).
- Anticipate that chloride levels will increase, causing bicarbonate levels to decrease.

- Anticipate that increased potassium levels will allow the kidneys to shift to excretion of potassium ions and retention of hydrogen ions.
- Anticipate orders for a venous blood sample, and report results to the medical team. A bicarbonate level > 35 mEq/L confirms metabolic alkalosis.
- Anticipate orders for routine or 24-hour urine specimen:
  - Discuss levels of urine chloride < 20 mEq/L, confirming alkalosis secondary to volume depletion.
  - Discuss levels of aldosterone, indicating hyperaldosteronism.
  - Anticipate orders for administration of spironolactone, dexamethasone, or angiotensin-converting enzyme inhibitors.
  - Anticipate preparation for surgery if a tumor is the primary cause.
  - Discuss levels of urine-free cortisol to confirm Cushing's syndrome.
  - Anticipate orders for potassium-sparing diuretics.
  - Discuss other endocrine urine levels as ordered to distinguish other potential metabolic dysfunctions or syndromes.
  - Anticipate orders for imaging studies for assessment for potential tumors of the adrenal glands or structural renal problems:
    - Inquire as to potential for pregnancy in premenopausal women.
    - Review results of urine pregnancy test before sending premenopausal women for radiological studies.
    - Review allergies to screen for allergy or sensitivity to radiological dye or seafood.
    - Screen patients for interfering metal implants and shrapnel, and discuss with the medical team before sending them for MRI.
  - Anticipate orders to assist in other metabolic testing to identify other genetic or metabolic syndromes as causes of alkalosis.

Systems Assessment and Actions

If laboratory values are pending but metabolic alkalosis is suspected, proceed with a systems assessment. Immediately consult with the medical team

MED INFO

Spironolactone (Aldactone) has an adult dosing of 50–100 mg orally every 6 hours. Dexamethasone has an adult dosing of 0.5–4 mg orally twice a day. Angiotensin-converting enzyme inhibitors include captopril, enalapril, and lisinopril. Captopril has an adult dosing of 6.25–50 mg orally twice a day; enalapril has an adult dosing of 2.5–20 mg orally daily; and lisinopril has an adult dosing of 5–20 mg orally daily.

at the onset or worsening of any of the symptoms that are listed in the following section.

Neurological

Perform frequent neurological assessments for decreased level of consciousness or mental status changes. If mental status changes, weakness, or if the potential for seizures occurs, then:

- Anticipate frequent measures of neurological status using the Glasgow Coma Scale.
- Maintain safety measures including keeping the bed low, padded side rails in place, and the call bell in reach.
- Continually reevaluate the patient's ability to follow instructions.
- Consult the medical team to discuss the need for one-on-one supervision.
- Institute safety precautions, and assist with all activities of daily living, transfers, and ambulation.

If mental status changes decline, take emergency measures, and ensure a secure airway.

CV

If there are signs of volume depletion, anticipate orders for intravenous fluid replacement with normal saline solution (0.9% NaCl) or half-normal saline solution (0.45% NaCl).

If symptoms of volume excess are present, carefully consult the medical team before routinely administering prescribed diuretics, as they may worsen metabolic alkalosis. In the presence of low chloride alkalosis, anticipate orders for replacement of chloride with potassium chloride rather than sodium chloride.

If hypocalcemia or hypokalemia is present or if pH is near or >7.55, then:

- Anticipate orders for continuous cardiac monitoring.
- Anticipate orders for replacement of low potassium with potassium chloride in the presence of low chloride alkalosis.
- Discuss with the medical team the best electrocardiogram (ECG) leads to monitor for signs and symptoms of cardiac dysrhythmias associated with electrolyte changes as described in the hypocalcemia section of Chapter 3A and the hypokalemia section of Chapter 3E.

Respiratory

If respiratory depression or insufficiency is present, then:

- Anticipate orders to place the patient on continuing oxygen saturation pulse oximetry.
- Anticipate orders for supplemental oxygen support.

If oxygen levels drop < 93% or below the patient's oxygenation baseline, or if respiratory support or mechanical ventilation is required, anticipate reassuring the patient that support is temporary while the underlying condition is corrected. If the patient is placed on mechanical ventilation, then:

- Explain to the patients the need for the ventilation support.
- Inform patients who are ordered to receive NIPPV, such as bi-pap or c-pap, the need to wear a tight mask over their face until carbon dioxide levels return to normal or until underlying conditions are corrected.
- Inform the patient requiring endotracheal intubation that speech is temporarily inhibited, and provide tools for the patient to communicate such as a picture board or pencil and paper.
- Anticipate orders to modify tidal volume and respiratory rate, and carefully monitor oxygen saturation, neurological changes, and respiratory effort response to changes in mechanical ventilation.

GI

If vomiting occurs, then:

- Carefully measure and document the volume and color of the emesis.
- Anticipate orders for antiemetic medication. Observe for neurological symptoms associated with Compazine (prochlorperazine), if ordered.

If gastric suctioning is required, then anticipate orders for histamine-blocking agents or proton pump inhibitors to decrease gastric secretions.

If licorice ingestion is the cause, provide potassium-sparing diuretics, as licorice enzyme shifts take up to 2 weeks to resolve.

GU

If fluid overload is present and diuresis must be stimulated, anticipate substitution of thiazide or loop diuretics with potassium-sparing diuretics or acetazolamide:

- Potassium-sparing diuretics include:
  - Triamterene (Dyrenium), with adult dosing of 100 mg orally twice a day.
  - Spironolactone (Aldactone), with adult dosing of 50–100 mg orally every 6 hours.
- Acetazolamide (Diamox), a carbonic anhydrase inhibitor, inhibiting the renal resorption of sodium bicarbonate:
  - Adult dosing is 250–500 mg orally every 6 hours or 5 mg/kg intravenously daily.
  - Caution must be used to prevent hyperkalemia.

Musculoskeletal

If increased reflexes, spasms, or tetany occurs, then:

- Institute standard safety precautions.
- Maintain the patient on bedrest.
- Assist patient with all activities of daily living, ambulation, and transfers.

Prevention

Teach patients to read medication labels carefully and to discuss the use of over-the-counter medications with care providers, especially antacids including magnesium, calcium carbonate, and bicarbonate. Patients should also learn to:

- Avoid taking antacids with milk to avoid milk alkali syndrome.
- Eat licorice sparingly and to keep it out of the reach of children and adults with mental disabilities.

Bulimic patients and patients with other chronic GI losses should be taught the signs of dangerous levels of metabolic alkalosis, including hypoventilation and changes in mental status.

Patients who use chewing tobacco should be taught that it is carcinogenic for head and neck cancers and can cause life-threatening metabolic changes.

 CLINICAL SCENARIO

DIAGNOSIS: METABOLIC ALKALOSIS RELATED TO ANTACID TOXICITY

Mrs. North was a patient with chronic GI upset related to a hiatal hernia. Her primary care nurse practitioner had prescribed a proton pump inhibitor, but Mrs. North lost her health insurance with a job layoff and could no longer afford her prescription medications. Mrs. North turned to inexpensive, over-the-counter antacids.

Overall, the antacids were ineffective, and she began to feel weak and confused. She reported to the emergency room with uncertain symptoms. However, her blood work showed potassium at 3.3 mEq/L and a hemoglobin level of 8.3. After intravenous hydration, her potassium level and her hemoglobin level dropped even further. Her potassium was replaced with intravenous potassium chloride, and—given her history of hiatal hernia and GI upset—she underwent an endoscopy. The results showed a bleeding gastric ulcer, contributing to low hemoglobin. She was placed on nothing-by-mouth status, an intravenous proton pump inhibitor, and low, intermittent gastric suction.

Continued

Her oxygen saturation showed 99% on room air after her endoscopy. However, after several hours of gastric suctioning, a spot check of her oxygen saturation showed a drop to 90%. The nurse noted that Mrs. North's breathing was shallow and about 8 breaths per minute. When Mrs. North was awakened and stimulated, she was disoriented, not remembering the name of the hospital. In consultation with the medical team, supplemental oxygen was provided to Mrs. North, and a blood gas test was ordered. Results showed metabolic alkalosis, with a pH of 7.50, an HCO_3^- of 27 mEq/L, and a return to her hypokalemia. Gastric suction was discontinued, and potassium chloride was once again ordered. A second blood gas test 4 hours later showed a marked resolution of her metabolic alkalois to a pH of 7.43 and an arterial HCO_3^- of 23 mEq/L.

1. Why was Mrs. North at risk for low potassium levels?
2. How can the nurse help Mrs. North prevent a recurrence of her alkalosis?
3. Besides ordered laboratory measures, what should the nurse measure to monitor potential electrolyte loss?

Metabolic Acidosis

Metabolic acidosis occurs when the body has an excess of circulating hydrogen ions or a loss of circulating bicarbonate molecules.

Laboratory Values (Arterial)
Arterial laboratory values for metabolic acidosis can be uncompensated or compensated:

- **Uncompensated:** $HCO_3^- < 18$ mEq/L; pH < 7.35; $P_{CO_2} = 35$–45 mm Hg
- **Compensated:** $HCO_3^- < 18$ mEq/L; pH $= 7.35$–7.45; $P_{CO_2} < 35$ mm Hg

ALERT

A pH of <7.10 can result in cardiac arrest. Symptoms of metabolic acidosis may begin to appear at bicarbonate levels <20 mEq/L.

Uncompensated metabolic acidosis means that blood bicarbonate levels are decreased, causing pH to be decreased, thus indicating acidosis. Values of partial pressure of carbon dioxide are within a normal range and have not yet begun to compensate for decreased levels of blood bicarbonate. With *compensated metabolic acidosis*, the levels of partial pressure of carbon dioxide have decreased, offsetting the decreased blood bicarbonate, to return the pH to a normal range.

Basic Concepts

Metabolic dysfunction can result in levels of bicarbonate in the bloodstream that are lower than normal. Metabolic problems can also cause increased acids either because of the kidneys' failure to excrete excess acids or because of increased production of lactic acids or ketones. Metabolic acidosis can also be related to toxic ingestion of anions. Lactic acid is associated with anaerobic metabolism of glucose when insufficient oxygen is present. Liver and renal dysfunction can prevent adequate excretion of excess lactic acid. Ketones are formed either when fatty acids rather than carbohydrates are used as an energy source or when alcohol is metabolized in the liver. With diabetes, ketosis can occur when not enough insulin is present to allow glucose to be directed into cells.

Respiratory response to metabolic acidosis includes deeper and more rapid breathing in order to discharge carbon dioxide. Partial pressure of carbon dioxide (Pco_2) decreases in a close ratio to the decrease in bicarbonate. For each mEq/L below normal serum bicarbonate, expect the lungs to attempt to decrease Pco_2 by 1–1.5 mm Hg. Renal response will be to increase hydrogen excretion and bicarbonate reabsorption. Renal disturbances can impair response to states of metabolic acidosis.

Etiology

Etiology of metabolic acidosis is evaluated using an anion gap measurement (see Chapter 6 formulas). A high anion gap, >12 mEq/L, indicates acid production or poisoning. With high ion gaps, bicarbonate levels go down because sodium binds to acids rather than to bicarbonate. A normal anion gap of 8–12 mEq/L indicates bicarbonate losses, or hyperchloremic acidosis, when chloride retention balances with bicarbonate loss. A low anion gap of <8 mEq/L also indicates bicarbonate losses, although the bicarbonate decreases due to unmeasured cation or anion changes. Changes in unmeasured anions or cations could be the result of decreased anion albumin or increased cations, IgG, and paraproteins related to multiple myeloma, lithium intoxication, or increased potassium, magnesium, or calcium. Conditions that cause low anion gaps include:

- Alcohol oxidation in the liver, causing ketoacidosis
- Aldosterone deficiency, causing renal secretion of acids
- Cancers, especially blood cancers increasing lactate production
- Diabetes with low insulin levels, resulting in ketoacidosis

- Diarrhea, ileostomy, and other lower GI fluid, increasing loss in bicarbonate
- Malnutrition or catabolism related to high metabolic need, causing ketosis and lactic acidosis
- Liver failure, increasing lactate levels and decreasing lactate excretion from other causes, such as ingestion of ethanol alcohol
- Renal dysfunction, which causes retention of acids (*Note:* Renal tubular acidosis may also decrease bicarbonate and increase retention of hydrogen.)
- Shock, which can cause a shift to anaerobic metabolism and a lack of ability to clear the lactic acid produced in a low oxygen state
- Poisoning or toxic ingestion of substances such as:
  - Ethylene glycol (antifreeze), lethal at 100 mL ingested
  - Methanol, which can be fatal when absorbed through the skin, ingested, or inhaled
- Thyrotoxicosis or hyperthyroidism, resulting in severe cellular catabolism
- Iatrogenic causes, which may include:
  - Aluminum chloride, causing excess chloride
  - Aspirin or salicylate (wintergreen) overingestion
  - Cholestyramine
  - Citrates (medications or related to blood transfusions)
  - Ether
  - Fluorides
  - Isoniazid
  - Iron
  - Metformin
  - Nothing by mouth orders (prolonged)
  - Potassium-sparing diuretics
  - Small-bowel resection or jejunoileal bypass related to carbohydrates passing directly to the colon
  - Sodium chloride administration
  - Sulfa medications
  - Total parenteral nutrition
  - Theophylline
  - Xylitol

ALERT

Aspirin or salicylate overingestion can be fatal. Methyl salicylate (i.e., oil of wintergreen) is commonly found in candies, topical muscle analgesics, and mouthwashes.

Symptoms

Symptoms of metabolic acidosis may appear when bicarbonate levels are < 20 mEq/L. Symptoms include:

- **Neurological:** Confusion, dizziness, headache, lethargy leading to coma, ringing in the ears (salicylate poisoning), vision disturbances, weakness
- **CV:** Cardiac pain or palpitations, edema, fatal arrhythmia (at pH of 7.2), fluid overload, hypotension, shock, venous distention
- **Respiratory:** Dyspnea at rest, fruity breath, Kussmaul's respirations (deep and rapid), pulmonary edema
- **Integumentary:** Cool and clammy during early stages of acidosis, evolving with increasing acidosis to warm and flushed resulting from lack of sympathetic stimulation
- **GI:** Diarrhea, nausea, pain, vomiting
- **GU:** Fluid volumes of < 400 mL over 24 hours
- **Musculoskeletal:** Bone pain, muscle weakness, osteomalacia, pathological fracture, diminished deep tendon reflexes

Assessment and Actions

Management of acidosis is related to identifying its source and treating it while attempting to correct the imbalance.

Fluid, electrolyte, and acid-base imbalances can rapidly cause life-threatening neurological, cardiac, and respiratory compromise, requiring immediate notification of the medical or rapid response team. Consult the medical team if any new onset occurs or if worsening symptoms or vital signs occur that are outside the normal range. If neurological, respiratory, or cardiac compromise occurs, call for assistance from the rapid or urgent response team or, if outside an acute care setting, call community EMS.

Patient History

Review for clues as to cause. The following conditions may be associated with or cause metabolic acidosis:

- Ingestion or toxic absorption of methanol and ethylene glycol
- If patient has a history of personal or familial diabetes leading to diabetic ketoacidosis
- Iatrogenic causes, including:
  - Shortened, resectioned, or bypassed small bowel, which can lead to D-lactic acidosis.

- Salicylate toxicity, which requires administration of activated charcoal or dialysis:
  - Activated charcoal is administered at a normal dose of 1–2 g/kg.
  - Anticipate orders for gastric lavage or whole-bowel irrigation with recent ingestion.
  - Anticipate orders for hemodialysis with high toxicity levels or chronic absorption.
  - See dialysis precautions in Chapter 2.

Laboratory Assessment and Actions

If the patient has signs and a disease history that point to acidosis, anticipate orders for an arterial blood draw for blood gas evaluation and venous blood draw for anion gap assessment:

- If pH is <7.35, consult the medical team to evaluate anion gap and collaborate for management.
- If anion gap is normal, then:
  - Anticipate the medical team may order bicarbonate orally or intravenously.
    - Anticipate frequent arterial blood draws to assess for effect of intravenous bicarbonate.
    - Anticipate order for oral sodium bicarbonate mouthwashes to neutralize oral acids, if the patient has a patent airway.
  - If anion gap is high, then:
    - Anticipate that measures other than sodium bicarbonate may be ordered.
    - Anticipate orders for fluid and oxygen resuscitation to improve oxygen delivery to the cells.

If the patient has a history of personal or familial diabetes, then:

- Anticipate assessment of blood glucose by finger stick and serum blood draw to assess for diabetic cause, lactic acid, and serum ketone levels.
- Anticipate orders for intravenous saline with potassium supplementation to reverse dehydration.
- Anticipate discussion with medical team for intravenous or subcutaneous regular insulin.

MED INFO Ⓡ

Many medical teams will withhold bicarbonate as a last-resort medication if the underlying disorder has not been identified or corrected. This is because bicarbonate is *not compatible* with most other intravenous medications and therefore should be delivered via a dedicated intravenous line. Carefully check for compatibility before running concurrent intravenous medications with bicarbonate. Intravenous bicarbonate will be ordered in measured doses of 50–100 mEq in an effort to raise pH to >7.20.

- Once glucose levels fall to 250 mg/dL, anticipate orders for glucose administration to prevent rebound hypoglycemia.
- Anticipate orders to draw a serum specimen for lactic acid level:
  - Note that lactic acid preservation requires special laboratory tubes and handling of serum specimen, either gray-topped sodium fluoride or green-topped lithium heparin, transported in an ice slurry to slow acid production.
- Discuss results with the medical team.
- If lactate concentration is >4 mEq/L, anticipate orders for a low-carbohydrate diet and orders to treat.
- Types of lactic acidosis include:
  - Type A, which occurs with decreased oxygenation of tissues
  - Type B, which occurs with renal or hepatic disease, drug toxicity, alcoholic acidosis, malignancy, and inborn errors of metabolism
  - Type D, which occurs with shortened bowel surgery; treatment requires administration of antibiotics targeted at the large bowel and lactic acid–producing organisms
  - Type L, which occurs with anaerobic metabolism with fluid resuscitation and efforts to promote reperfusion of tissues
- Anticipate orders to draw a serum specimen for osmolar gap calculation (see Chapter 6 for calculation):
  - Discuss with the medical team results of calculations derived from serum sodium, glucose, and blood urea nitrogen.
  - If the osmolar gap is >15, anticipate treatment for ingestion or toxic absorption of methanol and ethylene glycol:
    - Anticipate orders for intravenous fluids and hemodialysis.
    - Ethanol may also be ordered in some cases. Ethanol competes with the enzymes that metabolize methanol and ethylene glycol so that these more toxic alcohols can be dialyzed out of the blood before they are metabolized into acids.
- Anticipate orders for serum specimen salicylate levels:
  - Discuss results with the medical team.
  - If plasma levels are >40 mg/dL, anticipate administration of activated charcoal or dialysis (see charcoal precautions in the section of this chapter on respiratory alkalosis).

- Anticipate orders for serum specimen iron levels, and discuss results with the medical team:
  - If plasma levels are >300 mg/dL, then:
    - Anticipate orders for administration of deferoxamine intramuscularly or intravenously under the guidance of a toxicologist.
    - Anticipate orders for polyethylene glycol bowel preparation (GoLYTELY, Colyte) laxative under the guidance of a toxicologist.
  - Anticipate orders for intravenous hydrating normal saline solution or lactated. Ringer's solution to prevent hypovolemia.

Systems Assessment and Actions

If laboratory test results are pending but metabolic acidosis is suspected, proceed with a systems assessment. Immediately consult the medical team at the onset or worsening of any of the symptoms listed in the following section.

Neurological

Perform frequent neurological assessments for decreased level of consciousness, mental status, personality, or memory changes. If mental status changes occur, then:

- Anticipate frequent measures of neurological status using the Glasgow Coma Scale.
- Maintain safety measures including keeping the bed low, padded side rails in place, and the call bell in reach.
- Continually reevaluate the patient's ability to follow instructions.
- Consult the medical team to discuss need for one-on-one supervision.
- Institute safety precautions, and assist with all activities of daily living, transfers, and ambulation.
- If mental status declines, take emergency measures, and ensure a secure airway.

CV

If hyperkalemia is present or if pH is near or >7.20, then:

- Anticipate orders for continuous cardiac monitor.
- Anticipate orders for medications to lower potassium levels as described in the hyperkalemia section of Chapter 3E.
- Discuss with the medical team the best ECG leads to monitor for signs and symptoms of cardiac dysrhythmias associated with

electrolyte changes as described in the hyperkalemia section of Chapter 3E.

If chest pain or symptoms of impending cardiogenic shock occur, consult the medical team to initiate transfer of the patient to an intensive care environment:

- Anticipate orders for 12-lead ECG.
- Anticipate orders to treat potential myocardial ischemia, including administration of intravenous morphine.
- Anticipate orders for placement of large-bore intravenous lines and rapid infusion of fluid to correct hypotension.
- Anticipate orders for medications that will cause vasopressive effects (see Chapter 2 for management of shock).

If symptoms of fluid overload are present, then anticipate administration of intravenous diuretics and careful measurement of intake and output (see Chapter 2 for management of fluid excess states).

Respiratory

If hyperventilation is present, then:

- Anticipate orders to place patient on continuing oxygen saturation pulse oximetry.
- Anticipate orders for supplemental oxygen support.

If oxygen levels drop below 93% or below the patient's oxygen baseline, or if respiratory support or mechanical ventilation is required, then:

- Explain to the patient the need for the ventilation support.
- Inform the patient who is ordered to receive NIPPV, such as bi-pap or c-pap, the need to wear a tight mask over the face until carbon dioxide levels return to normal or until underlying conditions are corrected.
- Inform patients requiring endotracheal intubation that speech is temporarily inhibited, and provide tools for the patient to communicate, such as a picture board or pencil and paper.
- Anticipate orders to modify tidal volume and respiratory rate, and carefully monitor oxygen saturation, neurological changes, and respiratory effort response to changes in mechanical ventilation.

Integumentary

If the patient's skin becomes cool and clammy, then:

- Discuss with medical team suspicion of initial stages of acidosis.
- Provide a change of linens to keep skin dry and sufficient blankets to keep patient at normal body temperatures.

If the patient's skin becomes warm and flushed, then:
- Immediately inform medical team of decline to severe acidosis related to lack of sympathetic stimulation.
- Prepare for emergent respiratory and CV support.

GI

If nausea or vomiting occur, then:
- Anticipate administration of antiemetics. Caution for neurological side effects should be exercised if Compazine (prochlorperazine) is ordered.
- Anticipate placement of a nasogastric suction tube to remove gastric secretions.

If diarrhea occurs, then anticipate orders for antidiarrhea medications to prevent further loss of bicarbonate.

GU

If patient has fluid volumes of < 400 mL over 24 hours, then:
- Consult the medical team because the patient may be descending into renal failure.
- Anticipate hydration with crystalloid solutions.
- Anticipate repeated urine samples to assess effect of fluid loss on electrolyte imbalance:
  - If urine specimens are ordered, use caution to avoid contamination with water or soap.
  - If drawing from a catheter, make certain to draw urine from the collection tube rather than the collection bag, because the bag is where urine will start to degrade biologically.

Musculoskeletal

If weakness or decreased protective reflexes are assessed, then:
- Maintain safety measures including keeping the bed low, padded side rails in place, and the call bell in reach.
- Consult the medical team to discuss the need for one-on-one supervision.
- Institute safety precautions, and assist with all the activities of daily living, transfers, and ambulation.

Prevention

Keep all alcohols and medications away from children and adults with decreased mental capacity. Teach diabetic patients the signs and symptoms of diabetic acidosis, and caution them in administration of correct insulin doses.

CLINICAL SCENARIO

DIAGNOSIS: METABOLIC ACIDOSIS RELATED TO DIABETES MELLITUS

Mr. Sanert had a strong family history of diabetes, but he was not diagnosed with diabetes until he was in his late seventies. By that time, diabetes had affected his peripheral and retinal nerves, and he had difficulty seeing and manipulating his finger-stick meter and insulin syringe. He also had difficulty modifying his diet. He presented to the hospital for a routine colonoscopy after ingestion of a bowel laxative preparation regime.

On arrival to the outpatient desk, he seemed to be confused about his reason for coming and presented the nurse with his parking ticket when asked for his prescription. After a few minutes, the nurse assessed that Mr. Sanert was not himself and called for the clinic resident to assist her in assessing Mr. Sanert. A blood glucose finger stick was obtained and showed a blood glucose of 425. Mr. Sanert's breath had a distinct fruity odor, and he complained of blurry vision. He was taken to the emergency department, where he was provided with hydrating fluids, intravenous insulin, and intravenous potassium.

After several hours, Mr. Sanert's pH had returned to normal levels from an initial pH of 7.25. After his treatment, he was admitted for observation and inpatient colonoscopy. The diabetes nurse educator met several times with Mr. Sanert during his stay and arranged for a home care assessment to help create a regimen for diet, exercise, and safe administration of insulin. His finger-stick meter and insulin needles were changed to a product that allowed him to see a large-print readout and dial his insulin into a pen rather than draw up doses into a syringe.

1. Based on Mr. Sanert's initial presentation, how does the nurse suspect Mr. Sanert has been managing his insulin?
2. Why was Mr. Sanert's colonoscopy care plan changed from outpatient to inpatient?
3. In addition to his fruity breath, what breathing characteristics would the nurse anticipate with metabolic acidosis?

Review Questions

1. When an acid-base imbalance occurs, what is the first body system to respond?
2. What is the meaning of "pH" in an arterial blood gas measurement?
3. Which electrolyte values are associated with electrolyte alkalosis?
4. Acid-base imbalance can be associated with poisoning. What agency should be contacted to direct management of known or suspected poisoning?

5 Common Disease Processes and Metabolic Disturbances Associated with Fluid, Electrolyte, and Acid-Base Imbalances

Common Disease Processes and Metabolic Disturbances Associated With Fluid, Electrolyte, and Acid-Base Imbalances

Many common diseases and disorders are linked to fluid, electrolyte, and acid-base imbalances. This chapter discusses 13 common ailments: burns, cancer and nonmalignant tumors, chronic obstructive pulmonary disease (COPD), diabetes, other endocrine disorders, heart failure, infection and sepsis, liver failure and biliary and pancreatic dysfunction, gastrointestinal malabsorption, mental status changes, orthopedic disorders, renal disease and dysfunction, and trauma. Awareness of the role of electrolyte, fluid, and acid-base imbalances with these health problems enables the health team to anticipate and create a treatment plan for them.

Burns

A/B, $F(^+/^-)$, $Ca(^-)$, $K(^+)$, $Mg(^+/^-)$, $Na(^-)$, $Ph(^+/^-)$

The effect of- burns on fluids and electrolytes depends on the depth and area of skin damage. Fluid rapidly shifts from the intravascular area into the interstitial area because of cellular damage from the burn; fluid also

Table 5–1 Symbols in This Chapter

SYMBOL	MEANING
(-)	Deficit; for example, F(-) means fluid deficit
(+)	Excess; for example, F(+) means an excess of fluid
A/B	Acid/base
Ca	Calcium
Cl	Chloride
F	Fluid
K	Potassium
M	Minerals
Mg	Magnesium
Na	Sodium
Ph	Phosphorus

leaks out of the vascular space during the acute phase of the burn, which is when capillaries are more permeable. This acute period can continue for days after the burn.

Electrolyte shifts are a critical problem in burn patients. Calcium and sodium shift out of the vascular space into the area around the cells, with sodium pulling fluid along into the interstitial space. In the early hours after a burn, magnesium, phosphorus, and potassium shift out of cells into the vascular and interstitial spaces because of cellular destruction. If renal function is not decreased, potassium may clear, and levels may remain normal. However, diuresis may also contribute to hypokalemia. If burns cause kidney damage and potassium is not cleared well, hyperkalemia may occur.

Possible Imbalances During Treatment

Initial treatment may require massive fluid resuscitation in order to maintain vascular capacity and blood pressure. During recovery, patients may experience fluid overload if they are unable to mobilize the excess fluid that has been infused. Fluid overload combined with stress-induced catecholamine release can result in elevated blood pressure.

If blood transfusions are given, the preservative citrate may further decrease calcium levels.

During recovery from burns, phosphorous stores may be decreased by an increased metabolic demand. Depending on the extent of the burns, dressings can be extensive. Patients with extensive burns whose dressings include mafenide acetate are at risk for metabolic acidosis.

Cancer and Nonmalignant Tumors

A/B, $F(^+/^-)$, $Ca(^+/^-)$, $K(^+/^-)$, $Mg(^-)$, $Na(^-)$, $Ph(^+/^-)$

Certain types of cancer and cancer treatments can cause fluid and electrolyte shifts. For example:

- Malignant tumors can be associated with loss of calcium from bones into the blood, with resulting high blood calcium levels.
- Intracranial tumors can cause cerebral salt-wasting syndrome, in which the kidneys are unable to conserve sodium, resulting in hyponatremia.

Pituitary tumors can cause either an excess or deficiency of antidiuretic hormone–arginine vasopressin (ADH-AVP). Excess ADH-AVP is called syndrome of inappropriate antidiuretic hormone (SIADH) and leads to high fluid volume and low blood sodium levels because of vascular dilution (rather than actual sodium losses). A lack of ADH can result in diabetes insipidus (DI), which is characterized by excessive renal fluid loss that results in low fluid volume and sodium retention. More information on DI is in the Diabetes Insipidus section.

Endometrial or uterine cancers can be associated with high levels of blood loss and accompanying fluid deficit.

Parathyroid tumors can secrete excess parathyroid hormone (PTH), causing loss of bone calcium and increased serum calcium with resulting low phosphorus.

COACH CONSULT

The severity of a burn determines the extent of fluid and electrolyte shifts. Patients with extensive burns will be transported to specialized burn centers, where staff members have undergone training on the techniques of burn resuscitation and where sterile burn units are prepared to manage the severe immunocompromise that accompanies the loss of skin. At times, however, patients who experience smaller burns will be cared for in an acute care facility. For these patients, the risk of fluid and electrolyte shifts is less; however, the risk of immunocompromise is still high, and care must involve strict adherence to aseptic technique.

Thyroid tumors can increase calcitonin to extremely high levels, causing hypocalcemia.

Acute leukemia and some lymphoma tumors consume phosphorus, causing low phosphorous levels. Some leukemias are also associated with a drop in potassium.

It is therefore important to be familiar with the shifts associated with specific tumors and treatments so that these potential shifts can be anticipated and included in the treatment plan.

Possible Imbalances During Treatment

Cancer treatment can also cause fluid and electrolyte shifts. Tumor lysis syndrome, in which cells are destroyed in response to chemotherapy and radiation, causes potassium and phosphorus to leak out of damaged cells and move into the vascular space; in turn, high-serum phosphorus stimulates a reciprocal drop in calcium. Anorexia, diarrhea, or vomiting can be associated with chemotherapy and cause losses of fluids, sodium, magnesium, and potassium. Diarrhea and poor absorption related to either mucosal damage or scarring can be caused by radiation for abdominal or pelvic tumors.

Depending on the prescribed chemotherapy regimen, patients may experience electrolyte shifts with each dose of medication and require "rescue" fluids or electrolytes before or after prescribed chemotherapy. Some chemotherapy treatments cannot be administered until electrolytes have been repleted because they will cause severe electrolyte shifts during infusion. Although administration is performed by chemotherapy-certified nurses, nurses who care for patients before and after treatment must be alert for these potential shifts.

Similar effects may be seen with surgery that interrupts the gastric system, which decreases the volume of normal digestive fluids and the surface area for absorption. Alkalosis and acidosis can accompany loss of gastrointestinal fluids through preoperative bowel preparations, surgery, drains, and fistulas. If hysterectomy or removal of ovaries occurs, then calcium levels can be depleted, and patients may need to add a calcium and vitamin D supplement to their regular dietary intake to prevent bone losses.

Patients with gastrointestinal surgeries and other malnutrition risks may receive total or partial parenteral nutrition. Shifts in electrolytes and fluid can occur with this high-glucose, high-volume preparation. Caution should be used to ensure that electrolytes, fluid, and mineral levels stay within the normal range during therapy. Typically, the medical team will order an assessment of electrolytes and minerals daily or every other day until the patient has become stabilized on a routine dose, and then the orders may be based upon weekly assessments.

Chronic Obstructive Pulmonary Disease

A/B, F($^+$/$^-$)

Chronic obstructive pulmonary disease (COPD) is a group of diseases that includes chronic emphysema, chronic bronchitis, and chronic asthma. Emphysema causes mucous plugging and lack of elasticity of the lower airway, resulting in destruction of alveolar walls. Patients with chronic respiratory illness are also at high risk for acute respiratory illness. Infections can cause dehydration because of fever and increased metabolic demands. Rehydration is required not only to prevent extension of acute illness but also to allow for the chronic mucus that is formed with emphysema to stay liquid enough to be mobilized out of the lungs. Some patients may require intravenous fluids, whereas others may be sufficiently hydrated by a humidifier.

Bronchitis is centered in the mucous membranes of the larger airways. Inflammation of these tissues is related to chronic damage of epithelial cells and their cilia and can be further aggravated by an acute respiratory illness. Patients with emphysema and patients with bronchitis require careful monitoring of hydration and blood gases. Chronic bronchitis and emphysema can lead to right-sided heart failure and pulmonary hypertension. Patients with concurrent underlying chronic cardiac issues should be monitored for fluid excess.

Asthma is a reactive airway dysfunction in which inflammation is induced by triggers of environmental, physiological, and emotional origin. Smooth muscles of the upper airway spasm, and the airway closes down. Like emphysema and chronic bronchitis, chronic asthma causes increases in mucous production and fluid demand. Decreased airway exchange and periods of hyperventilation can cause acid-base imbalance.

COACH CONSULT

Cancer treatment is varied and is based on the staging, type, and location of tumor and whether the tumor has metastasized to other locations. Treatment can vary from pill chemotherapy to radiation to intensive chemotherapy to palliative care and may include novel or trial therapies. The staging of the tumor and the intensity of treatment determine which facility is best suited to patient care. Patients may be seen in home care, acute care, or hospice settings or as outpatients. Care providers in any setting need to be aware of the special characteristics of tumors and treatment to monitor for fluid and electrolyte shifts.

Patients with chronic respiratory illness are at risk for respiratory acidosis because of prolonged reduced airway gas exchange and the inability to clear carbon dioxide. In states of anxiety or decreased oxygenation, patients may have periods of hyperventilation and tachypnea, resulting in a loss of fluids and acid-base imbalance toward respiratory alkalosis, which is reflected in low carbon dioxide blood levels.

Possible Imbalances During Treatment
Each form of COPD has a different presentation and different medical treatment protocols, depending on cause and treatment practices. These treatments may include antibiotic therapy, oxygen therapy, bronchodilator or steroid therapy, surgery, or evolving medical therapies. Fluid and electrolyte shifts can occur with any of these treatments and should be considered when planning care.

Diabetes Mellitus and Diabetes Insipidus

A/B, $F(^+/^-)$, $Cl(^-)$, $K(^+/^-)$, $Mg(^+)$, $Na(^+/^-)$, $Ph(^+/^-)$

Diabetes insipidus (DI), diabetes mellitus (DM), hyperglycemic hyperosmolar nonketotic syndrome (HHNK), and diabetic ketoacidosis (DKA) can cause fluid and electrolyte shifts. DM and DI are characterized by polyuria (excessive urination) and polydipsia (excessive thirst). Both are diagnosed through blood tests, urine tests, and symptom presentation. Serum glucose levels >160 mg/dL cause osmotic diuresis. Fluid losses may cause increased serum magnesium, phosphorus, and potassium. Sodium and chloride losses occur through excessive diuresis.

 NURSE-TO-NURSE TIP

COPD can be managed so that patients remain stable on their medications and supportive treatments (e.g., oxygen) and continue to lead relatively normal lives. However, patients with chronic illness can slowly descend into ill health because of subtle shifts in their metabolism, diet, or activities. They are also at high risk for sudden shifts into acute health crisis because of the effects of seasonal illnesses, cardiovascular or neurological accidents, or other unanticipated stressors. Management of chronic illness requires care providers to educate patients and families on the health risks and signs and symptoms associated with fluid, acid-base and electrolyte shifts. If patients experience an acute stressor or acute exacerbation of their chronic disease, the medical team needs to plan care with knowledge of the risks associated with these illnesses.

DM: Type 1

DM is a disorder of insulin production or use, causing altered glucose metabolism. Type 1 DM is a result of the destruction of or the congenital absence of the pancreatic beta cells that produce insulin. Type 1 patients may also suffer from polyphagia (increased hunger) related to higher metabolic need. Patients with type 1 are treated with insulin replacement.

Possible Imbalances During Treatment

Treatment of DM involves administration of insulin, which tends to drive phosphorus and potassium from serum into cells. During treatment, phosphorous and potassium levels should be closely monitored.

DM: Type 2

Type 2 DM can occur through a variety of pathological mechanisms that result in low insulin availability or cellular resistance to insulin, which ultimately hinders glucose's movement into cells. Type 2 is more common in U.S. populations and may require activity and dietary changes, oral medication therapy, insulin, or a combination of all of these to control glucose levels.

Possible Imbalances During Treatment

Treatment of DM involves administration of insulin, which tends to drive phosphorus and potassium from serum into cells. During treatment, phosphorous and potassium levels should be closely monitored.

DKA

Patients with type 1 DM are at the highest risk for DKA, in which cells catabolize fats and proteins for energy because no glucose is available to them. Acidosis occurs because of an increased breakdown of fats, causing the liver to produce more ketones than can be excreted easily through urine. Because no insulin is present to carry glucose into cells, serum glucose is often >250 mg/dL, leading to osmotic diuresis.

During DKA, fluid and electrolyte losses occur from increased urination, vomiting, and rapid breathing. Potassium and water leave cells, causing hyperkalemia and cellular dehydration. Excess water in the vascular space causes low serum sodium levels. Lethargy, tachycardia, gastrointestinal pain, vomiting, polyuria, polydipsia, and a fruity-smelling breath from the excess ketone production are symptoms of DKA. Kussmaul's sign (rapid, deep breathing) occurs as an effort to decrease acidosis.

Possible Imbalances During Treatment

Treatment of DKA involves slow, careful administration of insulin, fluids, and replacement of depleted electrolytes in order to prevent rebound hypoglycemia or dangerous shifts of electrolytes. During treatment with insulin, phosphorus and potassium should be closely monitored to monitor for hypophosphatemia and the more common occurrence of hypokalemia.

Hyperosmolar Hyperglycemic State

Hyperosmolar hyperglycemic state (HHS) is similar to DKA. It is more common with type 2 DM and when a patient has serum glucose levels >600 mg/dL. Although serum osmolality is high—at >310 mmol/kg—acidosis is not expected. This high osmolality pulls fluid out of brain cells and causes central neurological symptoms from lethargy to coma. HHS can cause thrombotic stroke, but sometimes it causes neurological symptoms that may also mimic stroke symptoms. If neurological symptoms are assessed, the medical team may initiate stroke treatment protocols while working up a differential diagnosis.

Possible Imbalances During Treatment

Treatment of HHS involves fluid replacement because patients can lose up to 10 L of fluid through diuresis. Insulin and depleted electrolytes may also be used with caution, and serum glucose and electrolyte levels must be monitored frequently to prevent rebound hypoglycemia or dangerous shifts of electrolytes.

DI

DI is related to a deficiency of the hormone arginine vasopressin, also known as ADH-AVP. This is termed *central neurogenic* DI and can occur with head trauma, neoplasms, stroke, aneurysm, infection, brain surgery, and sometimes pregnancy. It can also occur as *nephrogenic* DI if the kidneys do not respond to circulating ADH. Nephrogenic DI can be genetically linked or it can be caused by low potassium or chronically elevated calcium. It can also be caused by lithium, demeclocycline, methoxyflurane, and amphotericin. The causes of about half the cases of DI are unknown. Blood levels of ADH and radiology or magnetic brain scans are used to differentiate between neurogenic and nephrogenic causes of DI.

If some ADH is still being secreted by the hypothalamus, patients may be able to balance fluid loss with fluid intake. These patients are most at risk when subjected to fluid restrictions or if they are unable to obtain water independently. Desmopressin acetate, a synthetic vasopressin, may be prescribed for patients with neurogenic DI as a subcutaneous injection, a nasal spray, or orally. Thiazide diuretics may also be prescribed for either neurogenic or nephrogenic DI. Although these diuretics may seem to counteract ADH, their effect is related to increasing water reabsorption by the kidneys. Nephrogenic DI is also treated with oral dosing of indomethacin, a nonsteroidal prostaglandin inhibitor.

With DI, fluid losses can be > 1 L/hr. Patients at greatest risk are those who are unable to obtain fluids independently. Patients may have a decreased sense of thirst and therefore should be encouraged to drink enough fluid to meet fluid losses. Urine osmolality is < 250 mOsm/L, whereas serum osmolality is > 300 mOsm/L. Electrolyte shifts may occur related to fluid losses and hemoconcentration.

Possible Imbalances During Treatment
DI is not treated with insulin because DI is not related to pancreatic beta cells. It is treated with a synthetic form of the hormone vasopressin. The major concern with DI is electrolyte shifts associated with fluid shifts.

Other Endocrine Disorders

Endocrine disorders—such as Addison's disease, Cushing's syndrome, hyperthyroidism, hyper/hypoparathyroidism, and SIADH—have been found to cause fluid and electrolyte imbalances.

Addison's Disease (Adrenal Insufficiency)
$F(^-)$, $Ca(^+)$, $Cl(^-)$, $K(^+)$, $Na(^-)$
Addison's disease, or adrenal insufficiency, causes low aldosterone, cortisol, and androgen. This condition can be caused by damage to the adrenal glands from infection, trauma, autoimmune response, and unknown sources. Adrenal insufficiency can also be linked to a pituitary or hypothalamic disorder, which decreases the formation or release of adrenocorticotropic hormone (ACTH). However, adrenal insufficiency does not

 NURSE-TO-NURSE TIP

Once it has been diagnosed, DM is a manageable chronic illness with a strict regimen of blood sugar measurement, diet, exercise and—if necessary—medication, including insulin. However, unanticipated metabolic or health stressors can cause a shift to a crisis of DKA or HHS. DKA and HHS also occur frequently prior to the diagnosis of DM and the first incident may lead to diagnosis. DI can occur with acute or chronic onset. Care providers must teach patients who need to manage chronic illnesses the risks for, prevention of, and signs of electrolyte and fluid imbalances. Given the rise in diabetes in the general population and in children, care providers in schools and other institutions, such as adult day care centers, need to be aware of the potential for fluid and electrolyte shifts.

usually affect aldosterone production. Without aldosterone, the kidneys do not retain sodium and chloride, and thus excess fluid is lost. With the loss of sodium, there is a concurrent retention of potassium. Dehydration also contributes to relatively high potassium and calcium levels.

Possible Imbalances During Treatment

Treatment may include administration of fluids, glucose, corticosteroids, and mineralocorticoids. Sodium and chloride are repleted, whereas potassium and calcium levels need to be lowered to correct electrolyte abnormalities associated with adrenal insufficiency.

Cushing's Syndrome

F($^+$), Ca($^+$), K($^-$)

Cushing's syndrome occurs when the adrenal cortex secretes too much glucocorticoid hormone or when a patient receives excess glucocorticoid medication. The primary cause is linked to adrenal tumors that cause excess cortisol production. A secondary cause can be overstimulation of the adrenal glands, which results from problems with the pituitary gland, which yields overproduction of ACTH. In high concentrations, cortisol can mimic mineralocorticoids, leading to potassium shifts into cells and excess excretion of potassium through the kidneys. An associated chronic electrolyte imbalance relates to increased metabolism, which causes calcium to leave the bones, which can result in osteoporosis.

Possible Imbalances During Treatment

Treatment may be focused on surgical removal of tumors, the medical suppression of excess steroids, or the tapered decrease in glucocorticoids. With a shift away from excess glucocorticoids, potassium, calcium, and fluid levels should return to normal.

Hyperthyroidism

Ca($^+$), K($^-$)

Hyperthyroidism has an effect on most body systems. Graves' disease is associated with chronic stress on the heart and other organs. Thyrotoxicosis (thyroid storm) causes high blood calcium levels and excess potassium excretion.

Possible Imbalances During Treatment

Treatment is centered on supplying extra oxygen, fluids, and calories to meet the high demands of an overstimulated metabolism and suppressing excess thyroid and sympathetic hormones with medication. As the hyperthyroid state is corrected, calcium and potassium levels should return to normal, and less fluid support will be required.

Hypoparathyroidism
Ca($^-$), Ph($^+$)

Low magnesium or damage to the parathyroid glands can cause decreased secretion of parathyroid hormone, which in turn causes hypoparathyroidism. There are also unknown causes of hypoparathyroidism, but two or more thyroid or neck surgeries dramatically increase incidence.

Hypoparathyroidism can cause high serum phosphorus and low calcium. It is associated with parathyroid hormone levels of < 10 pg/dL, serum calcium of < 8.5 mg/dL, and ionized calcium of < 4.5 mg/dL. Calcium and vitamin D supplementation are often required. Severe calcium deficiency can be exacerbated if alkalosis is also present. If alkalosis is related to loss of carbon dioxide, then sedation may be given to decrease respirations.

Possible Imbalances During Treatment

Treatment of hypocalcemia is a focus of treatment for hypoparathyroid presentations. Treatment may also include supplementation with vitamin D.

Hyperparathyroidism
Ca($^+$), Ph($^-$)

Hyperparathyroidism, which is associated with benign or malignant tumors, can cause elevated calcium and a reciprocal low phosphorous level. Chronic excess secretion of PTH causes bone demineralization and weakness. It can also cause calcium deposits in soft tissues, such as the kidneys, resulting in organ failure. The most frequent incidence is related to benign neoplasm of the parathyroid glands. Tumors in other locations can also be implicated; for example, pituitary and pancreatic tumors cause a decrease in calcium, which stimulates an overproduction of PTH. PTH levels are elevated in most cases in excess of 65 pg/mL. Serum calcium may be > 10.5 mg/dL, and ionized calcium may be > 5.5 mg/dL.

Possible Imbalances During Treatment

Reducing the impact of hypercalcemia is key to treatment of hyperparathyroidism, through the use of intravenous sodium chloride dilution and subsequent use of diuretics. Calcitonin can also be used to decrease circulating calcium. Surgery or drugs to block the parathyroid effects can be used. If they are effective, then calcium and phosphorous levels should return to normal.

SIADH
F($^+$), Ca($^{+/-}$), K($^{+/-}$), Na($^-$), Ph($^+$)

SIADH causes increased circulating ADH and resulting fluid retention. SIADH is associated with tumors that produce excess ADH, central neurological infections or trauma, and lung diseases including tuberculosis and pneumocystis pneumonia. Patients with immunosuppression are at increased risk for SIADH because of potential for respiratory and neurological infections. Iatrogenic causes include some analgesics and anesthetics or thiazide diuretics. Stress or temperature changes related to surgery can also induce SIADH.

Increased ADH secretion causes excess fluid retention, electrolyte dilution, and concurrent excretion of sodium by the kidneys. Critical hyponatremia is the primary concern for SIADH. Urine sodium at >20 mmol/L with concurrent serum sodium of <135 mEq/L can indicate SIADH. Blood and urine may be measured for osmolality, with serum levels <275 mOsml/L and urine levels >100 mOsml/L.

Possible Imbalances During Treatment

COACH CONSULT

Prior to diagnosis of endocrine imbalance, a patient is at high risk for electrolyte and fluid imbalance. Electrolyte and fluid imbalance may be the reason for hospitalization. Once the illness is diagnosed and a treatment plan is developed, care providers must educate patients on the risks, prevention, and signs associated with the underlying disorder and associated treatments. Chronic diseases may develop subtle signs over time, or they may accompany an acute stressor that causes an acute exacerbation of the illness. Care providers in primary care, long-term care, and acute settings need to be aware of the potential for these imbalances.

Treatment choices for SIADH are based on the cause and ongoing system and laboratory assessments; they are modified based on the patient's response to treatment. Typically, a nephrologist is asked to direct treatment with the medical team. Most frequently, the medical team is focused on decreasing fluid volumes through fluid restriction and the use of diuretics; treatment also focuses on preventing complications of serum hyponatremia and diluted levels of other electrolytes. Diuretics can be associated with decreased potassium levels. Overall, electrolytes should be measured frequently when fluid restriction is in place to ensure that sodium, potassium, calcium, and phosphorus imbalances (which can be associated with SIADH or the underlying causes of SIADH) do not result.

Heart Failure

F($^{+}$), K($^{-}$), Mg($^{-}$), Na($^{+}$/$^{-}$)

Heart failure, acute or chronic, is associated with fluid and electrolyte imbalances. For patients with chronic failure, the goal is to manage their illness and prevent fluid and electrolyte shifts. Acute failure is usually associated with unexpected illness or event. Heart failure is differentiated from other causes of fluid overload by evaluation of B-type-natriuretic peptide (BNP). The Fluid Excess section of Chapter 2 discusses the role of BNP in detail.

In both acute and chronic heart failure, the heart is unable to circulate blood appropriately, which causes fluid to build up vascularly and extravascularly. Symptoms of this process typically include increased heart rate and elevated blood pressures. As fluid builds up in the lungs, cyanosis, shortness of breath, rales/crackles, and even frothy sputum can occur with severe failure. Edema and weight gain can be symptoms of failure and will increase as failure worsens. Hemodilution can cause low levels of extracellular electrolytes. Plasma sodium can either be high, causing fluid retention and exacerbation of heart failure, or may become low because of the hemodilution caused by fluid retention.

Possible Imbalances During Treatment

Treatment is centered on efforts to decrease fluid through diuretics and to support the heart with medications that enhance cardiac function. Oxygen support may be necessary to treat associated hypoxemia. Positioning is important, including raising the head of the bed to support breathing. For patients who are able to mobilize and diurese excess fluids and who have sufficient cardiac output, elevation of the extremities to support venous return to the renal system may be ordered by the medical team. Continuous cardiac monitoring is typically ordered in acute exacerbation of heart failure to observe for electrical changes induced by electrolyte and fluid shifts and potential worsening of cardiac functioning. Daily weight, which is an essential measure of fluid balance along with intake and output measures, must be observed to monitor response to diuresis. Potassium can drop dramatically with the administration of potassium-wasting diuretics, such as furosemide, and must be monitored cautiously.

 NURSE-TO-NURSE TIP

Heart failure is very common in the elderly, but it can also occur in younger populations. Typically, it is managed as a chronic illness, requiring that care providers educate patients and families on potential fluid and electrolyte imbalance. Electrolyte and fluid ingestion have a strong correlation between disease management and disease exacerbation. Treatment may require acute admission, but treatment might be managed at home or in a chronic care environment. The shift of fluid and electrolytes typically depends on the extent of the underlying disease, concurrent factors (e.g., renal disease), and the aggressiveness of the treatment prescribed by the medical team. Some of the most commonly used medications associated with heart failure are antihypertensives and diuretics. Along with management of diet and exercise, care providers must be aware of the association of these medications with fluid and electrolyte shifts.

Infection and Sepsis

A/B, F(‾)

Fluid losses are common in infection because of excess respirations, sweating related to fever, and a generally increased metabolic requirement for production of immune system proteins like white blood cells.

Sepsis is a systemic inflammatory response associated with a bacterial, viral, or fungal infection and is characterized by a fever > 101.3°F (38.5°C) or < 95°F (35°C), a heart rate > 90 bpm, respirations > 20 breaths per minute, and a confirmed or presumed infection. Severe sepsis includes the preceding with an additional complication of organ dysfunction such as mottled skin, decreased renal output, mental status change, drop in platelet count, respiratory distress, or cardiac dysfunction. Septic shock is diagnosed with a significant decrease in blood pressure. Sepsis and similar syndromes, such as systemic inflammatory response syndrome, cause capillaries to leak fluids from the vascular space to the interstitial spaces.

Possible Imbalances During Treatment

Emergent fluid resuscitation is often required to prevent circulatory collapse. Frequent, large-volume fluid boluses can result in dilution of serum electrolytes and increased levels of sodium and chloride. Cellular destruction can result in potassium leaking out of cells and increasing electrochemical instability of the cardiac muscle. Acid-base imbalance is strongly associated with circulatory collapse as metabolic and respiratory sources combine to cause life-threatening acidosis. If a patient recovers from sepsis, diuresis of fluid given during resuscitation will occur if the kidneys recover from the insult. Loss of electrolytes through urine may occur to an extent that requires replacement.

Liver Failure, Biliary Dysfunction, and Pancreatic Dysfunction

F(‾⁺), Ca(‾), Cl(‾), K(⁺/‾), Mg(‾), Na(⁺/‾), Ph(‾)

Liver failure and cirrhosis cause problems with fluid backing up in the highly vascular hepatic system. A diseased liver cannot produce albumin, so this protein is not present in high enough amounts to retain fluid in the vascular space. Lack of albumin causes a shift of fluids into the extravascular space, including the abdominal cavity. This excess fluid is known as *ascites* and may need to be eliminated with needle paracentesis. Sodium moves into the interstitial and intracellular spaces. Potassium then shifts out of cells. However, dilution of intravascular fluid by these shifting fluids can also cause low calcium, low chloride, low magnesium, and low potassium levels. A vitamin D deficiency causes a decrease in calcium absorption and a resulting decrease in serum phosphorus.

Biliary duct blockage may contribute to fluids backing up into the hepatic system, and it can also cause pancreatitis. Pancreatitis is associated with low albumin levels, which accounts for low calcium levels because a percentage of calcium is bound to albumin. The relationship to albumin and calcium is explained in Chapter 3A.

Possible Imbalances During Treatment

Treatment may involve sodium and fluid restrictions to prevent worsening of ascites. Sterile-needle paracentesis or diuretics may be used to decrease ascites that compromises respiratory function.

However, dehydration is a hallmark of pancreatitis, which requires intensive intravenous fluid resuscitation while the patient is restricted from taking any foods or fluids by mouth.

Gastrointestinal Malabsorption

$F(\ )$, $Ca(\ )$, $K(\ )$, $Mg(\ )$, $Ph(\ )$

Gastrointestinal malabsorption is associated with Crohn's disease, anorexia, bowel surgery, starvation, and wasting from alcohol abuse, and it can decrease absorption of calcium, magnesium, and phosphorus. Low magnesium absorption prevents potassium absorption. Low albumin, which results from poor nutrition, lowers albumin stores. Because the kidney excretes potassium even without dietary intake, low potassium results when diet is restricted or when food is not properly digested and absorbed.

COACH CONSULT

Liver, biliary tract, and pancreatic disease can be chronic or acute. Obstruction of the biliary tract can create a fluid overload, but at times the patient may also have metabolic needs that require fluid resuscitation, such as in the case of acute pancreatitis. Chronic care requires education of the patient and family. Caregivers need to be alert for electrolyte shifts that accompany fluid shifts.

Possible Imbalances During Treatment

Hospitalized patients may be prescribed oral or tube feeding to help them recover from malnutrition. When malnourished patients begin to absorb high carbohydrate loads, refeeding syndrome may occur, which is when already depleted serum phosphorus can fall rapidly. Shifts related to metabolizing nutrition may consume phosphorous stores, so phosphorous supplementation is required to prevent hypophosphatemia. This syndrome is discussed in Chapter 3D.

COACH CONSULT

Chronic malabsorption syndromes often require supplementation of electrolytes—such as calcium, magnesium, and phosphorus—daily. As with all chronic diseases, care providers need to facilitate education for patients and their families on the risks, prevention, and signs of electrolyte and fluid imbalance. Acute exacerbations of these conditions put the patient at high risk for electrolyte and fluid imbalance and may require hospitalization during the acute phase of illness and through the initial recovery. Patients may already use alternative mechanisms to obtain nutrition, such as intravenous or gastric tube feedings.

Mental Status Changes

F($^+$/$^-$), Ca($^-$), K($^-$), Mg($^-$), Ph($^-$)

Mental status changes can occur as a result of cerebral vascular accident (stroke), head trauma, brain neoplasms, metabolic disorders, poisoning, and the use of medications and drugs such as sedatives, stimulants, hallucinogens, antidepressives, antipsychotic agents, analgesics, and anesthesia agents. Change in level of consciousness or decline in neurological function may also occur as part of the continuum of mental disorders that is related to congenital or acquired developmental delay, dementia, or mental health disorders and diseases. Changes may be subtle or may present as delirium, psychosis, or coma.

Fluid and electrolyte imbalance may occur as a result of a disorder or the imbalance may cause or exacerbate the underlying disorder. Because of the complexity of the spectrum of mental disorders and the impact that interventions may have on improving or worsening the relationship between mental disorders and a fluid or electrolyte imbalance, it is essential to assess and monitor patients closely.

Patients with mental status changes may not be able to access fluids and nutrition, or they may not be able to follow medical instructions fully for the restriction of fluids or certain foods. Patients with chronic mental disorders who live independently in the community are at special risk for poor regulation of fluid and nutritional needs. If patients and their caregivers are unable to meet basic metabolic needs, then any new illness or worsening of the underlying condition may further exacerbate a fluid or electrolyte imbalance. Patients in acute or chronic care settings may be restricted from adequate nutrition because of the use of restraints or an inability to eat or drink at the time that food and fluids are provided to them.

Some patients with a change in mental status may find intravenous or nasogastric intubation noxious and may not be able to tolerate the medical devices that allow for supplementation. In these cases, the medical team may order physical restraints in the short term to allow for correction of critical imbalances. Each institution will have specific regulations as to when, how, and by whom restraints may be ordered and what care and supervision is required while restraints are in place to maintain patient safety. However, a longer-term plan that does not include restraints needs to be developed that can meet these patients' nutritional and hydration needs.

COACH CONSULT

Patients may suffer from chronic or acute mental status changes. In the acute phase, patients and their families need to understand the risk of nutritional and fluid deficits and be educated on how to ensure proper access to and ingestion of electrolytes. Care providers must be cautious to observe for worsening of mental status decline that might further decrease the patient's ability to access essential fluids and electrolytes from diet, supplements, and medication.

Possible Imbalances During Treatment

The medical team, along with family or legal representatives, may have to make short- and long-term decisions for patients who are unable to make safe decisions for themselves. This may include implantation of a long-term peripheral intravenous central catheter or percutaneous gastrostomy tube. Patients who have suffered a stroke or other neurological deficit to their oral cavity or esophagus may also have dysphagia and be ordered for a modified diet, including fluid restriction, or their swallowing deficit may be so great that they will not be able to take anything by mouth and need alternative nutrition access. Nurses must be cautious to ensure that patients with alternative methods of nutrition are receiving sufficient free water and a proper ratio of electrolytes through their diet or supplementation to prevent dehydration or electrolyte deficiencies. Patients who have not been able to take in sufficient nutrition or fluids may experience fluid and electrolyte shifts once they begin receiving nutrition and hydration, such as the drop in serum potassium, phosphorus, and magnesium associated with refeeding syndrome. Serum electrolytes may also become diluted if the patient receives intravenous fluids for rehydration that do not contain electrolyte repletion.

Orthopedic Disorders

$Ca(^+/^-)$, $Ph(^+/^-)$

Osteomalacia, osteopenia, osteoporosis, and other disorders of low bone mass are associated with low overall calcium. These problems can be associated with low estrogen levels after menopause or hysterectomy. At times, acute bone loss can be associated with high serum calcium, such as during periods of prolonged immobility. Acromegaly and Paget's disease (which is the adult form of rickets) can be associated with high circulating calcium levels. In general, low calcium states result in high serum phosphorus, and high calcium states result in low serum phosphorus. For more information on the interdependent relationship of calcium and phosphorus in bone loss and development, see Chapters 3A and 3D.

Possible Imbalances During Treatment

Low bone calcium can be associated with high serum calcium. Efforts to supply enough dietary calcium and to enhance gastrointestinal absorption of calcium through the use of medications or supplementation with vitamin D may result in bone resorption of calcium and transient serum hypocalcemia. Calcium and phosphorous levels should be measured to assess short- and long-term effects of therapy.

COACH CONSULT

Management of calcium deficiency can be difficult because low calcium states can sometimes be masked by the body's ability to mobilize calcium from bone. Calcium deficiency may remain undiagnosed until after fractures occur. Care providers must educate and screen at-risk patients and ensure patients understand the need to follow prescriptions for calcium and vitamin D.

Renal Disease and Dysfunction

A/B, $F(^+)$, $Ca(^-)$, $K(^+/^-)$, $Mg(^-)$, $Na(^+)$, $Ph(^+/^-)$

Renal failure, acute or chronic, is a common cause of fluid and electrolyte imbalance. Renal failure can be caused by infection, exposure to medications, dehydration, cancer, poisoning, blood diseases, diabetes, cancers, trauma, urinary tract diseases or obstructions, autoimmune disease, hypertension, congenital or genetic disease, and other disease processes. There are many changes that can occur with a diseased kidney; for instance, with nephrosis and glomerulonephritis, proteins are lost in the urine, causing low levels of proteins in the bloodstream and resulting in fluid shifts to the extravascular space. Polycystic kidney disease is associated with blood or cystic material in the urine. Most forms of kidney disease are associated with some fluid and electrolyte shift. Renal tubular acidosis is a chronic disorder in which there are tubular defects that prevent bicarbonate reabsorption or hydrogen secretion, resulting in a chronic metabolic acidosis.

Renal failure is usually categorized as acute or chronic; however, acute failure can result in chronic failure if treatment is not successful. Acute failure is characterized by a progression from low urine output with accompanying increase in fluids in the vascular space to a high urine output phase. During the low output acute stage, excretion of potassium is limited, which raises serum levels.

Possible Imbalances During Treatment

Chronic failure requires careful management by patients, caregivers, and the medical team. At end-stage failure, when the kidneys are functioning at low levels, patients require either peritoneal dialysis or hemodialysis to maintain fluid and electrolyte balance. They also require careful limits on fluid and electrolyte intake. If sodium, potassium, or phosphorous levels are high, then they may need to be restricted. High phosphorous levels can cause decreased calcium levels. Phosphorous binders are prescribed to help regulate the high electrolyte intake. Magnesium levels can be low in patients with end-stage failure if the kidney tubules are unable to reabsorb magnesium.

Recovery from acute renal failure is known as the diuretic phase, and serum electrolytes that were elevated during the low urine output phase may now drop as fluid is excreted through the kidneys. Patients who undergo renal transplant may also lose calcium and phosphorus when they regain kidney function and have increased urine production.

Trauma/Ischemic Bowel/Rhabdomyolysis

A/B, $F(\bar{\ })$, $Cl(\bar{\ })$, $K(^+)$, $Na(\bar{\ })$

Trauma care is usually divided into acute care and recovery. The acute period is typically 2–3 days. Trauma from falls, motor vehicle accidents, weapon wounds, industrial accidents, and other assaults can cause life-threatening, massive fluid loss with hemorrhage or leaking from the vascular space into

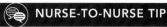
the interstitial space. Electrolytes can be lost from blood and fluid losses or may shift from cellular or vascular space into interstitial space. After the initial trauma, sepsis, acute respiratory distress syndrome, compartment syndrome, and rhabdomyolosis (lysis of muscle cells) can cause further destruction of cells. Ischemic bowel and rhabdomyolysis can occur in outpatient and inpatient settings and may be associated with surgery, trauma, cancer, and other diseases.

With cellular destruction, intracellular electrolytes, potassium, and phosphorus leak into vascular and interstitial space. With the disruption of blood vessels from trauma, neoplasms, or vascular disease, sodium and chloride move into cells, and the sodium and potassium pump may be disrupted. Cellular destruction also commonly results in a shift toward acidosis. Patients with serious infections or injuries may not be able to compensate for acidosis and may require treatment with ventilator support, alkalosing medications, and hydration. Chapter 6 describes these imbalances and treatments.

Possible Imbalances During Treatment

Treatment of trauma, crushing injuries, and sepsis usually includes massive fluid resuscitation and may include use of blood products. Because of the permeability of damaged vascular wall capillaries, much of the infused crystalloid fluids may shift out of the vascular space. In addition, fluid follows sodium either into the interstitial space or into the cells. The loss of vascular fluid causes an increase in the concentration of those electrolytes that are left in the vascular space, including chloride and calcium. A patient may retain fluid in extravascular spaces and cells for hours to days. Although many injuries of this type can be life-threatening, if a patient survives, then a diuretic phase will typically occur during the acute stage of recovery, in which fluid shifts back into the vascular space and fluid loss through the kidneys may once again create electrolyte imbalances. This process may also interrupt the kidney's ability to assist with acid-base regulation. Electrolyte levels, fluid status, and acid-base balance should be measured continually during recovery.

 NURSE-TO-NURSE TIP

Trauma is most likely to occur outside of institutions, but it can occur in hospitals or care centers. Serious trauma patients will typically be transported to a designated trauma center, where staff members are specially trained to manage trauma, including creating a care plan for fluid, electrolyte, and acid-base imbalance. Trauma and ischemic destruction of cells is a critical medical condition and is typically managed in a critical care setting. Care providers need to be aware of the potential of shifts through the acute and recovery phases.

6 Tools

CHAPTER 6

Tools

Common calculations, charts, procedures, and scales are in this section.

Calculations

Calculations included are anion gap, osmolar gap, body surface area (DuBois and DuBois), fractional excretion of magnesium, and fractional excretion of sodium.

Anion Gap

The common formula used to calculate anion gap is:

$$(Na^+) - [(Cl^-) + (HCO_3^-)] = anion\ gap$$

There is another formula used to estimate this gap that adds potassium to the sodium side of the equation:

$$[(Na^+) + (K^+)] - [(Cl^-) + (HCO_3^-)] = anion\ gap$$

With either formula:
- A *high* anion gap, >12 mEq/L, indicates acid production or poisoning. HCO_3^- levels go down because sodium binds to acids rather than bicarbonate.
- A *normal* anion gap of 8–12 mEq/L indicates HCO_3^- losses, or hyperchloremic acidosis, when chloride retention balances with bicarbonate loss.
- A *low* anion gap of <8 mEq/L also indicates HCO_3^- losses, although the bicarbonate decreases as a result of unmeasured cation or anion changes. Changes in unmeasured anions or

cations could be the result of decreased anion albumin or increased cations IgG and paraproteins related to multiple myeloma, lithium intoxication, or increased potassium, magnesium, or calcium.

Osmolar Gap
The osmolar gap is calculated by subtracting the calculated serum osmolarity from the measured serum osmolarity. The following steps can be used to calculate osmolar gap:

1. Calculate serum osmolarity using the following formula:

$$\text{Serum osmolarity} = (2 \, [\text{Na}] + [\text{glucose}]) / 18 + \text{BUN}/2.8 + \text{blood alcohol}/5$$

2. Subtract the calculated osmolarity from the measured osmolarity:

$$\text{Osmolar gap} = \text{Measured osmolarity} - \text{Calculated osmolarity}$$

If the osmolar gap is >10, the difference may indicate either excess toxins in the body or osmotically active molecules.

Body Surface Area: DuBois and DuBois Formula
The DuBois and DuBois formula used to estimate body surface area (BSA) is:

$$\text{BSA} = ([\text{weight kg}]^{0.425} \times [\text{height cm}]^{0.725}) \times 0.007184$$

Fractional Excretion of Magnesium
Fractional excretion of magnesium (FE_{Mg}) can be calculated using this formula:

$$\text{FE}_{\text{Mg}} = (\text{Urine Mg} \times \text{plasma creatinine}) / [(0.7 \times \text{plasma Mg}) \times (\text{urine creatinine}) \times 100]$$

Fractional excretion of Mg >2 indicates renal losses.

Fractional Excretion of Sodium
Fractional excretion of sodium (FE_{Na}) can be calculated using the following steps:

- **Step 1:** Multiply urine sodium and plasma creatinine.
- **Step 2:** Multiply plasma sodium and urine creatinine.
- **Step 3:** Divide Step 1's result into Step 2's result (result Step 1/result Step 2).
- **Step 4:** Multiply Step 3's result by 100.

FE_{Na} can also be expressed using the following equation:

$$FE_{Na} = (\text{Urine Na} \times \text{Plasma creatinine})/ (\text{Plasma Na} \times \text{Urine creatinine}) \times 100$$

Dehydration will be reflected by a ratio of < 1. Renal dysfunction will be reflected by a ratio > 2. Other causes of a fractional excretion of sodium can be related to renal vasoconstriction or inflammation from liver dysfunction, congestive heart failure, sepsis, infection, damage from NSAIDs, contrast dyes, or vasoconstricting medications.

Charts

The following charts show normal electrolyte levels and imbalances.

Normal Electrolyte Levels

Normal Electrolyte Levels			
	WEIGHT PER mEq	EXTRACELLULAR FLUID SERUM	INTRACELLULAR FLUID
Bicarbonate		24–28 mEq/L	7–10 mEq/L
Calcium	40 mg/2 mEq	8.2–10.2 mg/dL	<1 mEq/L
Chloride	35 mg/1 mEq	97–107 mEq/L	27 mEq/L
Glucose		90–120 mg/dL	
Magnesium	24 mg/2 mEq	1.32–2.14 mEq/L	20–40 mEq/L
pH		7.35–7.45 *arterial*	6.9–7.2
Phosphorus		2.4–4.5 mg/dL	100 mEq/L
Potassium	39 mg/1mEq	3.5–5 mEq/L	130–150 mEq/L
Sodium	23 mg/1 mEq	135–145 mEq/L	10–20 mEq/L
Urea nitrogen		8–21 mg/dL	10–20 mg/dL

Imbalance Charts

The following five charts show common disorders and effects of fluid, electrolyte, and acid-base imbalance. Because imbalances do not occur strictly in one direction metabolically, a decrease or increase in one area may cause a decrease or increase in another. An imbalance may also occur at one time in a disease process but then shift once treatment or physiological compensation is under way. Common symptoms, disease processes, and treatments related to fluid, electrolyte, and metabolic shifts are indicated. Given the complexity of the effects of these imbalances on the metabolism, the charts do not indicate all possible relationships. Even if a relationship is not represented in the charts, it may still exist in the course of illness and recovery.

Symptoms of Fluid, Acid-Base, and Electrolyte Imbalance

IMBALANCE (RIGHT)/ SYMPTOMS (BELOW)	Fl		pH		Ca		Cl		Mg		Na		Phos		K	
	←	→	←	→	←	→	←	→	←	→	←	→	←	→	←	→
Neurological																
Agitation/irritability/ restlessness	*		*	*	*		*	*		*	*	*		*	*	
Anxiety	*		*			*										
Babinski's sign										*						
Cataracts					*		*		*							*
Coma/Level of consciousness decreased–mental status changes	*		*	*	*	*				*	*	*	*			*
Confusion/Memory loss	*		*	*		*						*				
Conjunctiva-yellow													*			
Convulsions/posturing	*					*		*		*		*	*			

Continued

Symptoms of Fluid, Acid-Base, and Electrolyte Imbalance—cont'd

IMBALANCE (RIGHT)/ SYMPTOMS (BELOW)	Fl		pH		Ca		Cl		Mg		Na		Phos		K	
	→	←	→	←	→	←	→	←	→	←	→	←	→	←	→	←
Dizziness	*		*						*							
Fear of impending doom			*	*												
Hallucinations/delirium									*						*	
Headache		*	*	*	*	*		*			*			*		
Lethargy/fatigue/ drowsiness/apathy	*	*	*	*		*	*	*	*	*	*			*	*	*
Mood changes/depression					*										*	
Neuronal sensitivity increased					*											
Nystagmus									*							
Pain			*	*												
Paralysis													*		*	*
Parasthesias (tingling)							*						*	*	*	*
Personality changes				*					*							

	1	2	3	4	5	6	7	8	9	10	11	12	13	14	15	16	17	18
Reflexes (diminished)								*									*	*
Reflexes (increased)						*	*				*							*
Seizures	*					*	*	*			*	*	*	*	*			*
Speech difficulties																	*	
Tinnitus (ringing in ears)		*						*			*							
Twitching-tremors							*	*			*	*	*					
Visual disturbances			*			*	*		*									
Weakness				*			*				*		*	*				
Respiratory																		
Acidosis					*		*	*	*	*							*	*
Alkalosis						*	*		*	*						*	*	
Arrest/apnea/bradypnea							*	*		*	*						*	*
Bronchospasm/stridor/collapsed airway								*			*		*	*				
Cystic fibrosis												*						

IMBALANCE (RIGHT)/ SYMPTOMS (BELOW)	Fl		pH		Ca		Cl		Mg		Na		Phos		K	
	←	→	←	→	←	→	←	→	←	→	←	→	←	→	←	→
Deep breathing			*	*			*				*	*			*	
Dyspnea at rest/short of breath		*	*	*							*	*				*
Exertion—increased work of breathing Use of accessory muscles		*														
Fruity breath				*												
Irregular respirations	*			*							*			*		*
Kussmaul's respirations				*			*									
Rales, crackles/ pulmonary edema/moist cough	*	*	*	*				*		*	*	*				
Rhonchi/sputum		*	*	*				*								
Shallow respirations				*					*			*		*		
Tachypnea	*	*	*	*			*				*					

	1	2	3	4	5	6	7	8	9	10	11	12	13	14	15	16
Wheezing			*	*												
Cardiovascular																
Albumin (deficit)																
Anemia		*	*	*		*								*		
Arrest	*	*	*	*	*	*			*	*		*			*	*
Arteriole necrosis				*									*			
Bradycardia			*	*					*						*	*
Clotting delayed						*										
Dehydration	*	*			*		*	*	*		*	*	*		*	
Dysrhythmia	*	*	*	*									*	*		
—Depressed T waves																*
—Elevated T waves									*						*	
—Diminished P waves															*	
—Premature ventricular complex										*						

Symptoms of Fluid, Acid-Base, and Electrolyte Imbalance—cont'd

IMBALANCE (RIGHT)/ SYMPTOMS (BELOW)	Fl		pH		Ca		Cl		Mg		Na		Phos		K	
	←	→	←	→	←	→	←	→	←	→	←	→	←	→	←	→
—Prolonged PR interval									*							
—Prolonged QT interval						*							*		*	
—Shortened QT interval					*											
—Prolonged ST segment						*										
—Shortened ST segment					*											
—Supraventricular tachycardia										*						
—Torsades de pointes										*						
—U wave																*
—Ventricular tachycardia/ fibrillation			*	*		*				*						*
—Widened QRS									*						*	
Edema (peripheral)	*											*				
Fever		*	*	*				*			*	*				

Hypertension	*			*				*		*		*		*	*		
Hypotension		*	*	*	*	*	*	*	*	*	*	*		*	*	*	*
Immune dysfunction																*	
Palpitations	*		*											*	*	*	
Tachycardia	*	*	*				*	*	*		*					*	
Warmth (generalized)								*									
Weight gain (rapid)	*											*					
Integumentary																	
Cool, clammy			*														
Decreased turgor	*										*	*					
Mucous membranes dry	*																
Sweat/diaphoresis	*				*			*			*	*			*		*
Warm, flushed	*		*														

Continued

Symptoms of Fluid, Acid-Base, and Electrolyte Imbalance—cont'd

IMBALANCE (RIGHT)/ SYMPTOMS (BELOW)	Fl ←	Fl →	pH ←	pH →	Ca ←	Ca →	Cl ←	Cl →	Mg ←	Mg →	Na ←	Na →	Phos ←	Phos →	K ←	K →
Gastrointestinal																
Abdominal spasm/cramps	*					*									*	
Anorexia/nausea		*	*	*	*	*		*	*	*	*	*		*		*
Ascites	*		*	*		*		*								
Constipation		*			*	*							*			*
Diarrhea/fistula		*		*				*	*	*		*				*
Dysphagia					*	*				*						
Encephalopathy (hepatic)			*													
Foul breath													*			
Jaundice			*		*											
Laryngeal spasm/ swallowing problems													*			
Pancreatic enzymes elevation	*												*	*		

Assessment Finding	1	2	3	4	5	6	7	8	9	10	11	12	13	14	15	16	17	18
Thirst, dry tongue, cracked lips	*	*														*	*	*
Tongue coating					*													
Tongue twitching		*							*									
Vomiting/gastric suction		*			*	*	*	*								*		*
Vomit (phosphorescent)					*													
Genitourinary																		
Acidosis				*		*	*	*	*						*	*		
Alkalosis	*	*					*			*					*		*	
Oliguria						*		*								*		
Polyuria	*				*		*	*						*				*
Musculoskeletal																		
Bone pain				*														
Bone weakness (fractures)														*				
Chvostek's/Trousseau's sign											*		*					

Continued

IMBALANCE (RIGHT)/ SYMPTOMS (BELOW)	Fl →	Fl ←	pH →	pH ←	Ca →	Ca ←	Cl →	Cl ←	Mg →	Mg ←	Na →	Na ←	Phos →	Phos ←	K →	K ←
Cramping/spasms/contractions				*			*		*					*		
Deep tendon reflexes diminished			*							*						
Deep tendon reflexes increased					*		*									
Joint stiffening													*			
Leg swelling		*									*					
Muscle weakness			*						*	*				*		
Staggering/ataxia									*				*			
Tetany				*			*		*					*		
Tremors					*											

↑ = increased; ↓ = decreased

IMBALANCE (RIGHT)/ DISEASE PROCESS BELOW	Fl		pH		Ca		Cl		Mg		Na		Phos		K	
	←	→	←	→	←	→	←	→	←	→	←	→	←	→	←	→
Neurological/Psychiatric/ Dependency																
Alcoholism	*	*		*		*	*			*				*		*
Brain attack (cerebrovascular accident)	*	*	*			*				*				*		*
Brain trauma (bleed)		*		*			*									
Central nervous system infection (myelinolysis)											*	*				
Cerebral salt wasting syndrome												*				
Guillain-Barré syndrome				*								*				
Pain			*	*												

Continued

IMBALANCE (RIGHT)/ DISEASE PROCESS (BELOW)	Fl		pH		Ca		Cl		Mg		Na		Phos		K	
	←	→	←	→	←	→	←	→	←	→	←	→	←	→	←	→
Cardiovascular																
Albumin (deficit)						*										
Altitude (elevations)			*	*												
Anemia			*	*		*					*			*		
Arrest			*						*	*						
Congenital heart disease			*	*		*										
Congestive heart failure	*		*	*				*		*	*	*				*
Eosinophilia												*				
Hyperglycemia	*											*				
Hyperlipidemia	*											*				
Hyperproteinemia	*											*				
Sepsis		*	*	*			*			*						
Shock	*	*	*	*									*		*	*

Condition																	
Sickle cell disease																*	
Respiratory																	
Anoxia			*	*														
Asthma/bronchitis/COPD/ emphysema			*	*		*	*	*		*			*					*
Bronchitis					*													
Histoplasmosis						*												
Influenza/pneumonia				*	*				*									
Obesity hypoventilation syndrome				*	*		*											
Pneumothorax/ thoracic trauma			*	*	*						*							
Poison gases				*	*													
Pulmonary abscess															*			
Pulmonary edema		*		*	*		*			*								
Pulmonary embolism				*	*													

Continued

IMBALANCE (RIGHT)/ DISEASE PROCESS (BELOW)	Fl →	Fl ←	pH →	pH ←	Ca →	Ca ←	Cl →	Cl ←	Mg →	Mg ←	Na →	Na ←	Phos →	Phos ←	K →	K ←
Respiratory distress syndrome			*													
Sarcoidosis			*		*							*				
Thoracic skeletal deformity			*		*											
Tuberculosis			*			*					*					
Cancer	*	*	*	*	*	*			*		*	*	*	*	*	*
Bone														*		
Brain			*	*								*				
Endometrial	*										*					
Leukemia			*			*							*	*	*	
Lung				*												
Lymphoma			*			*							*	*		
Metastasis						*										
Multiple myeloma			*			*					*		*			

	C1	C2	C3	C4	C5	C6	C7	C8	C9	C10	C11	C12	C13	C14	C15
Nasopharyngeal					*										
Paraneoplastic					*										
Parathyroid			*	*								*			
Pituitary					*										
Prostate					*										
Renal											*				
Squamous cell carcinoma											*				
Thyroid										*					
Tumor lysis		*		*						*					
Ureter					*										
Uterine														*	
Endocrine															
Acromegaly								*		*	*	*			
Adrenal insufficiency/Addison's disease		*			*			*			*	*		*	

Continued

Tools **301**

IMBALANCE (RIGHT)/ DISEASE PROCESS (BELOW)	Fl ←	Fl →	pH ←	pH →	Ca ←	Ca →	Cl ←	Cl →	Mg ←	Mg →	Na ←	Na →	Phos ←	Phos →	K ←	K →
Cushing's disease/ Hyperaldosteronism/ Adrenalism	*		*		*		*				*	*				*
Diabetes insipidus	*	*	*	*			*	*	*		*	*	*	*	*	*
Diabetes mellitus	*	*	*	*		*		*	*	*	*	*	*	*	*	*
Diabetic ketoacidosis	*	*		*				*	*	*		*	*	*		
Hyperosmolar hyperglycemic state	*	*	*	*			*	*	*		*	*	*	*	*	*
Hyperparathyroidism					*									*		
Hyperthyroidism/ thyrotoxicosis			*									*	*			*
Hypoparathyroidism										*			*	*		
Hypothyroidism				*				*				*				
Syndrome of inappropriate antidiuretic hormone												*				

Gastrointestinal

	1	2	3	4	5	6	7	8	9	10	11	12	13	14	15
Anorexia	*	*	*	*	*		*		*		*			*	
Bulemia				*	*	*	*		*		*			*	*
Celiac disease							*								
Colitis							*								
Ischemic bowel		*		*	*				*				*	*	*
Liver disease/Failure/Cirrhosis	*				*								*	*	
Malabsorption (malnutrition, Crohn's disease, failure to thrive, starvation)			*				*		*	*	*		*		*
Reflux			*												
Obstruction (bowel)			*												
Pancreatitis			*	*											
Polydipsia					*										

IMBALANCE (RIGHT)/ DISEASE PROCESS (BELOW)	Fl ←	Fl →	pH ←	pH →	Ca ←	Ca →	Cl ←	Cl →	Mg ←	Mg →	Na ←	Na →	Phos ←	Phos →	K ←	K →
Genitourinary																
Azotemia											*					
Fanconi's syndrome					*											*
Glomerulonephritis						*				*						
Nephritis						*		*				*				
Pyelonephritis										*						
Renal failure (insufficiency)	*	*		*		*	*		*	*	*	*	*	*	*	*
Renal tubular acidosis				*			*			*						*
Integumentary																
Burns		*						*	*	*	*	*	*		*	
Musculoskeletal																
Fractures (pathological)				*												
Immobilization					*								*			

↑ = increased; ↓ = decreased

Muscular dystrophy											*		
Myesthenia gravis											*		
Osteomalacia											*		
Paget's disease										*	*		
Rhabdomyolysis	*		*	*		*			*		*		*	
Rickets										*			
Reproductive														
Lactation				*										
Pregnancy					*									*
Pregnancy-induced hypertension						*								

Fluid, Acid-Base, and Electrolyte Imbalance Caused by Medications

IMBALANCE (RIGHT)/ MEDICATION (BELOW)	Fl →	Fl ←	pH →	pH ←	Ca →	Ca ←	Cl →	Cl ←	Mg →	Mg ←	Na →	Na ←	Phos →	Phos ←	K →	K ←
Antacid																
Aluminum-based						*							*			
Aluminum chloride			*					*								
Calcium-based				*		*			*				*			
Magnesium-based				*	*					*			*			
Sodium bicarbonate				*			*		*		*	*			*	
Antibiotics																
Aminoglycosides																*
Gentamicin									*			*				
Methicillin					*											*
Penicillin															*	
Tetracycline					*											

	1	2	3	4	5	6	7	8	9	10	11	12	13	14	15	16	17
Anticholesterol																	
Cholestyramine															*		
Colestipol															*		
Anticonvulsants						*											
Carbamazepine													*				
Carvedilol													*				
Antifungals																	
Amphotericin											*	*	*	*			*
Carbenoxolone												*					
Chemotherapy																	
Carboplatin													*				
Cisplatin						*					*	*					*
Mithramycin						*											
Tamoxifen					*												
Vincristine													*				

Continued

Tools **307**

Fluid, Acid-Base, and Electrolyte Imbalance Caused by Medications—cont'd

IMBALANCE (RIGHT)/ MEDICATION (BELOW)	Fl ←	Fl →	pH ←	pH →	Ca ←	Ca →	Cl ←	Cl →	Mg ←	Mg →	Na ←	Na →	Phos ←	Phos →	K ←	K →
Diuretics																
CD diuretics (sodium channel blockers, potassium-sparing [amiloride, triamterene, spironolactone])		*	*				*					*	*		*	
Distal collecting tube (sodium chloride inhibitors, thiazide and thiazide-like [hydrochlorothiazide, metolazone])		*	*	*	*			*		*		*				*
Loop diuretic (Na+, K+, Cl inhibitor, bumetanide, ethocrinic acid, furosemide, torsemide)		*		*				*		*	*	*			*	
Osmotic diuretics (mannitol)	*										*	*			*	

Proximal diuretics (carbonic anhydrase inhibitor, acetazolamide)			*										*			
Iatrogenic																
Blood transfusion			*		*											
Bowel radiation											*					
Gastric suction/surgery			*						*							
Hard water for hemodialysis								*								
Ileostomy				*												
Mechanical ventilation			*													
Nasogastric suction								*	*		*					
Nothing-by-mouth orders	*			*												
Paracentesis								*								
Radiology contrast agents				*											*	
Tube feeding with insufficient free water																*

Continued

Fluid, Acid-Base, and Electrolyte Imbalance Caused by Medications—cont'd

IMBALANCE (RIGHT)/ MEDICATION (BELOW)	Fl		pH		Ca		Cl		Mg		Na		Phos		K	
	←	→	←	→	←	→	←	→	←	→	←	→	←	→	←	→
Immunosuppressants																
Basiliximab												*				
Cyclophosphamide												*				
Other																
Acetazolamide																*
Albuterol						*										
Amiodarone				*												
Ammonium chloride												*				
Angiotensin											*					
Aspirin																
Bisacodyl																*
Captopril																*
Cholestyramine				*												*

Citrate										*									
Colchicines	*															*			
Dextrose 5% in water			*											*	*				
Digitalis			*																*
Ether												*							
Fluorides												*							
Fluoxetine														*					
Gamma globulin																			
Glucagon						*													
Glucose		*				*									*	*			*
Insulin						*										*			*
Isoniazid												*							
Isoproterenol						*													
Lactated Ringer's solution											*								
Laxatives						*						*			*	*			*

Fluid, Acid-Base, and Electrolyte Imbalance Caused by Medications—cont'd

IMBALANCE (RIGHT)/ MEDICATION (BELOW)	Fl ←	Fl →	pH ←	pH →	Ca ←	Ca →	Cl ←	Cl →	Mg ←	Mg →	Na ←	Na →	Phos ←	Phos →	K ←	K →
Licorice (Glycyrrhiza glabra)			*													*
Lithium		*			*						*					
Metformin				*												
Metoprolol															*	
Nicardipine												*				
Propranolol															*	
Salicylates			*	*			*									
Saline >0.9% solution	*									*	*					
Saline <0.9% solution	*									*		*				
Sedatives				*												
Selective serotonin reuptake inhibitor												*				
Sodium bicarbonate			*					*		*	*					

Continued

	1	2	3	4	5	6	7	8	9	10	11	12	13
Sodium chloride		*			*		*	*					
Sodium polystyrene					*								
Succinylcholine												*	
Theophylline		*							*				*
Trazodone	*			*									
Steroids													
Corticosteroids	*	*	*	*				*		*		*	*
Corticosteroids (withdrawal)										*			
Mineral (aldosterone)		*	*					*					*
Surgery													
Abdominal (bowel)		*											
Renal transplant	*		*							*			
Small-bowel resection							*				*		
Thoracic		*											

Fluid, Acid-Base, and Electrolyte Imbalance Caused by Medications—cont'd

IMBALANCE (RIGHT)/ MEDICATION (BELOW)	Fl ←	Fl →	pH ←	pH →	Ca ←	Ca →	Cl ←	Cl →	Mg ←	Mg →	Na ←	Na →	Phos ←	Phos →	K ←	K →
Tourniquet for blood draw					*										*	
Total or partial parenteral nutrition with lactate or acetate			*	*												
Total or partial parenteral nutrition with low magnesium										*						
Vitamin supplements																
Vitamin A					*											
Boron (excess)				*												
Calcium carbonate			*		*					*				*		
Citrates						*										
Magnesium						*		*		*						
Phosphorus						*							*			*

↑ = increased; ↓ = decreased

Fluid, Acid-Base, and Electrolyte Imbalances Caused by Nutrition-Based Shifts

IMBALANCE (RIGHT)/ NUTRITION SHIFT (BELOW)	Fl →	Fl ←	pH →	pH ←	Ca →	Ca ←	Cl →	Cl ←	Mg →	Mg ←	Na →	Na ←	Phos →	Phos ←	K →	K ←
Foods																
Calcium (high milligrams)									*							
Contamination with mineral salts										*						
Decreased solutes combined with excess fluids											*					
Fiber supplements					*											
Fruits																*
Licorice				*	*										*	
Oxalic acid					*											
Phosphorus (high milligrams)					*									*		
Phytic acid					*											

Proteins (high milligrams)													
Sodium (high milligrams)													
Vegetables													
Oral Fluids													
Alcohol (ethanol													
Caffeine													
Ethanol ingestion													
Excess beer													
Excess water													

↑ = increased; ↓ = decreased

Fluid, Acid-Base, and Electrolyte Imbalances Caused by Additive and Illicit Substances

IMBALANCE (RIGHT)/ SUBSTANCE (BELOW)	Fl ←	Fl →	pH ←	pH →	Ca ←	Ca →	Cl ←	Cl →	Mg ←	Mg →	Na ←	Na →	Phos ←	Phos →	K ←	K →
Barbiturates				*												
Benzodiazepines				*												
Ethylene glycol (antifreeze)	*			*			*									
MDMA (ecstasy)												*				
Methanol	*			*			*									
Opiates				*												
Oral tobacco			*													

↑ = increased; ↓ = decreased

Procedures

Procedures included are arterial blood gas (ABG) collection, urine collection, and nasogastric tube placement.

ABG Collection

The medical team may order ABGs. Before communicating an ABG order to the personnel who will perform the draw, the nurse must assess the patient's arterial function. Any decrease in pulse should be reported to the medical team before attempting to obtain the sample.

Most facilities have restrictions on which personnel may obtain a direct arterial serum sample. Often this practice is restricted to trained physicians and respiratory therapists. Some institutions permit this procedure to be performed by trained nurses.

Sites for Withdrawal

Common sites for arterial blood draw are the radial arteries and, if necessary, the femoral arteries. Disruption of these arteries can result in a decreased perfusion distal to the arterial needle stick. It is essential to follow the guidelines specified by your institution in order to preserve function of the limb below the stick. If the radial artery is to be assessed, Allen's test should be performed in addition to a pulse assessment. See Box 6–1 for more details on Allen's Test.

The Patient Post Withdrawal

After blood is collected, the person who drew the blood or the nurse caring for the patient will need to maintain pressure on the intake site for at least 5 full minutes. This time may be increased to 15 full minutes if the patient is on any form of anticoagulant, including aspirin. Observe the site carefully for any sign of bleeding, bruising, or swelling, and observe the patient for any neurological symptoms such as tingling or numbness immediately after the test and 15 minutes afterward. Apply a pressure bandage to the artery after completion of the test.

Storage and Transport of ABG Sample

Blood gases must be placed on ice immediately for transport and must be analyzed very quickly, at least within 60 minutes of collection. Alert the personnel who are responsible for performing laboratory assessments on the specimen in advance of both (1) the time that the specimen will be drawn and (2) the anticipated time of delivery. Personnel will also need to know an accurate body temperature of the patient at the time the sample was drawn in order to correct for the effect that fever has on the gases.

Interpreting ABGs

Normal measurements for the levels obtained through blood gas collections can be found in Table 6–1. Table 6–1 also provides values that point to acidosis or alkalosis.

The results of blood gas measurements are often used to help distinguish the reason for an alkalotic or acidotic state. Interpretation is often framed as a series of questions; see Box 6–2 for sample questions.

In addition to fever, factors that can interfere with accurate results include specimens that were not kept on ice, not analyzed soon enough after sampling, or that were collected too soon after a change in respiratory or metabolic process to allow for correction. Examples of these changes can be a recent blood transfusion, a recent change in the way or amount of oxygen delivery by external source or internal mechanical ventilation, and recent suctioning of the patient's airway. Other interfering factors can be too much heparin in the tube, a very high white blood cell count, high levels of carbon monoxide, and hemoglobin levels that are too high or too low.

Urine Collection

A urine specimen may be ordered as *random, first morning,* or *timed* or *second void.* Random urine collection occurs any time during the day. First

Table 6–1 Blood Gas Results for Acid-Base Interpretation and Normal Gas Values

	CRITICAL ACIDOSIS	ACID	NORMAL RANGE	BASE	CRITICAL ALKALOSIS
pH arterial	7.20	<7.35	7.35–7.45	>7.45	7.60
pH venous		<7.32	7.32–7.43	>7.43	
Arterial P_{CO_2}	>67 mm Hg	>45 mm Hg	35–45 mm Hg	<35 mm Hg	<20 mm Hg
Venous P_{CO_2}		>51 mm Hg	41–51 mm Hg	<41 mm Hg	
Venous CO_2		>29 mEq/L	23-29 mEq/L	<23 mEq/L	
Arterial HCO_3^-	<10 mmol/L	<18 mEq/L	18–23 mEq/L	>23 mEq/L	>40 mmol/L
Venous HCO_3^-		<24 mEq/L	24–28 mEq/L	>28 mEq/L	
Base excess arterial		<12 mEq/L	-2–+3 mEq/L	>3 mEq/L	
Anion gap		>12 mEq/L	8–12 mEq/L	<8 mEq/L	
Arterial P_{O_2}			80–95 mm Hg		
Venous P_{O_2}			20–49 mm Hg		
Arterial O_2 saturation			95%–99%		
Venous O_2 saturation			70%–75%		

Questions Concerning Blood Gas Measurement Results

Is the pH (7.35–7.45)?
1) If *No:*
   a. Is the pH <7.35, showing acidosis?
      i. Is the HCO_3^- low (<18 mEq/L), showing metabolic acidosis?
      ii. Is the P_{CO_2} high (>45 mm Hg), showing respiratory acidosis?
   b. Is the pH >7.45, showing alkalosis?
      i. Is the HCO_3^- high (>23 mEq/L), showing metabolic alkalosis?
      ii. Is the P_{CO_2} low (<35 mm Hg), showing respiratory acidosis?
2) If *Yes:* A normal pH does not mean there is no imbalance; it may mean
   that the imbalance is being adequately compensated by automatic
   buffering mechanisms. If the pH is normal, take another look at the P_{CO_2}
   and HCO_3^-. Respiratory mechanisms, such as rapid or slow breathing, are
   rarely able to return pH to normal.
   a. Is the HCO_3^- low (<18 mEq/L), showing metabolic acidosis?
      i. Is the P_{CO_2} low (<35 mm Hg), showing respiratory compensation?
   b. Is the HCO_3^- high (>23 mEq/L), showing metabolic alkalosis?
      i. Is the P_{CO_2} high (>45 mm Hg), showing respiratory compensation?
   c. Is the P_{CO_2} high (>45 mm Hg), showing respiratory acidosis?
      i. Is the HCO_3^- high (>23 mEq/L), showing that renal compensation is
         active?
   d. Is the P_{CO_2} low (<35 mm Hg), showing respiratory alkalosis?
      i. Is HCO_3^- low (<18 mEq/L), showing that renal compensation is active?

A discussion should be held with the medical team to ensure that the patient has enough physiological reserve to attempt to compensate while specific
measures are taken to correct acidosis or alkalosis. If compensation is already
under way, anticipate the necessity of protecting the airway and respiratory exchange so that the patient is not breathing too rapidly, deeply, slowly, or shal-
lowly and that intake of other gases, such as oxygen, is not compromised.
Consult the medical team to ensure the patient has sufficient renal function to
buffer the underlying acidosis or alkalosis.

morning urine specimens are normally concentrated urine samples.
Timed or second void refers to urine that has not been held in the bladder overnight and is thus less concentrated (since it has not been sitting
for hours); *24-hour urine collections* are used to measure renal clearance of
particular electrolytes and/or molecules. Although each institution has
guidelines for specimen collection and transportation, the following general principles will assist with appropriate collection.

Random Specimen Collection

A random urine sample may be ordered to evaluate for electrolytes. In this case, the collection need not be sterile. The patient may void directly into a sterile container, clean dry urinal, clean dry toilet collection device (hat), or clean dry bedpan.

First Morning Collection

First morning voids are ordered to evaluate the concentrated urine that has collected in the bladder overnight. Instruct the patient before going to sleep the night before to anticipate collection, and demonstrate use of the collection container. If interventions are required during the night, the nurse and assistive personnel should remind the patient that first morning void will be collected.

Second Void Collection

In general, patients who are able to accept hydration will drink 32 oz of water over 2 hours, void, then wait 1 hour and collect a specimen during this second void. A *sterile collection* is required for culture. This involves a clean catch into a sterile container, catheterization, or access from an indwelling catheter. Information about each of these methods follows. Each institution may have a particular antiseptic agent for use with clean-catch cleansing or catheterization, such as chlorhexidine or povidone-iodine. Patients should be asked about allergies before applying any topical antiseptics.

Clean-Catch Urine Specimen

Clean catch is a technique that can be performed with patients who are able to follow instructions and manipulate the specimen container so as to keep it sterile. If a patient is unable to follow instructions or to manipulate the specimen container, even with assistance, then the specimen cannot be considered a clean catch. Consult the medical team for alternative orders, such as straight catheterization. Each institution has a procedure for use of a unique collection container with specific antiseptic pad or wipes. Read directions from the container to ensure correct specimen technique.

In general, ask the patient to wash and dry the hands. Then, the opening of the urethra is cleansed from the meatus outward with three separate wipes with a clean antiseptic cloth. For women, the movement of wipes should be from the urethra opening toward the vaginal opening in order to avoid contamination. For uncircumcised men, the foreskin needs to be slightly retracted to cleanse the meatus thoroughly.

After cleansing the urethral opening, instruct the patient to make a few drops of urine into the toilet and then stop the flow of urine. This allows for bacteria at the opening of the urethra to be rinsed away. Then, the patient should continue to urinate directly into the sterile specimen cup, up to the level required by the laboratory (usually approximately 30 mL). Ask the patient not to overflow the cup and to finish voiding into the toilet.

Straight Catheterization

If a patient cannot follow directions or is unable to manipulate the specimen container without contamination, the medical team may order catheterization. To avoid introducing complications—such as infection and trauma, which are associated with indwelling catheters—a straight or nondwelling catheterization may be ordered for the purpose of collecting a urine specimen.

Each institution has a procedure for catheterization and equipment supplied for this purpose. In general, the patient should have the procedure thoroughly explained, including the potential sensation of discomfort associated with catheterization. The patient should agree to the procedure before proceeding.

The narrowest gauge of catheter should be used to prevent trauma. Antiseptic cleansing should be similar to that performed by the patient for a clean catch. The catheter should then be lubricated with a water-soluble lubricant.

The urethral opening can be identified by moving aside the labia for women and the foreskin of uncircumcised men with the nurse's *nondominant* hand. Once this hand has come in contact with the perineum, it is no longer sterile and should not come in contact with any of the sterile collection materials.

The catheters should be passed gently into the urethra opening until urine comes out of the distal end of the catheter. Once a few milliliters have passed, the required amount of urine (approximately 30 mL) should be collected into a sterile specimen cup. After the urine is collected, the patient should be informed that the catheter will be withdrawn so that the sensation is not unexpected.

Indwelling Catheter Collection

Collection of a sterile specimen can also be made via an indwelling catheter. Urine may not be drawn from the collection bag attached to the catheter, as it will have started to degrade.

In order to collect a fresh specimen, the tubing connected to the catheter should be clamped only for as long as necessary to obtain about 30 mL of urine in the tubing without leaving the patient unattended.

Most commercial collection devices currently have a needle-less system that allows for collection with a Luer-Lok syringe. Others may require that a needle be attached to a syringe for collection. Either type of port should be cleansed according the institutional policy and allowed to dry before urine is withdrawn.

After collection with a sterile syringe, the urine should be transferred into a sterile collection container. Be certain to release the clamp on the patient's catheter tubing to prevent harm to the patient and allow the free flow of urine into the collection bag. If a needle is used, ensure that sharps precautions are observed.

Specimen Transportation

Ensure the container lid is tightly closed, properly labeled, and placed in a biohazard bag before sending it to the laboratory for analysis. Each laboratory has a procedure for how quickly the specimen must arrive. In general, the urine should be transported immediately, unless collected in a container that contains a laboratory-specific fixative.

Documentation

The process and outcome of any specimen collection and teaching should be documented in the patient's medical record.

24-Hour Urine Collections

If a 24-hour urine sample is requested, obtain the correct container and preservative from the laboratory. Assess the patient's ability to follow procedures for a 24-hour collection. Following HIPAA guidelines, place a sign to remind the patient and caregivers that urine is being collected. Educate the patient on proper collection procedures, including not voiding directly into the laboratory collection container, but using a clean collection container and allowing nursing personnel to transfer the urine into the laboratory container. Remind the patient to avoid contamination of the urine with paper or stool.

Nasogastric Tube Placement

Most institutions have policies regarding which personnel may place what type of nasogastric (NG) device. Nurses who are permitted by their institution to place NG tubes should follow institutional guidelines. The following are some general steps for placing an NG tube.

- **Step 1:** Assess for patency of the nares.
- **Step 2:** Prepare appropriate water-soluble lubrication to protect the patient from disruption of mucous membranes.
- **Step 3:** Instruct patient to position his or her head as upright as possible, and ask patient to swallow small sips of water.
- **Step 4:** Apply nonsterile gloves, and measure tube length by measuring from the bridge of the nose to the earlobe and from the earlobe to the midpoint between the bottom of the sternum

and the umbilicus (xyphoid process). Mark that measurement with a permanent marker as a guide to the depth of insertion.

NG tube insertion is contraindicated for patients with facial trauma. Tube insertion should be halted if any signs of respiratory irritation or decline occur, because those signs mean that the tube was most likely passed into the airway.

Scales

The following scales are discussed: edema measure, Glasgow Coma, and the jugular venous distention scale.

Edema Measure

Peripheral edema is assessed by pressing a finger over the bony area of the radius or tibia. Practitioners commonly estimate edema, but a scale that indicates the depth of the depression remaining on the patient's limb can be helpful in describing edema more objectively. Figure 6-1 is an example of such a scale. Along with indicating the depth of depression and the duration of the induration, the practitioner should indicate at what level of the limb the edema is assessed, such as "at the level of the patella" or "one quarter of the way up the leg." This way, if diuretics or other measures to decrease third spacing are employed, the practitioner can assess whether the measure has been helpful in decreasing the edema.

Glasgow Coma Scale

The Glasgow Coma Scale, initially a tool for research at the Institute of Neurological Sciences, University of Glasgow, Glasgow, Scotland, has evolved into an internationally recognized tool for communication among

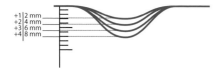

FIGURE 6-1: Using an edema scale can enhance communication between practitioners. Edema is usually estimated after pressure is applied briefly by one finger. For this scale an indentation over a bony area after brief pressure is graded from + 1 to + 4. + 1 edema: an indentation of about 2 mm; + 2 edema: an indentation of about 4 mm; + 3 edema is an indentation of about 6 mm; and + 4 edema is an indentation of about 8 mm.

caregivers for patients experiencing brain injury or metabolic disorders associated with decreased level of consciousness. Institutions may modify the language from the initial scale, based on the vast amount of research that has been conducted using the scale since it was developed in the 1970s and published in 1974 by Bryan Jennett and Graham Teasdale. Although the scale can be linked with the Glasgow Outcome Scale for predicting a patient's prognosis, the purpose of using the coma scale at the bedside is to enhance communication. As such, each institution may seek to ensure that education on the use of the scale crosses disciplines.

Glasgow Coma Scale

EYE OPENING RESPONSE	
Spontaneous. Indicates arousal, not necessarily awareness.	4
To speech. When spoken to–not necessarily the command to open eyes.	3
To pain. Applied to limbs, not face where grimacing can cause closure.	2
None.	1
VERBAL RESPONSE	
Oriented. Knows who, where, when; year, season, month.	5
Confused conversation. Attends and responds but answers muddled/wrong.	4
Inappropriate words. Intelligible words, but mostly expletives or random.	3
Incomprehensible speech. Moans and groans only–no words.	2
None.	1
MOTOR RESPONSE	
Obeys commands. Exclude grasp reflex or postural adjustments.	6
Localizes. Other limb moves to site of nailbed pressure.	5
Withdraws. Normal flexion of elbow or knee to local painful stimulus.	4

Continued

Glasgow Coma Scale—cont'd

MOTOR RESPONSE	
Abnormal flexion. Slow withdraw with pronation of wrist, adduction of shoulder.	3
Extensor response. Extension of elbow with pronation and adduction.	2
None.	1
Total (out of 15)	

Jugular Venous Distention

Jugular venous distention (JVD) can be a sign of increased fluids and can assist with estimating central venous pressures. For proper measure, the patient must be positioned at a 45° angle. A centimeter ruler is placed, with the bottom resting on the angle of Louis, which is the sternal angle. Another straight edge is extended from the point of highest visual pulsation of the internal jugular vein. The point where the two rulers cross allows for an estimation of JVD (Fig. 6-2). Because the angle of Louis is approximately 5 cm above the right atrium of the heart, the measure of centimeters from the angle of Louis to the internal jugular pulsation is added to 5 cm to estimate central venous pressures. For instance, a measure of 3 cm would be added to 5 cm and equal 8 mm Hg; 0–8 mm Hg is a normal mean resting value.

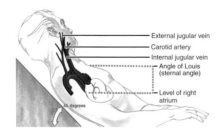

Figure 6-2: To measure JVD: Position the patient at a 45° angle, looking to the left; extend a centimeter ruler vertically upward from the angle of Louis; distinguish the highest point of pulsation of the internal jugular vein by having the patient look to the left; hold another ruler perpendicular to the first at the level of the pulsation; estimate the JVD by adding 5 to the height in centimeters of the pulsation.

ANSWER KEY

CHAPTER 2: FLUID BALANCE AND IMBALANCE

Clinical Scenario: Fluid Excess

1-A B-type natriuretic peptide level of 500 indicates that Mr. De Jesus' left ventricle is enlarged and that the cause of his shortness of breath is likely related to fluid overload.

2-Mr. De Jesus' sodium, chloride, and glucose values are elevated. The nurse should not assume the types of food that Mr. De Jesus consumed at his daughter's wedding but should be prepared to discuss the effect of food that is high in salt and sugar.

3-As the fluids in Mr. De Jesus' lungs diminish, the level at which the nurse is able to auscultate rales/crackles will fall lower. When documenting a respiratory assessment, it is helpful to document the anatomical level where fluid overload is heard, such as scapular, or sixth rib.

Clinical Scenario: Fluid Deficit

1-A gain of 2.2 lb, or 1 kg, represents a gain of about 1 L of fluid. Shortness of breath is a symptom that excess fluid is building up in Mrs. Artise's lungs because of worsening heart disease.

2-Mrs. Artise was likely to continue to take her diuretic and ACE inhibitor, even though she did not take in enough fluid to offset the heat in her home. This change in her normal environment caused her to need more fluid than she normally consumed with the fluid restriction prescribed for her heart failure.

3-Mrs. Artise is likely experiencing cold sepsis related to a urinary tract infection that has set in because of inadequate perfusion to her kidneys.

Review Questions

1-Patients and community members who cannot cool down adequately can lose up to 1 L of fluid per hour through sweat.

2-Dry stool can be a symptom of dehydration, whereas loose, watery stool can indicate excess fluid losses.

3-Serum osmolality is a measure of bicarbonate, chloride, glucose, sodium, and urea particles.

4-A 1% increase in hematocrit from the patient's baseline shows a loss of approximately 100 mL of intravascular fluid and 400 mL from interstitial fluid.

5-If a patient consumes >700 mL/hr, water toxicity can ensue. The medical team should be alerted to patients who are experiencing polydipsia so that an underlying cause can be established and a care plan can be created to protect the patient.

6-Patients who require IV fluids often have underlying medical conditions that prevent them from ingesting, regulating, or excreting fluids appropriately. They also have a higher likelihood of associated electrolyte and acid-base imbalance. Patient positioning, vascular stability, blood pressure, and other factors can increase or decrease the rate of fluid being delivered by an IV line that is only regulated by a roller clamp.

CHAPTER 3A: CALCIUM
Clinical Scenario: Hypocalcemia

1-Mrs. Albert would be at risk for bone weakness and fractures as well as nerve and immune system dysfunction.

2-Vitamin D also helps regulate normal phosphorous levels.

3-Because hypocalcemia can be linked to seizures, the medical team should be consulted to evaluate the adequacy of phenytoin, vitamin D, and calcium levels.

Clinical Scenario: Hypercalcemia

1-Mrs. Wood has a complex metabolic problem with hyperparathyroidism and poor calcium intake, both contributing to increased levels of blood calcium.

2-Mrs. Wood's lack of dietary calcium contributed to calcium loss from her bones into her bloodstream.

3-Weight-bearing exercise will help stimulate increased calcium absorption by her bones and normal blood calcium levels.

Review Questions

1-In low albumin states, the medical team will likely order ionized calcium to determine blood calcium.

2-Serum calcium has an inverse relationship with serum phosphorus. When calcium levels are high, phosphorous levels are low.

3-In acidotic states, calcium does not bond as well to serum proteins, causing an increase in free ionized serum calcium.

4-Of calcium, 98%–99% is stored in bones and teeth.

5-Calcium channel blockers decrease stimulation of vascular smooth muscle, thus lowering blood pressure.

6-Orders should not be written in milliliter or ampoule dosing; they should be written in mEq or g because calcium chloride contains approximately three times as much calcium as calcium gluconate in each gram.

CHAPTER 3B: CHLORIDE
Clinical Scenario: Hypochloremia

1-A temperature of 99°F, elevated heart rate in the 90s, and a decreased systolic blood pressure < 100 mm Hg should alert the nurse to the possibility that Mrs. Henninger is experiencing dehydration.

2-A larger-bore catheter can help prevent IV irritation with potassium chloride solution.

3-The nurse can consult the medical team to ensure the potassium chloride is well diluted, to decrease irritation with a smaller-gauge catheter, and to ask the team for orders to place a second, larger catheter once Mrs. Henninger has achieved increased hydration.

Clinical Scenario: Hyperchloremia

1-Tinnitus, a reported sensation of ringing of the ears, is a symptom of salicylate toxicity.

2-Mrs. Smyth's Alzheimer's disease puts her at risk for ingestion of inappropriate or dangerous poisons and requires high levels of monitoring by family and caregivers.

3-Mrs. Smyth must be supported emotionally and cognitively to help maintain her IV infusion and other invasive interventions such as arterial blood gas. Her husband may not be able to offer her enough support to protect her from further injury. Therefore, the nurse should institute one-on-one observation during her treatment.

Review Questions

1-Sodium chloride.

2-Sodium, potassium chloride, and bicarbonate.

3-Vomiting or loss of hydrochloric acid through gastric suctioning contributes to chloride loss.

4-Chloride loss through sweat is associated with cystic fibrosis.

5-Infusion of dextrose and water, which contains no chloride, can cause dilution of chloride and symptomatic hypochloremia.

6-Urinary potassium losses can be caused by low chloride levels.

CHAPTER 3C: MAGNESIUM
Clinical Scenario: Hypomagnesemia

1-Mrs. Daj's history of GI problems should alert the nurse to a problem with magnesium ingestion and possible wasting if she has lost any gastric secretions through vomiting or diarrhea.

2-The dextrose in the IV fluids that Mrs. Daj receives may be pulled out of urine into cells.

3-Symptoms of alcohol withdrawal can be overwhelming to patients and typically have an onset of 24 hours after the last drink, peaking between 24 and 36 hours.

Clinical Scenario: Hypermagnesemia

1-Cefazolin and lithium can cause renal insufficiency. Mr. Anderson's low urine output and flank pain also indicate renal problems.

2-The nurse should observe for bradycardia, a wide QRS complex, a long PR interval, and elevated T waves.

3-Mr. Anderson's hypotension is likely related to low calcium levels secondary to high magnesium. Until his high magnesium is reversed, the nurse may have difficulty placing a large-gauge IV line. After hydration and treatment of the high magnesium, the nurse should anticipate the potential need of future electrolytes or other emergency medications and obtain an order to place a large-bore IV line as soon as the patient's veins will accept it.

Review Questions

1-The body stores magnesium in bone, and the magnesium can be mobilized if magnesium levels in the blood drop below normal.

2-With low magnesium levels, the muscles are unable to relax.

3-Calcium, phosphorus, and sodium are affected by magnesium levels.

4-Coffee, tea, and cocoa can be dietary sources of magnesium.

5-Bone allows for magnesium stores to be used in low magnesium states.

6-The renal system will attempt to conserve magnesium when serum magnesium is low. Urine magnesium levels will be lower than normal.

CHAPTER 3D: PHOSPHORUS
Clinical Scenario: Hypophosphatemia

1-Alcohol decreases absorption of phosphorus and the activation of vitamin D in the intestines. Adequate levels of vitamin D are required for phosphorous absorption.

2-These patients often have decreased appetite and decreased ability to metabolize foods. Because phosphorus is supplied through foods, patients with malnutrition states are at risk for low phosphorus.

3-Alcohol withdrawal is considered a state of high-energy demand. In this state, phosphorus tends to move out of the blood and into cells.

Clinical Scenario: Hyperphosphatemia

1-Typically, high calcium levels result in low phosphorous levels, and low calcium levels result in high phosphorous levels.

2-Elevated calcium levels are likely related to bone calcium changes, putting Mrs. Ryan at high risk for stress fractures.

3-Mrs. Ryan has had several admissions for congestive heart failure, anemia, and hypertension. Although renal failure can be the cause of these problems, it is likely that Mrs. Ryan is also being treated medically to prevent worsening of these diseases. The nurse should review all Mrs. Ryan's medications with her on a regular basis to ensure that Mrs. Ryan is able to comply with her regimen and knows to discuss areas of concern with the medical team.

Review Questions

1-The bones and teeth, cellular DNA (or RNA), adenosine triphosphate, creatinine phosphate molecules, and cellular membranes.

2-Calcitriol and parathyroid hormone work together to regulate calcium and phosphorus.

3-In low phosphorous states, it is more difficult for oxygen to release from hemoglobin and transfer to the body's cells.

4-Vitamin D is required for intestinal absorption of phosphorus.

5-Caffeine and alcohol can interfere with maintenance of appropriate phosphorous levels.

6-Chvostek's and Trousseau's sign can be used to evaluate for both, as neurological symptoms may be caused by the decrease of serum calcium levels associated with high phosphorous levels.

CHAPTER 3E: POTASSIUM
Clinical Scenario: Hypokalemia

1-Paresthesias, mental status changes, heart palpitations, anorexia, thirst, vomiting, constipation, excessive urination, muscle cramping, and weakness.

2-Sodium chloride, and carbon dioxide to evaluate for alkalosis; urine potassium levels to check for ketoacidosis, aldosterone shifts, and elevated corticosteroids; and blood cell counts to evaluate for interfering factors such as elevated white blood cells or platelets.

3-Mr. Sarandon should monitor fluid intake, urine output, and daily weight. Weight should be measured every day at the same time, with the patient wearing similar clothing.

Clinical Scenario: Hyperkalemia

1-Mrs. Hapman should be alert for palpitations, decreased respiratory rate or depth, and weakness.

2-About 80%–90% of potassium is excreted through the kidneys. With decreased renal function, less potassium is excreted, resulting in hyperkalemia.

3-Fruits are typically high in potassium, with some exceptions, especially dried fruits and citrus. Legumes, including peanuts, coffee, and chocolate, are unexpected sources of potassium. Prepared foods may contain potassium, so Mrs. Hapman should read labels of food she normally purchases.

Review Questions

1-Because dehydration may increase potassium blood levels as fluid levels decrease and kidneys may no longer excrete excess potassium, the nurse should check any chemistry samples that have been drawn and discuss potassium orders with the medical team before giving potassium supplementation.

2-A too-rapid infusion of potassium can cause cardiac arrest. This is why vials of potassium are not stored on nursing units and potassium infusion is expected to be prepared in the pharmacy by a pharmacist.

CHAPTER 3F: SODIUM
Clinical Scenario: Hyponatremia

1-The nurse should anticipate orders for hydration with normal saline 0.9% solution for correction of hyponatremia.

2-The nurse should measure intake and compare that with output and observe carefully for symptoms of fluid overload, if Mr. Jones is unable to make sufficient urine once hydration has been corrected.

3-The Glasgow Coma Scale and a three-point orientation scale (full name, room number and name of hospital, and day with date) are considered evidence-based measures of neurological changes. However, the nurse should consistently ask and document the three points of orientation with each assessment so that subtle changes may be observed and reported to the medical team.

Clinical Scenario: Hypernatremia

1-Normal saline can be infused via a 24- or 22-gauge IV at a slow rate. Caution should be used to assess for movement of the catheter once the vein grows larger in diameter as Mr. Odam becomes more hydrated.

2-Mr. Odam was taking Lasix, despite his poor hydration. Mr. Odam's dementia put him at risk for managing safe fluid intake and controlling his environment.

3-High sodium levels will cause fluid to stay in the vascular space and may cause symptoms of fluid overload, including jugular venous distention. As sodium levels are corrected, some fluid will move into cells to correct cellular dehydration but, with CHF, fluid may also be retained in the interstitial space and produce edema and rales or crackles in the lungs.

Review Questions

1-People who consume water while losing sodium through sweat and fad dieting, those who drink beer in excess or take the recreational drug ecstasy, or people with psychiatric diseases or developmental delay who suffer from polydipsia are at risk. Patients with chronic or acute health problems and who retain water inappropriately without infusion or ingestion of sodium are at risk.

2-Central pontine myelinolysis, the loss of the myelin sheath of the brainstem, is associated with too rapid correction of hyponatremia. Neurological symptoms can be masked, because they are similar to the neurological symptoms associated with hyponatremia.

3-Hypotonic saline will cause further dilution of IV sodium and may stimulate sodium to leave cells rapidly by osmosis. Water will leave cells along with sodium, causing dangerous shrinkage of cells and eventual cellular dysfunction.

4-When the sodium balance is restored between vascular and intracellular compartments, water may rush across the cellular membrane rapidly and cause the cells to swell. This is particularly dangerous for brain cells, because the cranium will force the swollen brain downward against the brainstem.

5-Foods containing sodium bicarbonate, pickled or smoked foods, and foods preserved in cans often contain high levels of sodium. Patients at risk for hypernatremia should be taught to read labels to estimate the sodium content of foods.

6-Patients with untreated diabetes insipidus will lose high volumes of fluid through urine, up to 20 L/day.

CHAPTER 4: ACID-BASE BALANCE AND IMBALANCE

Clinical Scenario: Respiratory Alkalosis

1-Mrs. Aslam has salicylate toxicity, which is stimulating her rapid breathing.

2-Levels will likely peak about 4 hours later, so blood should be drawn close to 4 hours after the source is ingested.

3-Head or thoracic trauma, blood infection, and pulmonary embolus or respiratory pathology may all be life-threatening causes of rapid breathing.

Clinical Scenario: Respiratory Acidosis

1-Slow, shallow breathing should be an indication to observe for possible symptoms of developing acidosis.

2-Narcotics, sleeping medication, exhaustion, and abdominal or thoracic surgery can compromise deep and regular breathing.

3-Patients may have obesity-associated breathing problems such as sleep apnea or obesity hypoventilation syndrome. Hospitalized patients are at risk for immobility and respiratory compromise due to frequent supine positioning and medical devices that restrict movement.

Clinical Scenario: Metabolic Alkalosis

1-Mrs. North was probably not ingesting appropriate levels of potassium from her diet because of her abdominal pain and lost potassium via gastric suctioning.

2-The nurse should educate Mrs. North regarding over-the-counter antacids and contact social services to assist with funding prescription medications.

3-The nurse should measure and report gastric and urinary output to allow for monitoring of potential hydrogen, potassium, and chloride.

Clinical Scenario: Metabolic Acidosis

1-Based upon Mr. Sanert's initial glucose of 425 and signs of ketoacidosis, the nurse should suspect that the patient has not been receiving sufficient amounts of insulin.

2-Given Mr. Sanert's metabolic instability, undergoing an invasive procedure with sedation will increase Mr. Sanert's risk for increased complications. He will require a longer period of observation for metabolic changes.

3-In an effort to breathe off carbon dioxide, patients will frequently present with deep and rapid breathing. This breathing can be sustained only for a limited period until the patient becomes exhausted from the excess work of breathing.

Review Questions

1-Chemical buffer systems are constantly at work to prevent acid-base shifts. When a sudden shift occurs and the buffer systems are no longer able to modulate the imbalance, the respiratory system will respond. However, the respiratory system is limited in its ability to compensate. Hyperventilation, an attempt to blow off excess carbon dioxide, is limited by exhaustion, and hypoventilation, as an effort to retain carbon dioxide, is limited by the need to inhale oxygen.

2-pH represents hydrogen levels in the body. An arterial blood pH <7.35 indicates acidosis, whereas a pH >7.45 indicates alkalosis.

3-Low chloride and low potassium levels can be linked to metabolic alkalosis and must be corrected before alkalosis can be reversed.

4-The Poison Control Center at 1-800-222-1222 should be contacted to discuss evidence-based treatment of poisoning.

FIGURE CREDITS

Figures 1-1, 1-4, 3E-1, 3F-1, and 4-2 are from Scanlon VC and Sanders T. *Essentials of Anatomy and Physiology*, 5th ed. Philadelphia: F.A. Davis, 2007.

Figures 1-2, 4-1, and 6-2 are from Wilkinson JM and Van Leuven K, eds. *Fundamentals of Nursing*. Philadelphia: F.A. Davis, 2008.

Figures 1-3, 1-5, 2-4, 2-5, 2-6, 2-7, 3A-2, 3E-2, and 3E-3 are from Phillips, LD. *IV Therapy Notes: Nurse's Clinical Pocket Guide*. Philadelphia: F.A. Davis, 2005.

Figures 2-1, 2-2, and 2-3 are based on illustrations by Deirdre Cruice Cabanel. Redrawn with permission.

Figure 3C-1 is from Jones SA. *ECG Success: Exercises in ECG Interpretation*. Philadelphia: F.A. Davis, 2007.

Figure 4-3 is from Strasinger SK and Di Lorenzo MS. *Urinalysis and Body Fluids*, 5th ed. Philadelphia: F.A. Davis, 2008.

Figure 6-1 is from Dillon, PM, ed. *Nursing Health Assessment: A Critical Thinking, Case Studies Approach*. Philadelphia: F.A. Davis, 2003.

REFERENCES

General

Deglin, JH and Vallerand, AH. *Davis's Drug Guide for Nurses*, 11th ed. Philadelphia: F.A. Davis, 2009.

Dillon, PM, ed. *Nursing Health Assessment: A Critical Thinking, Case Studies Approach*. Philadelphia: F.A. Davis, 2003.

Kowalak, JL and Turkington, C, eds. *Lippincott Manual of Nursing Practice Series: ECG Interpretation*. Philadelphia: Lippincott Williams & Wilkins, 2008.

Porth, CM. *Essentials of Pathophysiology: Concepts of Altered Health States*, 7th ed. Philadelphia: Lippincott Williams & Wilkins, 2005.

Scanlon, VC and Sanders, T. *Essentials of Anatomy and Physiology*, 5th ed. Philadelphia: F.A. Davis, 2007.

Sommers, MS, Johnson, SJ and Beery, TA. *Diseases and Disorders: A Nursing Therapeutics Manual*, 3rd ed. Philadelphia: F.A. Davis, 2007.

Stanley, M, Blair, KA and Beare, PG. *Gerontological Nursing: Promoting Successful Aging With Older Adults*, 3rd ed. Philadelphia: F.A. Davis, 2005.

Strasinger, SK and Di Lorenzo, MS. *Urinalysis and Body Fluids*, 5th Edition. Philadelphia: F.A. Davis, 2008.

Van Leeuwen, AM and Poelhuis-Leth, DJ. *Davis's Comprehensive Handbook of Laboratory and Diagnostic Tests With Nursing Implications*, 3rd ed. Philadelphia: F.A. Davis, 2009.

Venes, D, ed. *Taber's Cyclopedic Medical Dictionary*, 21st ed. Philadelphia: F.A. Davis, 2009.

Wilkinson, JM and Van Leuven, K, eds. *Fundamentals of Nursing*. Philadelphia: F.A. Davis, 2008.

Chapter 1: General Principles of Fluid, Electrolyte, and Acid-Base Balance and Imbalance

Brosnan, JT and Brosnan, ME. The sulfur-containing amino acids: An overview. *The American Society for Nutrition Journal.* June 2006:136:1636S-1640S.

Frassetto, L, Morris, RC, Jr., et al. Diet, evolution and aging: The pathophysiologic effects of the post-agricultural inversion of the potassium-to-sodium and base-to-chloride ratios in the human diet. *European Journal of Nutrition.* October 2001:40:200-213.

Haber, D. *Health Promotion and Aging: Practical Applications for Health Professionals.* NY: Springer Publishing, 2007.

Hannan, E, Bernard, H, O'Donnell, JF, et al. Methodology for targeting hospital cases for quality of care record reviews. *American Journal of Public Health.* April 1989:79: 430-436.

Johnson, LR and Byrne, JH. *Essential Medical Physiology.* Maryland Heights, MO: Elsevier Science and Technology Books, 2008.

Marmarou, A, Sigoretti, S, et al. Predominance of cellular edema in traumatic brain swelling in patients with severe head injuries. *Journal of Neurosurgery.* May 2006:104(5):720-730.

Nakamura, H, Kajikawa, R and Ubuka, T. A study of the estimation of sulfur-containing amino acid metabolism by the determination of urinary sulfate and taurine. *Amino Acids.* 2002:23

Rosenthal, K. Intravenous fluids: The whys and wherefores. *Nursing.* July 2006:36(7):26-27.

Wells, JL and Dumbrell, AC. Nutrition and aging: Assessment and treatment of compromised nutritional status in frail elderly patients. *Aging.* March 2006:1(1):67-79.

Chapter 2: Fluid Balance and Imbalance

AGA Institute, Clinical Practice and Economics Committee. Management of acute pancreatitis. *Gastroenterology* May 2007:132(5):2019-2021.

Al-Khafaji, A. Fluid resuscitation. *Continuing Education in Anesthesia, Critical Care & Pain.* 2004:4(4):127-131.

American Red Cross. Practice guidelines for blood transfusion: A compilation from recent peer-reviewed literature, 2nd ed. Available at: http://www.redcross.org/www-files/Documents/WorkingWiththeRedCross/practiceguidelinesforbloodtrans.pdf; Retrieved April 2007.

Culp, K, Mentes, J and Wakefield, B. Hydration and acute confusion in long-term care residents. *Western Journal of Nursing Research.* 2003:25(3):251-266.

Goertz, S. Gauging fluid balance with osmolality. *Nursing.* 2006:36(10):70-71.

Hahn, S, Kim, Y and Garner, P. Reduced osmolarity oral rehydration solution for treating dehydration due to diarrhoea in children: systematic review. *British Medical Journal.* 2001:323:81-85.

Hankins, J, Lonsway, RA, Hedrick, C, et al. *Infusion Therapy in Clinical Practice,* 2nd ed. Philadelphia: Elsevier Health Sciences, 2001.

Jaquier, E and Constant, F. Water as an essential nutrient: The physiological basis of hydration. *European Journal of Clinical Nutrition.* 2009:64:115-123.

Mentes, JC. A typology of oral hydration problems exhibited by frail nursing home residents. *Journal of Gerontological Nursing.* 2006:32(1).

Monti, S and Pokorny, ME. Preoperative fluid bolus reduces risk of postoperative nausea and vomiting: A pilot study. *Internet Journal of Advanced Nursing Practice.* 2000:4(2).

Moore, K. Controversies in fluid resuscitation. *Journal of Trauma Nursing.* 2006:13(4):168-172.

Nussey, SS and Whitehead, SA. *Endocrinology: An Integrated Approach,* Oxford: BIOS Scientific Publishers, 2001.

Perilli, V, Sollazzi, L, Bozza, P, et al. The effects of the reverse Trendelenburg position on respiratory mechanics and blood gases in morbidly obese patients during bariatric surgery. *Anesthesia & Analgesia.* 2000:91:1520-1525.

Pestana, C. *Fluids and Electrolytes in the Surgical Patient,* 5th ed. Philadelphia: Lippincott Williams & Wilkins, 1999.

Rafael, AR. Body temperature regulation. Available at: Slideshare http://www.slideshare.net/rtrafaelmd/body-temperature-regulation; Retrieved April 2009.

Redden, M and Wotton, K. Clinical decision making by nurses when faced with third-space fluid shift: How well do they fare? *Gastroenterology Nursing.* 2001:24(4):182-191.

Shike, M. *Modern Nutrition in Health and Disease.* 10th ed. Philadelphia: Lippincott Williams & Wilkins, 2005.

Smartt S. The pulmonary artery catheter: Gold standard or redundant relic? *Journal of Peri-Anesthesia Nursing.* 2005:20(6):373.

Stevens, W. Fluid Balance and Resuscitation: Critical aspects of ICU care. *Critical Care Nursing.* 2008:3(2):12-21.

Talecris Biotherapeutics. Albumin (human) 5%, USP package insert. Available at: http://www.talecris-pi.info/inserts/Plasbumin5.pdf; Accessed April 2009.

Vincent, JL and Weil, M. Fluid challenge revisited. *Critical Care Medicine.* 2006:34(5).

Weinstein, S and Plumer, AL. *Plumer's Principles and Practice of Intravenous Therapy,* 8th ed.

Chapter 3A: Calcium

Ariyan, CE and Sosa JA. Assessment and management of patients with abnormal calcium. *Critical Care Medicine.* 2004:32(4S):S146-S154.

Chavan CB, Sharada K, Rao HB, et al. Hypocalcemia as a cause of reversible cardiomyopathy with ventricular tachycardia. *Annuals of Internal Medicine.* 2007:146(7):541-542.

Criddle, LM. Rhabdomyolysis. *Critical Care Nurse.* 2003:23:14-30.

Insel, P, Ross, D, et al. *Nutrition.* Boston: Jones & Bartlett Publishers, Inc., 2004.

Lefrandt, JD, Heitmann, J, et al The effects of dihydropyridine and phenylalkylamine calcium antagonist classes on autonomic function in hypertension: The VAMPHYRE Study. *American Journal of Hypertension.* 2001:14:1083-1089.

Lyma, D, Undiagnosed vitamin D deficiency in the hospitalized patient. *American Family Physician*, 2005: January 15.

Office of Dietary Supplements, NIH Clinical Center. *Dietary Supplement Fact Sheet: Calcium.* Available at: http://ods.od.nih.gov/factsheets/calcium.asp; retrieved June 15, 2009.

Shuey, KM and Brandt, JM. Hypercalcemia of malignancy: Part II. *Clinical Journal of Oncology Nursing.* 2004:8(3): 321-323.

Stewart AF. Clinical practice: Hypercalcemia associated with cancer. *New England Journal of Medicine.* 2005:352(4):373-379.

Tuma, R. Q&A with Stefan Feske, M.D. *Research Forefronts, New York University Langone Medical Center.* Available at: www http://www.med.nyu.edu/research_forefronts/current_articles/feske.html; retrieved June 2009.

Wilson, WC, Grande, CM and Hoyt, DB, eds.: *Critical Care*, vol. 2. London: Taylor & Francis, 2006.

Woods, SL, Motzer, SA and Froelicher, ESS. *Cardiac Nursing*. Philadelphia: Lippincott Williams & Wilkins, 2004.

Chapter 3B: Chloride

Chang, CH, Kuo, PH, Hsu, CH, et al. Persistent severe hypocapnia and alkalemia in a 40-year-old woman. *Chest.* 2000:118(1):242-245.

Eisenhut, M. Causes and effects of hyperchloremic acidosis. *Critical Care.* 2006: 10(3): 413

Grosse, SD, Boyle, CA, Botkin, JR, et al. (2004), Newborn screening for cystic fibrosis: Evaluation of benefits and risks and recommendations for state newborn screening programs. *Morbidity and Mortality Weekly Report Recommendations Reports.* 2004:53:1-36.

Hadaway, LC. How to safeguard delivery of high-alert IV drugs. *Nursing.* February 2001.

Kellum JA. Determinants of plasma acid-base balance. *Critical Care Clinics.* 2005:21(2):329-46.

Lennie, TA. Nutritional recommendations for patients with heart failure. *Journal of Cardiovascular Nursing.* 2006:21(4):261-268.

Lewis, J, Kaplan, LJ and Frangos, S. Clinical review: Acid-base abnormalities in the intensive care unit, part II. *Critical Care.* 2005:9:198-203.

Salyer, R. Improving medical/surgical practice with JCAHO's 2005 National Patient Safety Goals. *Nursing.* 2005:35:12-13.

Story, DA, Morimatsu, H and Bellomo, R. Hyperchloremic acidosis in the critically ill: One of the strong-ion acidoses? *Anesthesia Analgesia.* 2006:103(1):144-148.

Wiseman, AC and Linas, S. Disorders of potassium and acid-base balance. *American Journal of Kidney Disease.* 2005:45(5):941-949.

Chapter 3C: Magnesium

Agricultural Research Service USDA. Lack energy? Maybe it's your magnesium level. *Agricultural Research.* 2004. Available at: http://www.ars.usda.gov/is/AR/archive/may04/energy0504.htm?pf=1; accessed February 2010.

Food and Agricultural Organization of the United Nations. Human vitamin and mineral requirements: Magnesium. Available at: http://www.fao.org/DOCREP/004/Y2809E/y2809e0k.htm#bm20; accessed February 2010.

McKinley, MG. Alcohol withdrawal syndrome overlooked and mismanaged. *Critical Care Nurse.* 2005:25:40-48.

Merck Manual. Magnesium. Available at: http://www.merck.com/mmhe/sec12/ch155/ch155h.html; accessed February 2010.

Murphy, K. Managing the ups and downs of biopolar disorder. *Nursing.* 2006:36(10)58-63.

NIH Clinical Center. Magnesium. Available at: http://ods.od.nih.gov/factsheets/magnesium.asp; accessed February 2010.

Porth, CM. *Pathophysiology: Concepts of Altered Health States,* 6th ed. Philadelphia: Lippincott, 2002.

Ronco, C, Bellomo, R and Kellum, JA. Critical Care Nephrology, 2nd ed. Philadelphia: Elsevier Health Sciences, 2008.

Chapter 3D: Phosphorus

Achinger, SG and Ayus, JC. The role of daily dialysis in the control of hyperphosphatemia. *Kidney International.* 2005:67:S28-S32.

Brunelli, SM and Goldfarb, S. Hypophosphatemia: Clinical consequences and management. *Journal of the American Society of Nephrology.* 2007:18:1999-2003.

Charron, T, Bernard, F, Skrobik, Y, et al. Intravenous phosphate in the intensive care unit: More aggressive repletion regimens for moderate and severe hypophosphatemia. *Intensive Care Medicine.* 2003:29(8):1273-1278.

Cohen, J, Kogan, A, et al. Significant hypophosphatemia following major cardiac surgery: Incidence and consequences. *Critical Care.* 2004:Supp. 1.

Crook, MA. Management of severe hypophosphatemia. *Nutrition.* 2009:24(3):368-369.

Davis KG. Acute management of white phosphorus burn. *Military Medicine.* 2002:167(1):83-84.

Insel, P, Ross, D and Turner, E. *Nutrition.* Boston: Jones & Bartlett, 2004.

Kollef, MH, Bedient, TJ, Isakow, W, et al. *The Washington Manual of Critical Care.* Philadelphia: Lippincott, Williams & Wilkins, 2007.

Lopes, AA and Lopes, GB. Reducing serum phosphorus concentration in patients with end stage renal disease. *JAMA.* 2009:3301(23):2443-2444.

Mehanna, H, Nankivell, PC, Moledina, J, et al. Refeeding syndrome: Awareness, prevention and management. *Head and Neck Oncology.* 2009:1(1):4.

Moe, SM. Disorders involving calcium, phosphorus, and magnesium. *Primary Care: Clinics in Office Practice.* 2008:35(2):215-237.

NIH. Phosphates. Available at: http://www.nlm.nih.gov/medlineplus/druginfo/natural/patient-phosphorus.html; accessed August 2009.

NIH. Phosphorus. Available at: http://www.nlm.nih.gov/medlineplus/druginfo/natural/patient-phosphorus.html; accessed June 24, 2009.

Office of Dietary Supplements, NIH Clinical Center. Dietary supplement fact sheet: Calcium. Available at: http://ods.od.nih.gov/factsheets/calcium.asp; Retrieved June 15, 2009.

Qunibi, W, Hootkins, RE, et al. Treatment of hyperphosphatemia in hemodialysis patients: The calcium acetate renal evaluation. *Kidney International.* 2004:65:1914–1926.

Ronco, C, Bellomo, R and Kellum, J. *Critical Care Nephrology*, 2nd ed. Philadelphia: Elsevier Health Sciences, 2008.

Schiavi, SC and Moe, OW. Phosphatonins: A new class of phosphate-regulating hormones. *Current Opinion in Nephrology and Hypertension.* 2002:11(4):423-430.

Schwartz, A. Association between phosphatemia and cardiac arrhythmias in the early stages of sepsis. *European Journal of Internal Medicine.* 2002:13(7):34-43.

Sherwood, L. *Fundamentals of Physiology: A Human Perspective.* Pacific Grove, CA: Cengage Learning, Brooks Cole, 2005.

Slatopolsky, E. New developments in hyperphosphatemia management. *Journal of the American Society of Nephrology.* 2003:14:S297-299.

Somerman, MJ and McCauly, LK. Bisphosphonates: Sacrificing the jaw to save the skeleton? *BoneKEy-Osteovision.* 2006:3(9):12-18.

Thomas, N. *Renal Nursing.* Philadelphia: Elsevier Health Sciences, 2008.

Tuma, R. Q&A with Stefan Feske, M.D. *Research Forefronts, New York University Langone Medical Center.* Available at: www http://www.med.nyu.edu/research_forefronts/current_articles/feske.html; retrieved June 2009.

Wilson, WC, Grande, CM, and Hoyt, DB, eds. *Trauma: Critical Care*, vol 2. London: Taylor and Francis, 2006.

Woods, SL, Motzer, SA and Sivarajan Froelicher ES. *Cardiac Nursing.* Philadelphia: Lippincott Williams & Wilkins, 2004.

Chapter 3E: Potassium

Burger, C. Hypokalemia: Averting crisis with early recognition and intervention. *American Journal of Nursing.* 2004:104(11):61-65.

Cohn, JN, Kowey, PR, Whelton, PK, et al. New guidelines for potassium replacement in clinical practice: A contemporary review by the National Council on Potassium in Clinical Practice. *Archives of Internal Medicine.* 2000:160(16):2429-2436.

Criddle, LM. Rhabdomyolysis, pathophysiology, recognition, and management. *Critical Care Nurse.* 2003:23:14-30.

Davey, M. Calcium for hyperkalaemia in digoxin toxicity. *Emergency Medical Journal.* 2002:19(2):183.

Dharmarajan, T, Nguyen, T and Russell, R. Life-threatening, preventable hyperkalemia in a nursing home resident: Case report and literature review. *Journal of the American Medical Directors Association.* 2005:6(6):400-405.

Elkinton, JR. Whole-body buffers in the regulation of acid-base equilibrium. *Yale Journal of Biology and Medicine.* 1956:29(3):191-210.

Freeman, K, Feldman, JA, Mitchell, P, et al. Effects of presentation and electrocardiogram on time to treatment of hyperkalemia. *Academic Emergency Medicine.* 2008:15(3):239-249.

Garth, D. Hyperkalemia. *E-Medicine.* Available at: http://emedicine.medscape.com/article/766479-overview; accessed February 2010.

Garth, D. Hypokalemia. *E-Medicine.* Available at: http://emedicine.medscape.com/article/767448-overview; accessed February 2010.

Garth D. Hypokalemia. *E-Medicine on Medscape.* Updated Aug. 23, 2007. Available at: http://emedicine.medscape.com/emergency_medicine#endocrine

Position statement from the International Marathon Medical Directors Association. *Clinical Journal of Sports Medicine.* 2006:16:283–292.

Sweeney, J. What causes sudden hypokalemia? *Nursing.* 2005:35(4):12.

Tran HA. Extreme hyperkalemia. *Southern Medical Journal.* 2005:98(7):729-732.

Treatment of hyperkalemia and metabolic acidosis. *Clinical and Experimental Nephrology.* 2009:12(3):1342-1751.

Vacca, V. Hyperkalemia. *Nursing.* 2008:38(7):72.

Vacca, V. Hypokalemia. *Nursing.* 2009:39(7):64.

Vuckovic, K. Clinical rounds: Bradycardia induced by hyperkalemia. *American Association of Occupational Health Nurses Journal.* 2004:52(5).

Weisberg, LS. Management of severe hyperkalemia. *Critical Care Medicine.* 2008:36(12):3246-3251.

Chapter 3F: Sodium
Adrogue HJ, Madias NE. Hypernatremia. *New England Journal of Medicine.* 2000:342(20):1493-1499.

Adrogue, HJ, Madias, NE. Hyponatremia. *New England Journal of Medicine.* 2000:342(21):1581-1589.

Almond, CS, Shin, AY, Fortescue, EB, et al. Hyponatremia among runners in the Boston marathon. *New England Journal of Medicine.* 2005:352(15):1550-1556.

Chatterjee, K. Analytic review: Hyponatremia in heart failure. *Journal of Intensive Care Medicine.* 2009:24:347-351.

Goh, Kian-Peng. Management of hyponatremia. *American Family Physician.* May 15, 2004.

Goldberg, A, Hammerman, H, Petcherski, S, et al. Prognostic importance of hyponatremia in acute ST-elevation myocardial infarction. *American Journal of Medicine.* 2004:117(4):242-248.

Hew-Butler, T., Verbalis, J.G., and Noakes, T.D. , (2006), Updated Fluid Recommendation: Position Statement From the International Marathon Medical Directors Association (IMMDA), Clinical Journal of Sports Medicine 2006:16:283–292), available: www.aims-association.org/articles/IMMDA_Updated_Fluid_Recommendation.pdf

Institute of Medicine. Dietary reference intakes: Electrolytes and water. Available at: www.iom.edu/Object.File/Master/20/004/0.pdf

International Marathon Medical Directors Association. Revised fluid recommendations for runners and walkers. Available at: http://www.aimsworldrunning.org/guidelines_fluid_replacement.htm

Joint Commission on Accreditation of Healthcare Organizations. SBAR technique: Improves communication, enhances patient safety. 2005:5(2).

Kelleher, H and Henderson, SO. Severe hyponatremia due to desmopressin. Journal of Emergency Medicine. 2006:30(1):45-47.

King, CK, Glass, R, Bresee, JS, et al. Managing acute gastroenteritis among children: Oral rehydration, maintenance, and nutritional therapy. *National Guideline Clearinghouse.* Available at: www.guideline.gov

Kragh-Hansen, U, Roigaard-Petersen, H, Jacobsen, C, et al. Renal transport of neutral amino acids: Tubular localization of Na+ dependent phenylalanine and glucose transport. *Biochemical Journal.* 1984:220(1):15-24.

Kugler, JP and Hustead, T. Hyponatremia and hypernatremia in the elderly. *American Family Physician.* June 15, 2000.

Lab Studies in Renal Disease. National Kidney Foundation. Available at: http://www.kidney.org/kidneydisease/ckd/knowGFR.cfm

Lee, CT, Guo, HR and Chen, JB. Hyponatremia in the emergency department. *American Journal of Emergency Medicine.* 2000:18:264-268.

Metzger, RA, Vaamonde, LS, Vaamonde, CA, et al. Renal Excretion of sodium during oral water loading in man. *Nephron.* 1969:6:11-27.

Nzerue, CM, Baffoe-Bonnie, H, You, W, et al. Predictors of outcome in hospitalized patients with severe hyponatremia. *Journal National Medical Association.* 2003:95:335-343.

Chapter 3G: Essential Minerals and Elements

Agency for Toxic Substances and Disease Registry. Toxicological profile for manganese. Atlanta, GA: U.S. Department of Health and Human Services, Public Health Service, 2008.

Allen, LH. Anemia and iron deficiency: Effects on pregnancy outcome. *American Journal of Clinical Nutrition.* 2000:71:1280S-1284S.

Althuis, MD, Jordan, NE, Ludington, EA, et al. Glucose and insulin responses to dietary chromium supplements: A meta-analysis. *American Journal of Clinical Nutrition.* 2002:76(1):148-155.

Balk, EM, Tatsioni, A, Lichtenstein, AH, et al. Effect of chromium supplementation on glucose metabolism and lipids: A systematic review of randomized controlled trials. *Diabetes Care.* 2007:30:2154-2163.

Barclay, L. Excessive zinc supplementation may increase prostate cancer risk. *Journal of the National Cancer Institute.* 2003:95:1004-1007.

Berry, MJ and Ralston, NV. Mercury toxicity and the mitigating role of selenium. *Ecohealth.* 2008:5(4):456-459.

Cerhan, JR, Saag, KG, Merlino, LA, et al. Antioxidant micronutrients and risk of rheumatoid arthritis in a cohort of older women. *American Journal of Epidemiology.* 2003:157:345-354.

Connelly-Frost, A, Poole, C, Satia, JA, et al. Selenium, folate, and colon cancer. *Nutrition and Cancer.* 2009:61(2):165-178.

Craig, WJ and Mangels, AR. Position of the American Dietetic Association: Vegetarian diets. *Journal of the American Dietetic Association.* 2009:109(7):1266-1282.

Daley, B, Doherty, AT, Fairman, B, et al. Wear debris from hip or knee replacements causes chromosomal damage in human cells in tissue culture. *Journal of Bone and Joint Surgery—British.* 2004:86B:598-606.

Dennert, G and Horneber, M. Selenium for alleviating the side effects of chemotherapy, radiotherapy, and surgery in cancer patients. *Cochrane Database Systematic Review.* 2006:19(3); accessed October 2009.

Dietary Reference Intakes. Elements. Available at: http://www.iom.edu/Object.File/Master/7/294/0.pdf

Docherty, JP, Sack, DA, Roffman, M, et al. A double-blind, placebo-controlled, exploratory trial of chromium picolinate in atypical depression: Effect on carbohydrate craving. *Journal of Psychiatric Practice.* 2005:11(5):302-314.

Food and Nutrition Board, Institute of Medicine. Dietary reference intakes for vitamin A, vitamin K, boron, chromium, copper, iodine, iron, manganese, molybdenum, nickel, silicon, vanadium, and zinc. Washington, D.C.: National Academy Press, 2001.

Gaggelli, E, Kozlowski, H, Valensin, D, et al. Copper homeostasis and neurodegenerative disorders (Alzheimer's, Prion, and Parkinson's diseases and amyotrophic lateral sclerosis). *Chemical Reviews.* 2006:106(6):1995-2044.

Hulisz, D. Efficacy of zinc against common cold viruses: An overview. *Journal of the American Pharmacists Association.* November 2004.

Kazal, LA. Prevention of iron deficiency in infants and toddlers. *American Family Physician.* October 2002.

Levina, A, McLeod, A, Seuring, J, et al. Reactivity of potential anti-diabetic molybdenum (VI) complexes in biological media: A XANES spectroscopic study. *Journal of Inorganic Biochemistry.* 2007:101:1586-1593.

Marinella, MA Nocturnal pagophagia complicating gastric bypass. *Mayo Clinic Procedings.* 83:961-961.

Mayer, JE, Pfeiffer, WH and Beyer, P. Biofortified crops to alleviate micronutrient malnutrition. *Current Opinion in Plant Biology.* 2008:11(2):166-170.

Muszynska, A, Palka, J and Gorodkiewicz, E. The mechanism of daunorubicin-induced inhibition of prolidase activity in human skin fibroblasts and its implication to impaired collagen biosynthesis. *Experimental Toxicology Pathology.* 2000:52(2): 149-155.

Ramakrishnan, U. Prevalence of mircronutrient malnutrition worldwide. *Nutritional Reviews.* 2002:60(Supp 1):46-52.

Rucklidge, JJ, Johnstone, J and Kaplan, BJ. Nutrient supplementation approaches in the treatment of ADHD. *Expert Review of Neurotherapeutics.* 2009:9(4): 461-476.

Sandstrom, B. Micronutrient interactions: Effects on absorption and bioavailability. *British Journal of Nutrition.* 2001:85(Supp 2):S181-185.

Suzuki, KT and Ogura, Y. Biological regulation of copper and selective removal of copper: Therapy for Wilson disease and its molecular mechanism. *Journal of the Pharmaceutical Society of Japan.* 2000:120:899-908.

U.S. Department of Health and Human Services. Bone health and osteoporosis: A report of the Surgeon General. Rockville, MD: USDHHS, 2004.

Vincent, JB. Recent advances in the nutritional biochemistry of trivalent chromium. *Proceedings of the Nutrition Society.* 63(01):41-47.

White, PJ and Broadley, MR. Biofortification of crops with seven mineral elements often lacking in human diets—iron, zinc, copper, calcium, magnesium, selenium, and iodine. *New Phytology.* 2009:182(1):49-84.

Zeng, H. Selenium as an essential micronutrient: Roles in cell cycle and apoptosis. *Molecules.* 2009:14(3):1263-1278.

Chapter 4: Acid-Base Balance and Imbalance

Berry, BE and Pinard, AE. Assessing tissue oxygenation. *Critical Care Nurse.* 2002:22:22-40.

Bullock, J, Wang, M, et al. *National Medical Series.* Philadelphia: Lippincott Williams & Wilkins, 2001.

Calabrese, AT, Coley, KC, et al. Risk of lactic acidosis with metformin therapy. *Archives of Internal Medicine.* 2002:162:434-437.

Cham, GW, Tan, WP, Earnest, A, et al. Clinical predictors of acute respiratory acidosis during exacerbation of asthma and chronic obstructive pulmonary disease. *European Journal of Emergency Medicine.* 2002:9(3):225-232.

Criddle, LM. Rhabdomyolysis. *Critical Care Nurse.* 2003:23:14-30.

Duiverman, ML, Wempe, JB, Bladder, G, et al. Nocturnal noninvasive ventilation in addition to rehabilitation in hypercapnic patients with COPD. *Thorax.* 2008:63(12): 1052-1057.

Englehart, MS and Schreiber, MA. Measurement of acid-base resuscitation endpoints: Lactate, base deficit, bicarbonate, or what? *Current Opinion in Critical Care.* 2006:12(6): 569-574.

Epstein, SK and Singh, N. Respiratory acidosis. *Respiratory Care.* 2001:46(4):366-383.

Gillespie, GL and Campbell, M. Diabetic ketoacidosis: Rapid identification, treatment, and education can improve survival rates. *American Journal of Nursing.* 2002:102:13-16.

Hoo, GW, Hakimian, N and Santiago, SM. Hypercapnic respiratory failure in COPD patients: Response to therapy. *Chest.* 2000:117(1):169-177.

Kellum, JA. Disorders of acid-base balance. *Critical Care Medicine.* 2007:35(11): 2630-2636.

Kirsch, DB and Józefowicz, RF. Neurologic complications of respiratory disease. *Neurology Clinics.* 2002:20(1):247-264.

Lum, E. Valproic acid management of acute alcohol withdrawal. *Annals of Pharmacotherapy.* 40(3):441-448.

McCray, S, Parrish, CR and Walker, S. Much ado about refeeding. *Practical Gastroenterology.* 2005:30-44.

Medarov, BI. Milk-alkali syndrome. *Mayo Clinic Procedings.* 2009:84(3):261-267.

Muscari, ME. The role of the nurse practitioner in the diagnosis and management of bulimia nervosa: Physiologic management. *Journal of the American Academy of Nurse Practitioners.* 2007:5(5):19-24.

Nowbar, S, Burkart, KM and Gonzales, R. Obesity-associated hypoventilation in hospitalized patients: Prevalence, effects, and outcome. *American Journal of Medicine.* 2004:116(1):1-7.

Reddy, P and Mooradian, AD. Clinical utility of anion gap in deciphering acid-base disorders. *International Journal of Clinical Practice.* 2009:63(10):1516-1525.

Rocktasechel, J, Morimatsu, H, et al. Acid-base status of critically ill patients with acute renal failure: Analysis based on Stewart-Figge methodology. *Critical Care.* 2003:7:60-66.

St. John, RE. Airway management. *Critical Care Nurse.* 2004:24:93-97.

Taylor, A, and McGrath, RP. Team management of the chest trauma patient. *OR Nurse.* 2008:2(3):32-37.

Wiseman, AC and Linas, S. Disorders of potassium and acid-base balance. *American Journal of Kidney Disease.* 2005:45(5):941-949.

Chapter 5: Common Disease Processes and Metabolic Disturbances Associated With Fluid, Electrolyte, and Acid-Base Imbalances

Bourbeau, J. Activities of Life: The COPD Patient. *COPD: Journal of Chronic Obstructive Pulmonary Disease.* 2009:6(3):192-200.

Brandt, CP, Coffee, T, Yurko, L, et al. Triage of minor burn wounds: Avoiding the emergency department. *Journal of Burn Care and Rehabilitation.* 2000:21(1):26-28.

Criddle, LM. Rhabdomyolysis, pathology, recognition, and management. *Critical Care Nurse.* 2003:23:14-30.

Ferreri, R. Treatment practices of diabetic ketoacidosis at a large teaching hospital. *Journal of Nursing Care Quality.* 2008:21(2):147-154.

Flounders, JA. Syndrome of inappropriate antidiuretic hormone. *Oncology Nursing Forum.* 2003:30(3).

Gavi, SG, Henley, J, Cervo, F, et al. Management of feeding tube complications in the long-term care resident. *Annals of Long-Term Care.* 2008:16(4).

Gronkiewicz, C and Borkgren-Okonek, M. Acute exacerbation of COPD: Nursing application of evidence-based guidelines. *Critical Care Nursing Quarterly.* 2004:27(4):336-352.

Hoorn, EJ, Lindemans, J and Zietse, R. Development of severe hyponatraemia in hospitalized patients: Treatment-related risk factors and inadequate management. *Nephrology Dialysis Transplantation.* 2006:21(1):70-76.

Klien, MB, Hayden, D, Elson, C, et al. The association between fluid administration and outcome following major burn: A multi-center study. *Annals of Surgery.* 2007:245(4):622-628.

Kumar, S, Fowler, M, Gonzalez-Toledo, E, et al. Central pontine myelinolysis: An update. *Neurology Research.* 2006:28(3):360-366.

Latto, C. An overview of sepsis. *Dimensions of Critical Care Nursing.* 2008:27(5): 195-200.

McGraw, B. At an increased risk: Tumor lysis syndrome. *Clinical Journal of Oncology Nursing.* 2008:12(4):563-565.

National Institute of General Medical Science. Sepsis fact sheet: Taking aim at sepsis. *NGMS Publications.* Available at: http://www.nigms.nih.gov/Publications/ factsheet_sepsis.htm

Nobel, K. The stressed patient with diabetes mellitus. *Journal of Peri-Anesthesia Nursing.* 2005:20(5):354-360.

Noble, KA. Thyroid storm. *Journal of Peri-Anesthesia Nursing.* 2006:21(2):119-125.

Orr, PA, Case, Keiko, O and Stevenson, JJ. Metabolic response and parenteral nutrition in trauma, sepsis, and burns. *Journal of Infusion Nursing.* 2002:25(1)45-53.

Owens, B. A review of primary hyperparathyroidism. *Journal of Infusion Nursing.* 2009:32(2):87-92.

Papini, R. Management of burn injuries of various depths. *British Medical Journal.* 2004:329(7458):158-160.

Powers, KA, Burchell, PL and Sane, A. Sepsis alert, avoiding shock. *Nursing.* 2010:40(4):34-38.

Rai, A, Whaley-Connell, A, McFarlane, S, et al. Hyponatremia, arginine vasopressin dysregulation, and vasopressin receptor antagonism. *American Journal of Nephrology.* 2006:26(6):579-589.

Simmons, S. Flushing out the truth about diabetes insipidus. *Nursing.* 2010:40(1): 55-59.

Spain, M and Edlund, BJ. Geropharmacology: Pharmacological management of type 2 diabetes in newly diagnosed older adults. *Journal of Gerontological Nursing.* 2009:35(7).

Sprague, SM. A comparative review of the efficacy and safety of established phosphate binders: Calcium, sevelamer, and lanthanum carbonate. *Current Medical Research and Opinion.* 23:12:3167-3175.

Stelfox, HT, Ahmed, SB, Khandwala, F, et al. The epidemiology of intensive care unit–acquired hyponatraemia and hypernatraemia in medical-surgical intensive care units. *Critical Care.* 2008:12(6):R162.

van Berge-Landry, J. Serum electrolyte, serum protein, serum fat, and renal responses to a dietary sodium challenge: Allostasis and allostatic load. *Annals of Human Biology.* 2004:31(4):477-487.

Weber, J and McManus, A. Nursing committee of the International Society for Burn Injuries: Infection control in burn patients. *Burns.* 2004:30(8):A16-A24.

Yontz, LL. Congestive heart failure: Early recognition of congestive heart failure in the primary care setting. *Journal of the American Academy of Nurse Practitioners.* 6(6): 273-279.

DuBois, D and DuBois, EF. A formula to estimate the approximate surface area if height and weight be known. *Archives of Internal Medicine.* 1916:17:863-871.

Jennett, B. Development of Glasgow coma and outcome scales. *Nepal Journal of Neuroscience,* 2005:2(1):24-28.

Teasdale, G and Jennett, B. Assessment and prognosis of coma after head injury. *Acta Neurochirurgica.* 1976:34:45-55.

Teasdale, G and Jennett, B. Assessment of coma and impaired consciousness: A practical scale. *The Lancet.* 1974:2:81-88.

Index

Note: Page numbers followed by "b," "f," and "t" indicate boxes, figures, and tables, respectively.